Manual of
Parrot Behavior

Manual of Parrot Behavior

Andrew U. Luescher, Editor

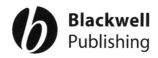

Blackwell
Publishing

Andrew U. Luescher, DVM, PhD, is Director of the Animal Behavior Clinic at Purdue University. He established the Animal Behavior Clinic in 1997 and is certified as an applied animal behaviorist by the Animal Behavior Society and is a diplomate of the American College of Veterinary Behaviorists. He has been treating animals with behavioral problems for more than 20 years.

Blackwell Publishing Professional
2121 State Avenue, Ames, Iowa 50014, USA

Orders: 1-800-862-6657
Office: 1-515-292-0140
Fax: 1-515-292-3348
Web site: www.blackwellprofessional.com

Blackwell Publishing Ltd
9600 Garsington Road, Oxford OX4 2DQ, UK
Tel.: +44 (0)1865 776868

Blackwell Publishing Asia
550 Swanston Street, Carlton, Victoria 3053, Australia
Tel.: +61 (0)3 8359 1011

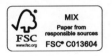
MIX
Paper from
responsible sources
FSC
www.fsc.org   FSC® C013604

First edition, 2006

Library of Congress Cataloging-in-Publication Data

Manual of parrot behavior / edited by Andrew U. Luescher.— 1st ed.
     p. cm.
  Includes bibliographical references and index.
  ISBN-13: 978-0-8138-2749-0 (alk. paper)
  ISBN-10: 0-8138-2749-3 (alk. paper)
  1. Parrots—Behavior. I. Luescher, Andrew U.

  SF473.P3.M27 2006
  636.6′865—dc22

                                    2005028547

Contents

Contributors

Numbers in brackets refer to chapters

Laurie Bergman, VMD, DACVB [7,19]
Co-ordinator Clinical Animal Behavior Service
University of California Veterinary Medical
  Center, San Diego

Bobbi Brinker [14]
Parrottalk.com

Brenda Cramton, MS, JD [12]
Arroyo Veterinary Hospital
Denair, CA

Robert J. Dooling, PhD [4]
Department of Psychology
University of Maryland, College Park

Ernesto C. Enkerlin-Hoeflich [2]
www.conanp.gob.mx/

Rebecca Fox [10]
Department of Animal Science
University of California, Davis

S.G. Friedman, PhD [14]
Department of Psychology
Utah State University, Logan

**Jennifer Graham, DVM, Diplomate, ABVP,
  Avian [4]**
Affiliate Assistant Professor, Department of
  Comparative Medicine,School of Medicine,
  University of Washington
Veterinary Specialty Center of Seattle,
  Lynnwood, WA
www.seattleveterinaryspecialists.com

Dominique G. Homberger [1]
Professor of Zoology, Dept. of Biological
  Sciences
Louisiana State University, Baton Rouge

**Ruediger Korbel, Prof. Dr. med. vet., Dr. med.
  vet. habil. [4]**
Director Institute of Avian Diseases, Ludwig-
  Maximilians-University Munich
Cert. Spec. Avian Medicine, Cert. Spec. Vet.
  Ophthalmol., Dipl. ECAMS. Univ.–Institut
  fuer Gefluegelkrankheiten

Elizabeth A. Koutsos [6]
Department of Animal Science
University of Missouri, Saint Louis

Phoebe Greene Linden, MA [11]
Santa Barbara Bird Farm
Santa Barbara, CA

**Andrew U. Luescher, DVM, PhD, DACVB
  [Editor, 11,18,20,26]**
Director of the Animal Behavior Clinic
Purdue University, West Lafayette, IN

Kenneth M. Martin, DVM [24]
Veterinary Behavior Consultations
New Orleans, LA

Scott George Martin, MS, DVM [9]
Animal Health Clinic
Jupiter, FL

Steve Martin [14]
Natural Encounters, Inc.
Winter Haven, FL

Kevin David Matson [6]
Department of Biology
University of Missouri, St. Louis

Cheryl Meehan, PhD [27]
Associate Director, Center for Animal Welfare
University of California, Davis

Joy Mench [27]
Professor and Director of the Center for Animal
    Welfare, Department of Animal Science
University of California, Davis

Charles A. Munn, PhD [3]
Chairman of the Board, Tropical Nature
Arlington, VA
www.tropicalnature.org

**Susan E. Orosz, PhD, DVM, Diplomate,
    ABVP, Avian, and Diplomate, ECAMS [17]**
Perrysburg Animal Care, Perrysburg, Ohio
Adjunct Professor, The University of Tennessee,
    College of Veterinary Medicine, Knoxville
Consultant, Lafeber Company, Cornell, Illinois

Irene M. Pepperberg [13]
Research Associate Professor, Dept. of
    Psychology, Brandeis University
Research Scientist, MIT School of Architecture
    and Planning

Ulrike S. Reinisch, DVM [7,19]
Resident–Clinical Animal Behavior Service
University of California, Davis

**April Romagnano, PhD, DVM, ABVP (Avian
    Practice) [9,22]**
Animal Health Clinic
Jupiter, FL

**Lynne M. Seibert, DVM, MS, PhD, Dipl
    ACVB [5,23]**
Veterinary Specialty Center of Seattle
Lynnwood, WA

Noel F.R. Snyder [2]
Portal, AZ

Tracey R. Spoon [8]
Department of Biology
University of Massachusetts, Boston

Fern Van Sant, DVM [21]
For the Birds
San Jose, CA

**Kenneth R. Welle, DVM, Diplomate, ABVP,
    Avian [15, 16, 18]**
All Creatures Animal Hospital
Adjunct Assistant Professor, University of
    Illinois College of Veterinary Medicine
Urbana, IL

James W. Wiley [2]
USGS-BRD
Maryland Cooperative Fish and Wildlife
    Research Unit, Princess Anne, MD

**G. Heather Wilson, DVM, Diplomate, ABVP,
    Avian [25]**
Assistant Professor Exotic Animal, Wildlife, and
    Zoological Medicine, Department of Small
    Animal Medicine, College of Veterinary
    Medicine
University of Georgia, Athens

Liz Wilson, CVT [16,20,26]
Parrot Behavior Consultant
Levittown, PA

Timothy F. Wright, PhD [4]
Genetics Lab, National Museum of Natural
    History, Smithsonian Institution, Smithsonian
    National Zoo
Washington, DC

Many have forgotten this truth, but you must not forget it. You remain responsible, forever, for what you have tamed.

—Antoine de Saint-Exupery

Preface

The untamed beauty of parrots has fascinated humans for centuries and keeps us in its spell to the present time. Parrots are beautiful, they can fly, they are different from us, they are intelligent, and they remain mysterious. However, our relationship with parrots has changed greatly over time. Once considered a plentiful natural resource worth exploiting, we now make great efforts to protect their dwindling natural populations. At the same time we have come a long way in how we keep parrots in our homes. They no longer are but brilliant exhibition pieces chained to a T-stand but have become members of our families whose sensitivities, cognitive abilities, and emotions we respect and try to understand.

Yet parrot-keeping is a challenging endeavor. We admire their wildness, yet we bring them into a very unnatural captive environment for which they have not evolved. We admire their flight, yet in most cases where we keep parrots as pets we need to clip their wings. We like them because they are social creatures, yet we frequently keep them as solitary birds so they will redirect their affection toward us, and in most cases we leave them alone for extended periods of time. We recognize their intelligence, yet maintain them in a very restricted and confining environment.

No wonder behavior problems in parrots are plentiful and the numbers of abandoned parrots ending up in sanctuaries is increasing. Stories of parrots relegated to small cages in the basement,

neglected, covered with a towel to keep them quiet, are much too common. Even normal parrot behavior such as vocalization, chewing, and being messy does not fit well with people's lifestyles and can result in a broken human-animal bond. This book is written by authors who understand and love parrots in order to help foster a mutually beneficial and enjoyable relationship between parrots and their humans. We hope it can set up new parrot-human relationships for success and rekindle the joy that should be inherent in such relationships in cases where it has been lost. We intend to promote a deepened understanding and responsible attitude toward parrots in the wild as well as in captivity. We hope this will contribute to the welfare of parrots and help develop a respect for and appreciation of these fascinating beings.

Although scientific interest in parrot behavior is growing, knowledge in this area is still limited. This is especially true for behavior problems of pet birds and their treatment. The information in this book is based on scientific principles and available publications but, where specific and proven information is not available, may reflect the opinion and the personal experience of the authors. Therefore, there may be some degree of contradiction or difference in interpretation between chapters. This inconsistency was intentionally maintained to offer the reader different perspectives.

I once had a sparrow alight upon my shoulder for a moment, while I was hoeing in a village garden, and I felt that I was more distinguished by that circumstance that I should have been by any epaulet I could have worn.

—Henry David Thoreau

Foreword

As a veterinarian I have spent most of my professional life trying to understand why parrots behave as they do as it did not take me long to understand that avian behavior and veterinary care are deeply entwined. One cannot effectively treat avian patients without a deep and thorough understanding of their natural behavior. Likewise, many bird owners struggle to develop and maintain a "healthy" relationship with their bird(s) for as we know, these amazing and beloved creatures are not simply dogs and cats with feathers. In many cases, success in establishing this relationship with a bird may be a testament to the bird's adaptability, not to the owner's understanding of their pet. This book provides information that will help improve many people's interactions with birds.

When asked to write the foreword for this book, I was very excited about the prospect of reading the manuscript penned by the distinguished list of authors. I was more than surprised and elated by the quality of the writing and wide variety and depth of information offered in the chapters. This book covers topics ranging from the classification of Psittaformes, conservation, reintroduction, behavior in the wild, behavior in captivity, the natural science of behavior, medical diagnostics and treatments for behavioral problems, development of neonates, housing, management and [all]welfare to name a few. Each chapter provides a unique insight into what makes psittacine birds the exceptional creatures we all love so much. I was especially appreciative of the scientific information debunking frequently held beliefs such as height dominance and positive punishment, common misconceptions that I have been fighting for years.

The avian veterinary practitioner will find this book to be overflowing with pertinent information on all aspects of behavior, medical conditions such as sexual behavioral problems and feather picking, diagnostic tools, and treatments. The avian behaviorist will find this book ripe with natural history information as well as solid behavior modification techniques based on the natural science of psittacine behavior in the wild. This book should also be of great interest for the advanced bird watcher, avian biologist and bird owner.

I have spent countless hours watching these magnificent creatures in their natural habitat, on my own, and in the company of some of the authors of these chapters. During those times of observation I was able to gain knowledge from these learned people and understand their unique perspective into the natural behavior of these splendid animals. I am thrilled by the invaluable observations, understandings and medical knowledge that have been brought together in this unique book.

In the end, we must take all the responsibility for parrot learning and understanding. It is not the parrot's job to understand human behavior and perform as we ask. To the contrary, it is our job to understand parrot behavior and work within their construct if we ever expect a lasting and beneficial bond based on trust to develop.

Thomas M. Edling, DVM, MSpVM
National Director, Veterinary Medicine
PETCO Animal Supplies, Inc.
San Diego, CA

Manual of
Parrot Behavior

1

Classification and Status of Wild Populations of Parrots

Dominique G. Homberger

THE ORDER PSITTACIFORMES AND ITS RELATIONSHIPS WITHIN THE CLASS AVES

The roughly 350 species in about 74 genera of parrots and cockatoos (Forshaw 1989; Collar 1997; Rowley 1997; Juniper & Parr 1998) are grouped within the Psittaciformes, one of the most distinctive and largest of the 28 avian orders (Brooke & Birkhead 1991). Parrot and cockatoo species are usually easily recognized as psittaciform (or "psittacine") birds because of their curved beaks, in which the tip of the maxilla projects beyond the shorter mandible, and their zygodactylous feet, in which the second and third toes point forward and oppose the first and fourth toes, which point caudally. Other characteristics include a usually colorful plumage; a very large brain; curiosity, lifelong capacity for learning, and adaptability to changing environmental conditions; distinctive vocalizations; a feeding ecology as seed predators; versatile feeding mechanisms; a complex social behavior; lifelong pair bonding; nesting in cavities; white eggshells; and nidicolous young.

In the past, there have been some attempts at identifying the avian orders that are most closely related to the Psittaciformes by looking for common features, but it has become clear that any such commonalities reflect traits that have evolved in adaptation to similar environmental conditions and not traits that have been retained from a common ancestor. Furthermore, most of the common features at the ordinal level resemble one another only superficially and are easily recognized as having evolved independently in various avian orders. For example, in the curved beak of owls (Strigiformes) and raptors (Falconiformes), the mandible points straight forward, and the hooked maxilla serves to get a grip when grabbing or tearing apart prey. In the zygodactyl feet of woodpeckers (Piciformes) and cuckoos (Cuculiformes), the limb musculature differs from that of Psittaciformes, and the scaly skin differs in the shape and number of the scales. These differences indicate that the zygodactyl feet reflect an adaptation to an arboricole lifestyle, which has evolved separately in the ancestors of each order, rather than one that has evolved in a common ancestor of all three orders.

THE EVOLUTIONARY ORIGIN OF PSITTACIFORMES

The evolutionary origin of the Psittaciformes can be reconstructed from a combination of functional morphological, ecological, phylogenetic, biogeographical, geological, and paleoecological data (Cracraft 2001; Homberger 1991, 2003). The zygodactylous feet that are especially adept at climbing tree trunks and the predominant nesting in tree cavities suggest that the Psittaciformes originated as forest birds. The white color of the eggshells indicates that the ancestral species incubated their eggs in cavities (probably of trees), where they would not need camouflaging color pattern to escape the attention of predators.

The functional morphology of their feeding apparatus provides additional support for a psittaciform origin from an ancestor that was adapted to living in forests (Homberger 2003). The quadratomandibular, or jaw, joint is uniquely shaped to allow lateral movements of the lower mandible relative to the upper maxilla. However, parrots and most cockatoos, such as the White and Pink Cockatoos (*Cacatua* spp., *Eolophus roseicapillus*, *Lophochroa leadbeateri*, *Plictolophus* spp.), the Cockatiel (*Nymphicus hollandicus*), the Yellow-tailed and White-tailed Black Cockatoos (*Calyptorhynchus* [*Zanda*]), and the Palm Cockatoo (*Probosciger aterrimus*), use this capacity only during bouts of bill honing and for minor adjustments when positioning food items between their mandible to bite into them. It is unlikely, therefore, that the psittaciform jaw articulation was evolved in conjunction with the bill movements observed in these species. It has long been suspected that it was a feature that originated in a psittaciform ancestor as part of a feeding behavior that differed from that which is common among extant parrots (Homberger 1981).

In contrast, the lateral deflection of the lower mandible is an integral part of the feeding mechanism in most Red-tailed Black Cockatoos (*Calyptorhynchus banksii* subspecies), the Glossy Black Cockatoo (*C. lathami*), and the Gang-gang Cockatoo (*Callocephalon fimbriatum*) (Homberger 2001, 2003). They align one of the paired, projecting corners of their V-shaped lower bill tip with their upper bill tip. They do this in order to use their beak as pincer-like pliers to tear apart woody branches to extricate wood-boring or gallicole insect larvae or to break apart woody-fibrous capsules to extract seeds (Homberger 2001, 2003). These species also possess a bony suborbital arch that juts out on the sides of their skull and is firmly buttressed against the postorbital and zygomatic processes of the cranium. The jaw muscles that attach to this suborbital arch assume an orientation that emphasizes transversely directed force components, which are instrumental for the lateral deflections of the mandible during feeding in these species. In this "calyptorhynchid" feeding apparatus, the shapes of the jaw joint, skull, and bill are structurally and functionally integrated with the feeding mechanism to tear apart food sources that are made of fibrous wood, which are prevalent in a wooded or forested environment (Homberger 2003). The tight functional integration of the features of the calyptorhynchid feeding apparatus also indicates that they are part of an ancestral condition for Psittaciformes. The calyptorhynchid feeding apparatus

may have originated in a psittaciform ancestor first to extract wood-boring or gallicole insect larvae and subsequently been applied with few, if any, modifications, to extract seeds from fibrous-woody fruits.

In the "psittacid" feeding apparatus of parrots and most cockatoos (except the Red-tailed Black Cockatoos, *Calyptorhynchus lathami* and most *C. banksii* subspecies, and the Gang-gang Cockatoo, *Callocephalon fimbriatum*), in contrast, the structure and function of the jaw joint does not fit the bill shape and feeding behavior. The psittacid feeding apparatus relies on specialized surface structures, such as the transverse step and filing ridges on the inside of the upper bill tip, to provide grip for seeds that are cut open with the cutting edge of the lower mandible (Homberger 1980a, 1980b, 2003). Psittaciforms with a psittacid bill (except the Pesquet's Parrot, *Psittrichas fulgidus*) remove the shells of all seeds before swallowing them, and they do so with a stereotypical seed-shelling mechanism that does not require lateral movement of the mandible. During this seed-shelling procedure, the tip of the tongue places and holds a seed against the corrugated upper bill tip and its transverse step, while the cutting edge of the mandible cuts open the seed-shell. The bony suborbital arch is generally absent so that the transverse component of the jaw muscles is much reduced in favor of the longitudinal and vertical force components. If a suborbital arch is present, as in many South American species, it is less massive and fused only with the postorbital process of the cranium (see Smith 1975). This functional dissociation of the various structural and functional features indicates that the shapes of the jaw joint, skull, and bill of parrots and cockatoos with a psittacid feeding apparatus have changed under the influence of a variety of selective regimes arising from environmental conditions that differ from those to which the psittaciform ancestor was adapted.

The most significant selective advantage of the psittacid feeding apparatus over the calyptorhynchid feeding apparatus is that the former can use both sides of the jaw musculature simultaneously to maximize the bite force of the mandible. This selective advantage, however, can be utilized only in environments in which plants with seeds enclosed in fruits that are not woody-fibrous predominate (Homberger 2003). Most of these fruits have a sclerotic endocarp (i.e., "stone") that can be split, or cracked open, by applying a focused pressure, such as by the cutting edge of the mandible, onto their preformed weak points or sutures that facilitate the germination of the seeds. The selective advantage of a psittacid feeding apparatus appears to be considerable because it has evolved multiple times in separate lineages of parrots and cockatoos, including among them some of the populations and subspecies of Red-tailed Black Cockatoos (*Calyptorhynchus banksii*). This convergent evolution of the psittacid feeding apparatus is made evident by the great variability of the individual components and features, such as the pattern and configuration of the filing ridges and corneous palate, the shape and expression of the transverse step, the shape of the cutting edge of the mandible, and the configuration and degree of the reduction of the suborbital arch (Homberger 1980a, 1980b, 2003).

The large brain of the Psittaciformes earned them the epithet "avian primates." As in primates, it is correlated with curiosity and exploratory behaviors and a lifelong capacity for learning (e.g., Mettke-Hofmann et al. 2002; Pepperberg 2002). This high degree of encephalization supports the hypothesis that the Psittaciformes originated from ancestors that were feeding on stationary food items that were hidden from sight (i.e., wood-boring or gallicole insect larvae and seeds within fruits) and, therefore, need to be located through indirect evidence and learning from experienced individuals. These arboreal food items further support the hypothesis that Psittaciformes originated in a forested environment.

Psittaciformess are concentrated in the continents and islands of the Southern Hemisphere with only limited expansions into the adjacent northern regions. Contrary to general impressions, Psittaciformes are not restricted to tropical regions, as several species occur in the colder regions of China, New Zealand, New Guinea, Tasmania, and South America. Such a distribution pattern can be understood only on the basis of past geological events. Biogeography has been suggestive of a psittaciform origin in the Southern Hemisphere (Boetticher 1959; Forshaw 1989) even before geological data could demonstrate that the southern continents were formed

through the disintegration of the Mesozoic southern continent called Gondwana and their subsequent migration northward toward the equator (Frakes & Vickers-Rich 1991; Schodde & Tidemann 1986; Stevens 1991).

Gondwana's climate in the Cretaceous was generally temperate to subtropical, and Gondwana itself was covered mostly with evergreen mesic forest and rain forest (White 1990). As the continents moved northwards, they tended to become more arid with the rising temperatures (Frakes & Vickers-Rich 1991; Stevens 1991; White 1994). The original plant communities that included southern gymnosperms (e.g., *Araucaria*), Casuarinas, Proteaceae (e.g., *Banksia*, *Protea*, *Grevillea*), Myrtaceae (e.g., ancestors of *Eucalyptus*), Podocarpaceae, Nothofagaceae (e.g., Southern beeches—*Nothofagus*), and so forth, adapted to the changing conditions, were replaced by other plant communities, or retreated to refugia in which the original Gondwanan conditions were retained or changed but little. Such Gondwanan refugia are found today in Australia along its eastern coast, the southeastern and southwestern corners, and in Tasmania; in New Zealand, New Caledonia, and Fiji; in the central highlands of New Guinea; in the Drakensbergs of eastern South Africa; and in the Valdivian and Patagonian rain forests along the eastern coast of southern South America and the cooler Atlantic rain forests in Southern Brazil.

In Australia, several of these seed plants (e.g., Casuarinas, Proteaceae, Myrtaceae) occur predominantly in the Gondwanan refugia (Schodde & Tidemann 1986) and bear complex inflorescences that mature into multi-seeded, fibrous-woody infructescences, called cones, cobs, or capsules. Several species have also become serotinous (i.e., they retain their mature fibrous-woody fruits for several years in their canopy instead of shedding their mature seeds), presumably in adaptation to their fire-prone environment (Homberger 2003). That the psittaciform species that possess a calyptorhynchid feeding apparatus (most Red-tailed Black Cockatoos, *Calyptorhynchus banksii* subspecies; the Glossy Black Cockatoo, *C. lathami*; and the Gang-gang Cockatoo, *Callocephalon fimbriatum*) not only occur in these refugia but also have a feeding apparatus that is specifically adapted to exploiting these plants supports the hypothesis that the calyptorhynchid feeding apparatus is the ancestral condition for Psittaciformes.

In the other southern continents and islands, the Gondwanan refugia are dominated by Gondwanan plants whose seeds are enclosed in thinner seed-shells (e.g., Araucariaceae, Nothofagaceae, some Podocarpaceae) or sclerotic endocarps with preformed weak points and sutures (e.g., some Podocarpaceae). The psittaciform species that feed on these seeds and are restricted to Gondwanan refugia can be surmised to have evolved their psittacid feeding apparatus already in adaptation to these plants before the breakup of Gondwana and were able to retain it because their environment changed little, if at all. This is probably the situation, for example, of the Austral and Slender-billed Conures (*Enicognathus ferrugineus* and *E. leptorhynchus*) in southern South America; the Vinaceous Amazon (*Amazona vinacea*) in southern Brazil; the Cape Parrot (*Poicephalus r. robustus*) in southeastern Africa; and the non-cacatuid psittaciforms with a psittacid feeding apparatus in the Australo-Pacific region.

The greatest diversity of Psittaciformes at the familial and subfamilial levels is found in the Australo-Pacific region (see Figure 1.1). This indicates that this part of Gondwana may have contained the greatest psittaciform diversity even before its separation from the remainder of Gondwana and further breakup into what is known today as Australia, New Guinea, New Zealand, New Caledonia, and Fiji.

THE SUBDIVISION AND CLASSIFICATION OF THE PSITTACIFORMES

The very ease with which psittaciforms can be identified as such is compensated by the difficulties that are encountered trying to subdivide this large order into smaller, hierarchically arranged taxonomic units that are united by common characteristics (i.e., families, subfamilies, tribes, genera). Such a classification creates order within the multitude of species, which is needed for scientific research (e.g., systematics, comparative morphology, evolutionary biology) and applied biology (e.g., evaluation of susceptibility to certain diseases, choice of foster parents for the management of endangered species). However, it must be kept in mind that every classification is only a

hypothesis that needs to be tested continuously as new data emerge and earlier interpretations are re-evaluated in light of new observations. Changes in the nomenclature of taxa and in the hierarchical levels of taxonomic subdivisions are, hence, reflective of intense scientific activity but are not an end in themselves.

Numerous classifications have been proposed over the last 200 years, but all have faced considerable difficulties. One of the underlying reasons for this situation is that the Psittaciformes represent a very old group that had to adapt to numerous environmental changes in the course of its long history dating back to the early Tertiary (ca. 60 million years ago). Because similar environmental changes (e.g., aridification, tropicalization, colonization of volcanic islands, etc.) have occurred in different regions, many derived features have been acquired independently and convergently by different psittaciform lineages in adaptation to these new environments. This prevalence of convergent (i.e., homoplastic) features among the Psittaciformes as a group has hampered earlier efforts in classifying this avian order, mainly because many convergent and other non-homologous features have been misidentified as homologous ones that would indicate evolutionary relationships (for discussions, see Homberger 1980a, 1991; Güntert 1981).

The distinction between homologous and convergent features is one of the most challenging tasks for evolutionary biologists, because the first step in this procedure requires the analysis of both the structure and function of the features, as well as their biological role in the natural environment. Two examples will illustrate the basic approach. The first example will use the bony suborbital arch to demonstrate the possible pitfalls in analyzing features in isolation. A recent functional-anatomical analysis of the bony suborbital arch in cockatoos revealed that it is a component of the feeding apparatus and as such cannot be used as a feature in isolation. It also revealed that its most complete configuration is intimately connected with lateral mandibular movements during feeding in Black Cockatoos that possess a calyptorhynchid feeding apparatus. Various configurations of less complete suborbital arches in different psittaciform lineages that possess a psittacid feeding apparatus can, therefore, be interpreted as derived remnants of the ancestral condi-

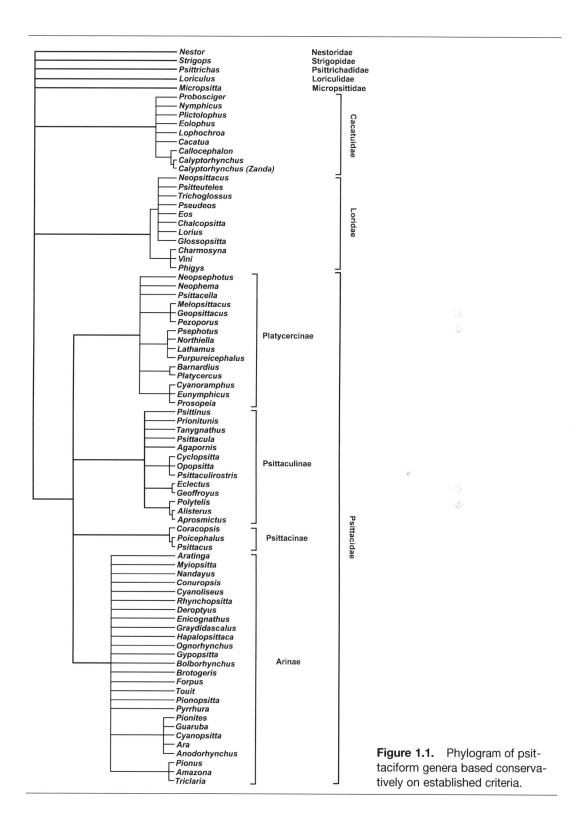

Figure 1.1. Phylogram of psittaciform genera based conservatively on established criteria.

tion that is still present in psittaciforms with a calyptorhynchid feeding apparatus. This reinterpretation of the evolutionary history of the bony suborbital arch is contrary to the original interpretation by Hofer (1950, 1953) and Zusi (1993), both of whom did not have access to observations of psittaciforms in their natural environment.

The second example will use the oral plate of the upper rhamphotheca (i.e., corneous sheath of the maxilla) to demonstrate that a particular structure may be composed of several features that provide different insights for the reconstruction of the evolutionary history of the Psittaciformes. The oral plate of the upper rhamphotheca consists of three parts: The inside of the upper bill tip, the transverse step, and the corneous palate. The inside of the upper bill tip of parrots that possess a psittacid feeding apparatus is corrugated by filing ridges. These filing ridges, however, are arranged in patterns and are formed by the underlying soft tissues in a manner that is highly variable among, but generally characteristic of, species. The inside of the upper bill tip of psittaciforms that possess a calyptorhynchid feeding apparatus is smooth and lacks any surface structure (Homberger 2003). The evolutionary transition from the ancestral to the derived condition of the inside of the upper bill tip is modeled by the various populations and subspecies of the Red-tailed Black Cockatoo (_Calyptorhynchus banksii_) and is clearly correlated with the derived seed-shelling behavior of psittaciforms with a psittacid feeding apparatus (Homberger 2003). In contrast, the surface structure of the corneous palate, which is the feature with the greatest diagnostic value for the identification of genera in psittaciforms, does not have any functional significance (Homberger 1980a).

Mosaic evolution, that is, the presence of primitive and derived characters in a single species as a result of asynchronous evolutionary changes, has been another source of difficulties for the classification of the Psittaciformes. Because of it, a phylogeny that is based on a particular set of features, such as the feeding apparatus, may not simply correspond to another phylogeny that is based on a different set of features. As a consequence, the evolutionary history of each lineage and species needs to be reconstructed by carefully analyzing, weighing, and integrating a variety of data and observations. A simplified example

taken from the Cacatuidae may illustrate such a case. Among birds in general, a large body size is a derived character, because flight has a much greater safety margin in small birds than in larger birds and, therefore, has probably originated in small avian ancestors whose flight apparatus may not have been perfected yet (Homberger & de Silva 2000; Homberger 2003). According to this criterion, the Cockatiel (_Nymphicus hollandicus_) could be considered the most ancestral cockatoo. This interpretation could be supported by its dark plumage color and pattern, which are similar to those of the Black Cockatoos (_Calyptorhynchus_ spp.) and clearly more ancestral than the plumage colors and patterns of the White and Pink Cockatoos. But the Cockatiel's psittacid feeding apparatus and its ecology in Australia's more arid woodlands indicate that it has also acquired derived characters in adaptation to the aridification of Australia. In contrast, the Red-tailed Black Cockatoos and the Gang-gang Cockatoo are characterized by ancestral plumage colors and patterns and by the ancestral calyptorhynchid feeding apparatus. At the same time, the Red-tailed Black Cockatoos are among the larger cockatoos, whose body size may have evolved in conjunction with their more massive bills to handle their diet of large fibrous-woody fruits (Homberger 2003).

At this point in time, the best classification of the Psittaciformes may be one that is based on a large number of features, whose biological and evolutionary significance has been analyzed and is well understood. Unfortunately, we are still far from this goal. The proposed classification (see Figure 1.1) is presented as a pragmatic proposal that combines simplicity and familiarity and avoids some of the errors of earlier classifications.

THE STATUS OF WILD POPULATIONS OF PARROTS

Over the millions of years since their origin in the early Tertiary, many psittaciform species have survived and continued to adapt successfully to changing environmental conditions, as we can conclude from their present geographical distribution and the number of existing species and individuals. Other species have not been able to do so and have become extinct, as we know from historical records or from fossils in regions, such as Europe, in which psittaciforms have been absent in historical times. Rates of extinction are difficult to estimate from the fossil record, because fossilization is a rare event in any case and especially so for organisms, such as the ancestral and many other Psittaciformes, that are relatively small and live in microorganism-rich forest environments with their characteristically rapid degradation of organic materials. Nevertheless, the large number of species that are known to have existed at least until the more recent rash of extinctions testifies to the success and probably net increase in number of species and individuals of the Psittaciformes over the course of their evolutionary history.

Although extinctions of species are a normal part of biological evolution, extinction must be counterbalanced by speciation, that is, the appearance of new species, if a taxon, or group of species, as a whole is to survive. The appearance of new species, however, is presently not occurring any longer, at least not naturally. This process normally starts when a certain portion of a population becomes separated from the rest of the population by the appearance of a geographical barrier, such as a river having changed direction, an area having been divided by the uplifting of a mountain or the formation of a desert, or a number of individuals having migrated permanently to an island. This separation, or isolation, prevents the exchange of genetic materials between the separate populations and provides the conditions for the two populations to accumulate distinctive mutations, undergo distinctive selective processes, and, thereby, acquire distinctive traits simply by themselves or in adaptation to distinct environmental conditions.

The main reason for natural speciation not to be initiated any longer is the accelerating and well-documented shrinking of the natural habitats, so that psittaciform populations cannot expand and subsequently be subdivided into non-interbreeding populations. However, the recent successful establishment of self-sustaining parrot populations from aviary and transport escapees in various urban and suburban places in regions that had been devoid of natural populations of psittaciforms may be considered an experiment in human-induced speciation. As we can extrapolate from earlier such experiments in the late 18th and early 19th centuries, during which European songbirds (e.g., House Sparrows, Starlings, Chaffinches, Blackbirds, European Goldfinches) were

transported to colonies in North America, Australia, and New Zealand by homesick European emigrants, the successful psittaciform expatriate populations in Germany, England, and North America may eventually become genetically distinct from their source populations. But modifications of external features will take many generations to become noticeable, as they did in the various domesticated psittaciforms, and these changes may reflect adaptations to the new environments or the lack of specific selection pressures (e.g., in cases of variable plumage colors), unless these mostly urban populations will be repeatedly swamped by new escapees and accidental releases. The possibility of such artificial speciation events may be a consolation, but hardly a compensation for the current progressive loss of the amazing diversity of psittaciform species in their natural environment.

There is no denying that the single-most threat to natural populations is the capture of individuals for aviculture and the pet market. Captive breeding of parrots by private individuals for conservation purposes should be recognized as the smoke screen that it is (Beissinger et al. 1991; Beissinger 2001; Snyder et al. 1997; Wright et al. 2001). Only a single psittaciform species, the Puerto Rican Amazon (*Amazona vittata*) (Wilson et al. 1994, Wunderle et al. 2003) has been brought back from the brink of extinction, which was made possible only through the lavish investment of governmental funding. The success of other governmental rescue programs for the Kaka (*Nestor meridionalis*) and Kakapo (*Strigops habroptilus*) in New Zealand (Beggs & Wilson 1991; Lloyd & Powlesland 1994) and the Orange-bellied Parrot (*Neophema chrysogaster*) in Australia (Drechsler 1998) is still uncertain. Such massive financial investments for the rescue of single species are beyond the possibilities of even very wealthy persons. Furthermore, although there have been successful reintroductions of captive individuals into the wild provided that these could be integrated with natural populations of the same species (Brightsmith et al. 2003), simple releases of captive-bred psittaciforms into natural environments, whose resources are characteristically seasonal and unpredictable, have not been successful (Snyder et al. 1994). The reason for these difficulties may well be based in the evolutionary origin of the Psittaciformes with their specialized diet of wood-boring and gallicole insect larvae, which could be detected only through indirect evidence and through learning from experienced individuals.

ACKNOWLEDGMENTS

I thank Andrew Luescher for his kind invitation to contribute to this volume and his excellent editorship. I also thank David Ray for designing the phylogram.

REFERENCES

Beggs, J.R., and P.R. Wilson. 1991. The kaka *Nestor meridionalis*, a New Zealand parrot endangered by introduced wasps and mammals. *Biol Conserv* 56 (1):23–38.

Beissinger, S.R. 2001. "Trade of live wild birds: Potentials, principles and practices of sustainable use." In *Conservation of exploited species,* ed. J.D. Reynolds, G.M. Mace, K.H. Redford, and J.G. Robinson, pp. 182–202. Cambridge: Cambridge University Press.

Beissinger, S.R., N.F.R. Snyder, S.R. Derrickson, F.C. James, F.C., and S.M. Lanyon, S.M. 1991. International trade in live exotic birds creates a vast movement that must be halted. *Auk* 108 (4):982–984.

Boetticher, H. von. 1959. *Papageien.* Wittenberg Lutherstadt, Germany: A. Ziemsen Verlag.

Brightsmith, D., J. Hilburn, A. del Campo, J. Boyd, M. Frisius, R. Frisius, F. Guille, and D. Janik. 2003. "Survival and reproduction of hand-raised scarlet macaws (*Ara macao*) in the wild." In *Abstracts of VII Neotropical Ornithological Congress, Termas de Puyehue, Chile: Program and book of abstracts,* p. 106. Chile: Neotropical Ornithological Society.

Brooke, M., and T. Birkhead. 1991. *The Cambridge encyclopedia of ornithology.* Cambridge: Cambridge University Press.

Collar, N.J. 1997. "Family Psittacidae (parrots)." In *Handbook of the birds of the world. Volume 4: Sandgrouse to cuckoos,* ed. J. del Hoyo, A. Elliott, and J. Sargatal, pp. 280–477. Barcelona: Lynx Edicions.

Cracraft, J. 2001. Avian evolution, Gondwana biogeography and the Cretaceous-Tertiary mass extinction event. *Proc R Soc Lond B* 268 (1466):459–469.

Drechsler, M. 1998. Spatial conservation management of the orange-bellied parrot *Neophema chrysogaster*. *Biol Conserv* 84 (3):283–292.

Forshaw, J.M. 1989. *Parrots of the world,* 3rd ed. Melbourne: Lansdowne Editions.

Frakes, L.A., and P. Vickers-Rich. 1991. "Palaeoclimatic setting and palaeogeographic links of Australia in the Phanerozoic." In *Vertebrate palaeontology of Australasia,* ed. P. Vickers-Rich, J.M. Monghan, R.F. Baird, and T.H. Tich, pp. 111–146. Melbourne: Monash University Publications Committee.

Güntert, M. 1981. Morphologische Untersuchungen zur adaptiven Radiation des Verdauungstraktes bei Papageien (Psittaci). *Zool Jahrb Anat* 106:471–526.

Hofer, H. 1950. Zur Morphologie der Kiefermuskulatur der Vögel. *Zool Jahrb Anat* 70 (4):427–556.

Hofer, H. 1953. Die Kiefermuskulatur der Papageien als Evolutionsproblem. *Biol Zentralbl* 62 (5/6): 225–232.

Homberger, D.G. 1980a. Funktionell morphologische Untersuchungen zur Radiation der Ernährungs und Trinkmethoden der Papageien (Psittacidae). [Functional morphological studies on the radiation of the feeding and drinking methods of the parrots]. *Bonner Zoologische Monographien,* No. 13, pp. 192.

Homberger, D.G. 1980b. "Functional morphology and evolution of the feeding apparatus in parrots, with special reference to the Pesquet's Parrot, *Psittrichas fulgidus* (lesson)." In *Conservation of new world parrots,* ed. R.F. Pasquier, pp. 471–485. International Council for Bird Preservation Technical Paper No. 1. Washington, DC: Smithsonian Institution Press.

Homberger, D.G. 1981. Morphological foundations of the bill honing behavior in parrots (Psittacidae). *Amer Zool* 21 (4):1039.

Homberger, D.G. 1991. "The evolutionary history of parrots and cockatoos: A model for evolution in the Australasian avifauna." Acta XX Congr Int Ornithol, pp. 398–403.

Homberger, D.G. 2001. "The case of the cockatoo bill, horse hoof, rhinoceros horn, whale baleen, and turkey beard: The integument as a model system to explore the concepts of homology and nonhomology." In *Vertebrate functional morphology: Horizon of research in the 21st century,* ed. H.M. Dutta and J.S. Datta Munshi, pp. 317–343. Enfield, NH: Science Publishers Inc.

Homberger, D.G. 2003. "The comparative biomechanics of a prey-predator relationship: The adaptive morphologies of the feeding apparatus of Australian black cockatoos and their foods as a basis for the reconstruction of the evolutionary history of the Psittaciformes." In *Vertebrate biomechanics and evolution,* ed. V.L. Bels, J.-P. Gasc, and A. Casinos, pp. 203–228. Oxford: BIOS Scientific Publishers.

Homberger, D.G., and K.N. de Silva. 2000. Functional microanatomy of the feather-bearing avian integument: Implications for the evolution of birds and avian flight. *Amer Zool* 40 (4):553–574.

Juniper, T., and M. Parr. 1998. *Parrots: A guide to parrots of the world.* New Haven: Yale University Press.

Lloyd, B.D., and R.G. Powlesland. 1994. The decline of

the kakapo *Strigops habroptilus* and attempts at conservation by translocation. *Biol Conserv* 69:75–85.

Mettke-Hofmann, C., H. Winkler, and B. Leisler. 2002. The significance of ecological factors for exploration and neophobia in parrots. *Ethology* 108 (3):249–272.

Pepperberg, I.M. 2002. *Alex studies: Cognitive and communicative abilities of grey parrots.* Cambridge, MA: Harvard University Press.

Rowley, I. 1997. "Family Cacatuidae (cockatoos)." In *Handbook of the birds of the world. Volume 4: Sandgrouse to cuckoos,* ed. J. del Hoyo, A. Elliott, and J. Sargatal, pp. 246–279. Barcelona: Lynx Edicions.

Schodde, R., and S.C. Tidemann. 1986. *Reader's Digest complete book of Australian birds.* Sydney: Reader's Digest.

Smith, G.A. 1975. Systematics of parrots. *Ibis* 117:18–68.

Snyder, N.F.R., S.R. Derrickson, S.R. Beissinger, J.W. Wiley, T.B. Smith, W.D. Toone, and B. Miller. 1997. Limitations of captive breeding: Reply to Gippoliti and Carpaneto. *Conserv Biol* 11 (3):808–810.

Snyder, N.F.R., S.E. Koenig, J. Koschmann, H.A. Snyder, and T.B. Johnson. 1994. Thick-billed parrot releases in Arizona. *Condor* 96:845–862.

Stevens, G.R. 1991. "Geological evolution and biotic links in the Mesozoic and Cenozoic of the southwest Pacific." Acta XX Congr Int Ornithol, pp. 361–382.

White, M.E. 1990. *The flowering of Gondwana; The 400 million year story of Australia's plants.* Princeton: Princeton University Press.

White, M.E. 1994. *After the greening: The browning of Australia.* Kenthurst, NSW: Kangaroo Press.

Wilson, M.H., C.B. Kepler, N.F.R. Snyder, S.R. Derrickson, F.J. Dein, J.W. Wiley, J.M. Wunderle, A.E. Lugo, D.L. Graham, and W.D. Toone. 1994. Puerto Rican parrots and potential limitations of the metapopulation approach to species conservation. *Conserv Biol* 8 (1):114–123.

Wright, T.F., C.A. Toft, E. Enkerlin-Hoeflich, J. Gonzalez-Elizondo, M. Albornoz, A. Rodríguez-Ferraro, F. Rojas-Suárez, V. Sanz, A. Trujillo, S.R. Beissinger, V. Berovides A., X. Gálvez A., A.T. Brice, K. Joyner, J. Eberhard, J. Gilardi, S.E. Koenig, S. Stoleson, P. Martuscelli, J.M. Meyers, K. Renton, A.M. Rodríguez, A.C. Sosa-Asanza, F. Vilella, and J.W. Wiley. 2001. Nest poaching in Neotropical parrots. *Conserv Biol* 15:710–720.

Wunderle, J.M., Jr., N.F. Snyder, S.R. Beissinger, J.M. Meyers, and J.W. Wiley. 2003. "Struggling out of the bottleneck: Puerto Rican parrot recovery from 1973 to 2000." In *VII Neotropical Ornithological Congress, Termas de Puyehue—Chile, October 5–11, 2003: Program and book of abstracts,* p. 155. Chile: Neotropical Ornithological Society.

Zusi, R.L. 1993. "Pattern of diversity in the avian skull." In *The skull. Volume 2: Patterns of structural and systematic diversity,* ed. J. Hanken and B.K. Hall, pp. 391–437. Chicago: University of Chicago Press.

2
Behavior of Wild *Amazona* and *Rhynchopsitta* Parrots, with Comparative Insights from Other Psittacines

Ernesto C. Enkerlin-Hoeflich, Noel F.R. Snyder, and James W. Wiley

Research on the behavioral characteristics of selected wild psittacines may be important in establishing management and conservation guidelines for these species, both in the wild and in captivity. An understanding of such behavioral characteristics may also have wider significance in aiding the interpretations of behavioral and natural history parameters in other psittacine birds. Prior to the 1970s, intensive biological studies of wild Neotropical parrots were nearly nonexistent. This gap in ornithological knowledge is now being rapidly remedied with numerous species under investigation throughout Central and South America and the West Indies. Yet to date there have been few attempts to integrate the information from various studies into coherent frameworks of biological understanding. In this offering, we provide a number of preliminary hypotheses about parrot behavior, based largely on studies of a variety of species, mainly in the genera *Amazona* and *Rhynchopsitta*. These hypotheses appear to have wide explanatory power, yet need to be tested in additional genera and species before their validity can be considered firm.

Our basic approach is the comparative one, looking at features of behavior that vary among species and attempting to correlate these differences with underlying ecological imperatives faced by the species under consideration. As raw materials for these comparisons, we rely heavily on intensive studies of (1) the Puerto Rican Parrot (*Amazona vittata*) by Snyder et al. (1987); (2) various subspecies of the Cuban Parrot (*Amazona leucocephala*) by Gnam (1991), Wiley (unpublished), and others; (3) the Hispaniolan Parrot (*Amazona ventralis*) by Wiley (unpublished); (4) the Jamaican Black-billed and Yellow-billed Parrots (*Amazona agilis* and *collaria*) by Koenig (1999); (5) the St. Lucia Parrot (*Amazona versicolor*), the Imperial Parrot (*Amazona imperialis*), the Red-necked Parrots (*Amazona arausiaca*) of the Lesser Antilles by Snyder, Koenig, and many others (unpublished); and (6) three species of amazons in northeastern Mexico by Enkerlin-Hoeflich (1995, unpublished)—the Red-crowned Parrot (*Amazona viridigenalis*), the Yellow-headed Parrot (*Amazona oratrix*), and the Red-lored Parrot (*Amazona autumnalis*). Studies of *Rhynchopsitta pachyrhyncha* and *terrisi* have been primarily carried out by Enkerlin-Hoeflich (unpublished), Cruz-Nieto et al. (1998), Snyder et al. (1999), Lanning and Shiflett (1981, 1983), and Lawson and Lanning (1982).

The particular behavioral features we consider here are (1) the values of intraspecific sociality in various species, (2) timing of nesting seasons, (3) site and pair fidelity, and nest reuse, (4) feeding behavior and rates, (5) relationships of species conspicuousness and nest accessibility to exploitation in the pet trade, and (6) deficits in breeding effort.

BACKGROUND

As generally understood, the genus *Amazona* includes 31 extant species limited largely to tropical areas of the Western Hemisphere. The various species occur from Argentina and Chile north through virtually all of mainland South America and Central America to northern Mexico (Juniper & Parr 1998). Feral populations of several species also exist in a number of southern cities of the United States, Mexico, and Puerto Rico (Enkerlin-Hoeflich & Hogan 1997; Mabb 1997). The West Indies have a particularly good *Amazona* fauna with nine extant species about evenly divided between the Greater Antilles and Lesser Antilles. Many *Amazona* species are now endangered, and most all are declining, threatened mainly by bird trade and habitat changes, but also in some cases by hunting, introduced exotic species, and other factors (Snyder et al. 2000). The various species of *Amazona* are far from monolithic in their behavior and ecology. Species vary in clutch and brood sizes, diets, feeding rates, degrees of sociality, reproductive effort, and reproductive success, to name just a few facets of interest.

The genus *Rhynchopsitta* has only two living species, both distributed in the highlands of northern Mexico in more or less "island-like" forest habitats. The Thick-billed Parrot (*R. pachyrhyncha*) is a tree-cavity nester inhabiting the Sierra Madre Occidental in western Chihuahua and eastern Sonora south through the mountains of Durango, Sinaloa, Nayarit, and Jalisco to Colima and Michoacan. It was also formerly a regular inhabitant of extreme southeastern Arizona and probably bred there until the early 20th century, although no historical records of nests exist for this region. The Maroon-fronted Parrot (*R. terrisi*) is a cliff-cavity nester that occurs in the Sierra Madre Oriental of northeastern Mexico in southeastern Coahuila, central western Nuevo León, and southwestern Tamaulipas (Juniper & Parr 1998). Like many of the *Amazona*, both extant species of *Rhynchopsitta* are globally threatened. In addition, on the basis of fossils, Rea (1997) recently described a third species of *Rhynchopsitta* (*R. phillipsi*), now extinct, that was apparently sympatric with both *pachyrhyncha* and *terrisi* in the Sierra Madre Oriental in the late Pleistocene. The former sympatry of *pachyrhyncha* and *terrisi* makes it quite clear that these two parrots are distinct species and not simply races of a single species, as they were considered by Forshaw (1990).

VALUES OF SOCIALITY AMONG *AMAZONA* AND *RHYNCHOPSITTA* PARROTS

In general, *Amazona* parrots tend to be highly social in foraging and roosting habits and somewhat social in nesting habits, but some conspicuous differences exist among species in these tendencies. Four species that stand out in their disinclination to travel in groups larger than family groups are the large amazons of the Lesser Antilles—the St. Lucia Parrot, the St. Vincent Parrot (*A. guildingii*), the Imperial Parrot, and the Red-necked Parrot. Although these species sometimes assemble in groups larger than family units at roosts and at rich food sources, they normally nest in relatively dispersed arrays and travel only as singles, pairs, or small family groups in moving from nests or roosts to foraging areas. In contrast, other amazons, including most of those in the Greater Antilles and Mexico, show clear tendencies toward clumped nesting, often travel in much larger groups, and typically feed in large aggregations. Low sociality in the Lesser Antillean species is also reflected in the fact that male and female adults often separate in foraging activities in the breeding season and often feed their young independently. Such independent provisioning of nests is virtually unknown in amazons of the Greater Antilles and the mainland Neotropics.

Are there any obvious ecological correlates to explain the relatively low sociality of the large amazons of the Lesser Antilles? One promising possibility is the fact that these species, essentially alone among species in the genus, live in habitats that are effectively free of predation threats from large raptors. Whereas most Greater Antillean amazons and essentially all mainland *Amazona* have to deal with threats from large raptors such as Red-tailed Hawks (*Buteo jamaicensis*), Peregrine Falcons (*Falco peregrinus*), and various *Accipiter* species, no large accipiters or buteos occur in the Lesser Antilles, and the Peregrine Falcons of these islands are largely wintering birds utilizing coastal areas separate from the rain forest habitats occupied by the Lesser Antillean parrot species.

The largest raptor in parrot habitats of most of

the Lesser Antilles is the Broad-winged Hawk, which is too small to represent a credible threat to the parrots and for which there are no records of parrot predation. The Red-tailed Hawk, on the other hand, is not a species to be underestimated in its capacities to take *Amazona* parrots. Records exist of it successfully dispatching a variety of *Amazona* and *Rhynchopsitta* species in the Greater Antilles and on the mainland.

Thus, to the extent that conspicuous flocking behavior has often been suggested as primarily an adaptation to reduce risks of avian predation, the Lesser Antillean amazons might be expected to gain little by flocking behavior and the tendency may never have evolved or may have disappeared in the evolutionary history of these species because of very low predation threats. Flocking behavior has often been envisioned as primarily a means to reduce predation via the increased vigilance possible when the combined sensory capacities of multiple individuals are available and when specific individuals can serve as sentinels for groups (see discussions in Snyder et al. 1987 and Yamashita 1987).

Only one of the Greater Antillean amazons shows social behavior similar to that of the Lesser Antillean species, the race of the Cuban Parrot on Cayman Brac (*Amazona leucocephala hesterna*). Like the Lesser Antillean species, the Cayman Brac Parrot rarely travels in groups larger than family groups, and its male and female adults often feed their young independently (Wiley, unpublished). And like the Lesser Antillean species, and as one might predict from the preceding discussion, this parrot lives in an environment free of significant avian predators. No Red-tailed Hawks or large accipiters occur on Cayman Brac, and the Peregrine Falcons that are seen there occasionally are mostly on the coast, posing no significant risks to the parrots.

The associations of low sociality with low predation risks and high sociality with high predation risks strongly suggest a causal connection of these features. Further reinforcing this conclusion is the fact that the race of the Cuban Parrot on Grand Cayman (*Amazona leucocephala caymanensis*) shows the typical *Amazona* tendency toward large flocks and apparently feeds its young as pairs. Significantly, there are Red-tailed Hawks on Grand Cayman, unlike nearby Cayman Brac. Thus the parrots of the various Cayman Islands in

themselves give strong evidence for the importance of avian predators in producing social tendencies among *Amazona* parrots.

We also call attention to the especially well-developed sociality of the Thick-billed and Maroon-fronted Parrots of Mexico. These *Rhynchopsitta* species are similar to the amazons in size and face predation risks from the same sorts of avian predators. In particular, these species face significant predation threats from both Red-tailed Hawks and Peregrine Falcons, and in the case of the Thick-billed Parrot, also from Apache Goshawks (*Accipiter gentilis apache*). In our experience, sociality in the *Rhynchopsitta* species is even more highly developed than in any *Amazona* species for which we have data. In fact, pairs of the Thick-billed Parrot often nest very close together, sometimes with more than one pair in the same tree, while Maroon-fronted Parrots typically nest in dense colonies in cliffs. Moreover, observations indicate that breeding males of the Thick-billed Parrot typically associate in combined flocks for foraging, often waiting for one another to leave the nesting areas as a group. Such coordinated male behavior has not been regularly recorded for any *Amazona* species.

Other explanations for the flocking and sociality of amazon parrots—for example, traditional arguments for advantages in food finding in birds (see Krebs 1974)—have difficulty in accounting for the variations in sociality seen in various *Amazona* species. That there might be any basic differences in food availability for the Cayman Brac Parrot and the Lesser Antillean species that could explain their low sociality is undocumented and does not seem intuitively likely. Available evidence suggests that they feed on much the same foods that are taken by other more social species in the genus.

Regardless of what factors are truly most important in producing the relatively high degree of sociality found in most *Amazona* and *Rhynchopsitta*, this characteristic is generally considered to be adaptive in the lives of these species. Modern circumstances, however, can produce situations where this is clearly not true. We call attention to a recent instance of mass drowning of *Rhynchopsitta terrisi* in an artificial water catchment where the species suffered a major population stress precisely because of its high degree of sociality. In this instance, in 1994, at least 52 *R.*

terrisi perished when they were unable to exit from an artificial cement water tank that they had apparently entered for drinking and/or bathing purposes. When one considers that the total population of this species is only about 3,000 birds and the annual recruitment of young is only about 200 individuals, this event was nothing short of catastrophic (Macías-Caballero et al. 2001).

As an aside, *Rhynchopsitta* parrots, like many species of Australian parrots, but unlike most Neotropical parrots inhabiting humid environments and consuming foods high in water content, come to water sources, such as waterfalls, to drink on a daily basis. This behavior has been documented in both species of *Rhynchopsitta* (Snyder et al. 1999; Macías-Caballero et al. 2001), and, like the parrot assemblages at clay licks of the Amazon basin, constitutes a marvelous spectacle. Unfortunately, man-induced changes in the environment have both reduced the availability of springs and waterfalls in the landscape and increased the presence of artificial water catchments that can pose inadvertent risks of mortality to the species.

Another species for which high sociality may have led to major population stress from human sources is the extinct Carolina Parakeet (*Conuropsis carolinensis*). Flocks of this species were exceedingly vulnerable to shooting, and the tendency of the species to roost together in large groups in hollow trees made it susceptible to heavy harvest for the pet trade, both of which factors were of presumed importance in the species' decline (Snyder & Russell 2002). The high sociality of this species may also have rendered it highly susceptible to the spread of exotic diseases.

Finally, as another aside, we note that the absence of any strong tendency for flocking in the Lesser Antillean and Cayman Brac *Amazona* is a factor that makes censusing of these species especially difficult. Although counts of large flocks entering and leaving roosts have proven an effective way to census many other *Amazona* species—for example, the Puerto Rican Parrot and the Bahama Parrot (*A. leucocephala bahamensis*)—it is not a practical option for species with low flocking tendencies.

TIMING OF NESTING SEASONS

In the West Indies, most amazon parrots begin egg laying in the late winter and early spring, with March usually the peak month. This timing is in general correlated with the dry season, and could be related primarily to minimizing risks of nest loss to flooding, although it could alternatively be keyed to seasonal aspects of food availability. Strongly suggesting the latter is the abnormally late egg-laying period seen in the Bahama Parrots of Abaco, which do not normally lay until late May and early June, just before onset of the rainy season in that region (Gnam 1991). Here, laying appears to be timed to take advantage of the abundance of poisonwood (*Metopium toxiferum*) fruits, wild guava (*Tetrazygia bicolor*) fruits and appropriate-aged pine (*Pinus caribea*) seeds in midsummer, the most important known foods for the species in provisioning young. The Bahama Parrots on Inagua Island apparently lay at a more typical time in the early spring, in line with other amazons of the West Indies (Snyder et al. 1982). Pine is absent from Inagua, and poisonwood is not nearly as conspicuous an element of the flora on this island as on Abaco.

Breeding seasons of mainland amazons have been especially closely studied in northeastern Mexico (Enkerlin-Hoeflich 1995) and are similar to most West Indian amazons, with peak laying in late March and early April (Table 2-1). The sympatric Red-crowned Parrot, Yellow-headed Parrot, and Red-lored Parrot have similar egg-laying dates. Food is abundant during spring and summer for Mexican *Amazona*. There is no clear-cut dry season, although spring and summer usually show peaks in rain and winter is normally dry. Their breeding season is earlier as one moves south and would indicate that it is more related to photoperiod or temperature than to food availability (Enkerlin-Hoeflich 1995, unpublished data).

Breeding seasons of the *Rhynchopsitta* species are extremely delayed relative to the *Amazona* species, and this delay is almost surely keyed to their specialized diets, primarily of various conifer seeds, which do not normally become abundantly available until midsummer, with early June being the low point in seasonal availability of seeds for the conifer species in the ranges of the species. The mean egg-laying date of the Thick-billed Parrot in Chihuahua has been mid-July, with most chicks fledged by the first or second week of October (Snyder et al. 1999). The Maroon-fronted Parrot starts somewhat later with

Table 2.1. Clutch initiation, incubation periods, feeding visits, and fledging age for *Amazona* parrots[a]

Descriptive statistics	*A. autumnalis* (n = 24)	*A. oratrix* (n = 6)	*A. viridigenalis* (n = 26)
Week (number of nests)			
1 = 19–24 March	3	1	1
2 = 25–31 March	4	3	7
3 = 1–7 April	10	1	10
4 = 8–14 April	5	1	2
5 = 15–21 April	1	0	5
6+ = after 22 April	1	0	1
"Mean" (week of initiation)[b]	3.00	2.33	3.23
Range (week of initiation)	1 to 6	1 to 4	1 to 6
Standard deviation	1.22	1.03	1.27
Coefficient of variation	0.41	0.44	0.39
Average initiation of clutch (date)[c]	2 April	31 March	5 April
Mean duration of incubation (days)	28[d]	28[d]	27 (n = 7)
Mean daily feeding visits to the nests[e]	2.09	2.18	2.08
Range of daily visits to the nest[e]	0–3	0–3	0–4
Mean age at fledging (days)	55 (n = 4)	57 (n = 2)	53 (n = 9)

[a]Based on nests inspected with a burrow probe in the 1993 and 1994 breeding seasons. For *A. oratrix,* two additional nests from the 1992 season were included to increase sample size; although no burrow probe was available in 1992, these two nests were shallow enough to be inspected directly.

[b]An index calculated from six categories (weeks) assigned based on day of initiation. A test using Kruskal-Wallis on this index showed no difference among species (KW = 2.5, df = 2, p < 0.281).

[c]Calculated from actual date of initiation for each nest.

[d]As reported in the popular captive breeding literature.

[e]Estimated by multiplying the average number of visits per observation session by two as justified in Enkerlin-Hoeflich 1995. The range of visits also refers to the observation sessions only.

most egg-laying in late July to early August and chicks fledging at the end of October through the first week of November.

Thus, the evidence for importance of diet in determining the timing of breeding is highly suggestive both in the Bahama Parrot and the *Rhynchopsitta* parrots, and diet may be the most important factor with the other *Amazona* as well, although this is less clear from available data. Future studies focused on crop sampling of nestlings of a variety of species to rigorously determine dietary relationships (Enkerlin-Hoeflich et al. 1999), combined with studies of seasonal availability of primary foods, may help solidify knowledge of the most important factors determining the timing of breeding.

NEST SITE AND PAIR FIDELITY, AND CAVITY REUSE

In general, nest site and pair fidelity tend to be high for psittacine birds (Snyder et al. 1987; Rowley & Chapman 1991), although there are variations to be seen among species. High pair fidelity, for example, has been found in two species of *Amazona* in northeastern Mexico—the Red-crowned and Yellow-headed Parrots (Enkerlin-Hoeflich 1995), and as with nest fidelity, may often be associated with improved productivity as the years of experience accumulate. In many studies, cases of divorce have been largely limited to instances of reproductive incompetence of one of the pair members (Snyder et al. 1987; Rowley & Chapman 1991).

Maroon-fronted Parrots nest in colonies ranging from one or two to more than 100 pairs. Pairs seem to have strong site fidelity, at least to the same colony, if not the same nest hole, as demonstrated by returns of birds carrying radio transmitters over periods of several years. Similarly, established pairs of most *Amazona* exhibit a marked degree of philopatry. For example, in northeastern Mexico in 1993, four pairs of visually distinctive *Amazona* that switched nest sites moved to new nests within a 50 m radius of their previous nests. In 1994, five pairs had new nests within a 50 m radius of their previous nests and two pairs moved within a radius of only 100 m. The attachment to specific nesting areas can be something that occurs rapidly: a female Red-crowned Parrot released with a radio collar established her nest sites in two successive nesting periods in trees within 200 m of the release cage (Enkerlin-Hoeflich 1995).

At least six pairs of Red-crowned Parrots and five pairs of Yellow-headed Parrots individually recognizable by feather characteristics showed mate fidelity between successive nesting periods, and at least three of each species exhibited fidelity for three nesting periods. Such high mate fidelity has also been documented in the Puerto Rican Parrot by Snyder et al. (1987) and may be generally true in the genus *Amazona*.

Fidelity to specific nest sites, however, is more variable. Enkerlin-Hoeflich's (1995) studies of Red-crowned and Yellow-headed Parrots in 1993 and 1994 revealed that fidelity to specific sites was low compared to that reported in other *Amazona* (Snyder et al. 1987; Gnam 1991; Rojas-Suárez 1994). In large measure, this difference may reflect species differences in cavity availability, with suitable cavities being considerably more abundant for the Red-crowned and Yellow-headed Parrots than for other amazons, although additional factors may well have been involved as well. Nest switching is standard in many cavity-nesting birds (e.g., Boreal Owls, *Aegolius funereus,* and California Condors, *Gymnogyps californianus*—see Hayward & Hayward 1993 and Snyder & Schmitt 2002), and may offer general advantages, such as reductions in parasite infestations, that need to be balanced against advantages that may result from maintaining site fidelity, especially in cavity-poor environments.

In many species, there is a tendency for pairs to switch nest sites after failures to fledge young and a tendency to stay with nest sites after success in fledging young (Saunders 1982). One pair of Puerto Rican Parrots studied over many years followed this pattern religiously, while other pairs exhibited strong nest-site fidelity regardless of success or failure in the sites over the years (Snyder et al. 1987). As an aside, until it was learned that the latter pattern was the more typical one for this species, efforts to multiple-clutch wild pairs were held in abeyance because of concerns that such efforts would drive pairs into using new nest sites for replacement clutches that might be vulnerable to predation by Pearly-eyed Thrashers (*Margarops fuscatus*). But once the strong tendency of pairs to stick with nest sites, despite failure in the sites, was established, multiple-clutching efforts were initiated with considerable success and without causing pairs to abandon sites.

Even with relatively low levels of nest reutilization, pairs of Red-crowned and Yellow-headed Parrots have exhibited greater tendencies to reuse sites in which they have succeeded than sites in which they have failed. Similarly, studies of Maroon-fronted Parrot nesting colonies indicate that cavities producing fledglings are generally the cavities most frequently reused over several-year periods.

Thus there are reasons to suspect that poaching of entire broods from nests of many species may not only remove immediate reproduction but may also affect future reproduction by stimulating pairs to move to new and untested nest sites, both because poachers frequently destroy nest sites in harvesting them and because they often stimulate the birds to move even if they do not harm the nest sites. If instead parrot trappers were to allow at least one young to fledge per nest and were not to harm nest sites in harvesting young, both parrots and trappers might ultimately benefit from greater overall parrot populations and nest success in the populations. Instituting such relatively prudent harvesting procedures, unfortunately, is unlikely in areas subject to unregulated harvest, because maximization of short-term benefits tends strongly to overbalance maximization of long-term benefits.

FEEDING BEHAVIOR AND RATES

Amazon parrots of the mainland, such as Red-crowned Parrots of northeastern Mexico, almost invariably feed their nestlings only twice a day, regardless of the age of the nestlings—once in early to mid-morning and once in late afternoon (Enkerlin-Hoeflich 1995). This pattern also applies to Lilac-crowned (*A. finschi*), Yellow-headed, Yellow-naped (*A. auropalliata*) , White-fronted (*A. albifrons*), and Red-lored Parrots of Mexico and Central America (personal observations; Renton & Salinas-Melgoza 1999). In contrast, amazon parrots of the West Indies, both in the Greater and Lesser Antilles, typically feed their young four to five times per day, a major difference. The Puerto Rican Parrot, for example, averages about 4.6 feeding trips per day during the nestling period (Snyder et al. 1987). Similarly, the Hispaniolan Parrot (*A. ventralis*) averages 4.3 feeding trips per day and the Cuban Parrot (*A. leucocephala*) averages 4.5 feeding trips per day (Wiley, unpublished). The differences among species in provisioning rates have potentially important consequences, for example with respect to vulnerabilities of adults and nests to predation, and it is of considerable interest to seek potential causes of the differences.

As studied by Enkerlin-Hoeflich (1995) in Red-crowned, Yellow-headed, and Red-lored Parrots, the overall commitment of mainland amazons to a regimen of two feedings per day at nests is extreme. The first feeding visit to nests usually takes place about one hour after sunrise, presumably after a foraging bout. The second visit occurs about one and a half hours before sunset, shortly before adults assemble in roosts. Other mainland Amazons exhibit similar patterns (e.g., Renton & Salinas-Melgoza 1999). In these studies, provisioning trips were highly stereotyped in timing even in cases where feedings were omitted at the expected time in the morning or were interrupted in the morning due to disturbance (e.g., presence of a predator) or other unknown factors. The birds did not attempt compensatory feedings during the middle of the day to make up for the missed feedings, and instead waited until the next normal evening feeding period to resume feeding the young. On a few occasions, we observed that as many as two consecutive feeding sessions were omitted, resulting in up to 36 hours of fasting for the chicks. Nevertheless, the chicks involved eventually fledged successfully. The pattern of visiting the nest only once in the morning and once in the evening

seems so highly ingrained in these species that they seem almost incapable of provisioning at other times of day.

In contrast, amazons of the West Indies characteristically make four to five feeding trips to their nests per day, including multiple trips during the midday hours, and this is true of both the large Lesser Antillean species and the much smaller Greater Antillean species. Somewhat intermediate is the Black-billed Parrot of Jamaica, with an average of 3.8 feeding trips per day (Koenig 1999).

What factors could explain the differences in provisioning rates between the mainland and island amazons? Two possible explanations come immediately to mind—differences in the nutritional quality of diets and different daily regimes of temperature stress. The mainland populations studied to date have essentially all been close to sea level in regions with high midday temperatures potentially offering stress for adults in foraging at that time of day, whereas the island amazon populations studied have mostly been relatively high-elevation rain forest populations that are spared comparable midday heat stress. But in addition, there appears to be a major difference in quality of foods offered to nestlings, with crop sampling of nestlings indicating very high proportions of seeds in the diet of mainland species (Enkerlin-Hoeflich 1995), and with most foods documented for the island species being various kinds of soft fruits (e.g., Snyder et al. 1987). As seeds are a much more concentrated form of nutrition than fruits, the differences in provisioning rates at nests could be largely a consequence of a necessity for the fruit eaters to process large volumes of food to compensate for the low nutritional quality of fruit foods.

These hypotheses are not mutually exclusive and surely are not the only explanations that could be offered for the feeding rate differences, but it is worth examining available data to see if both these hypotheses are consistent with existing information. Here, we caution that comprehensive determinations of diet fed to nestlings are difficult to achieve by observations of adult feeding behavior, as studies of Enkerlin-Hoeflich et al. (1999) have shown that crop sampling of nestlings often yields rather different evaluations of diet than observations of adults foraging. Nevertheless, where crop sampling has been employed most comprehensively—for mainland amazons—it appears that seeds are indeed the overwhelming food types given to nestlings. Much less crop sampling of nestlings has been performed with the island amazons, and although these data are generally consistent with a predominance of fruit feeding, the database is not nearly as good as for the mainland amazons.

With respect to temperature stress explanations, a precise quantification of environmental conditions faced by various species has not been achieved, and could also be related to timing of nesting as was discussed earlier. Nevertheless, we note that the Bahama Parrots of Abaco Island exist in a near-sea-level environment with high midday temperatures, yet also exhibit a high rate of provisioning at nests (averaging about five trips per day). Although these parrots have not been studied with comprehensive crop sampling, they do appear to take many fruits as breeding-season food, especially poisonwood and wild guava, although they also take substantial quantities of pine seeds. Thus the diet of this species on Abaco seems relatively similar to that of other Greater Antillean species and the high feeding rates of the Abaco parrots provide some apparent support for dietary explanations of provisioning rates and lack of support for major temperature effects. Similarly, studies of sea-level populations of the Cuban Parrot in Cuba have also yielded high provisioning rates (4.5 trips per day) in spite of potential temperature stresses. The latter also show overall diets with a substantial proportion of fruit (Gálvez-Aguilera et al. 1998).

Somewhat different conclusions apply to the Black-billed Parrot of Jamaica, with an intermediate feeding rate of about 3.8 trips per day to the nest. One might hypothesize that the Black-billed Parrots might be feeding relatively higher portions of seeds to their nestlings, but this has yet to be shown conclusively. The Jamaican Black-billed Parrots have been studied at mid-elevations, in relation to some other amazons of the West Indies, so they would presumably fall somewhere in the middle in temperature relationships, although this has not been carefully documented.

The *Rhynchopsitta* parrots also offer some potential for distinguishing food quality versus temperature effects on feeding rates. Crop sampling of Thick-billed Parrot nestlings indicates a high proportion of seeds in the diet, primarily pine seeds and, to a lesser extent, acorns, and yet the species occupies a relatively cool and temperate high-elevation range during the breeding season (Snyder et al. 1999). On the basis of a seed diet, one might anticipate only two feedings per day in Thick-bills, by comparison with the amazon species, but on the basis of temperature relationships, one would anticipate an absence of major midday temperature stress, and therefore the potential for more feeding trips per day. Data for the Thick-billed Parrot (Snyder et al. 1999) indicate a usual provisioning rate of three to four trips per day, an intermediate result apparently most consistent with temperature explanations but not entirely inconsistent with nutritional explanations, as the cool high-elevation habitats occupied by these species may increase food or energy needs relative to those of lowland seed-eating amazons. This is reinforced by the presence of brood reduction due to starvation of younger chicks in Thick-billed Parrots, rarely seen in *Amazona*.

Clearly, progress in resolving alternative hypotheses could be achieved by intensive crop-sampling efforts with nestlings of a variety of amazon species, showing a variety of feeding rate patterns, and by quantification of environmental conditions in nesting habitats of the various species.

RELATIONSHIPS OF SPECIES CONSPICUOUSNESS AND NEST ACCESSIBILITY TO EXPLOITATION IN THE PET TRADE

The three species of *Amazona* studied by Enkerlin-Hoeflich (1995) in northeastern Mexico—the Red-crowned, the Yellow-headed, and the Red-lored Parrots—offer an especially instructive look at the influence of behavior on the comparative vulnerability of parrots to exploitation by the pet trade, especially through nest robbing. For the three species, nests of the Red-crowned Parrot are by far the easiest to find, and this species has been so heavily exploited by poachers that it has been totally eliminated from many areas, especially in riparian habitats that are easily accessible (Iñigo-Elias & Ramos 1997; Clinton-Eitniear 1986). The Yellow-headed Parrot has also been very popular in trade because of its capacities to talk, and has also suffered greatly from poaching, although its nests are less easy to find. The most inconspicuous species, the Red-lored Parrot, is in contrast more abundant and widely distributed, and may even be increasing in numbers in the same region inhabited by the other two species. Even without the legal protection enjoyed by the Red-crowned Parrot and the Yellow-headed Parrot, this species has been captured and traded within Mexico to a considerably lesser extent. Its nest trees are as easy to climb as those of the Red-crowned Parrot and Yellow-headed Parrot, and it is abundant in some second-growth and agricultural landscapes, so the lesser degree of human impacts on the species deserves analysis.

Perhaps the most crucial factor in the success of the Red-lored Parrot is its overall wariness and inconspicuousness around nests, leading to major difficulties for humans in finding nests. Pairs of Red-lored Parrots are loud in the general vicinity of nests but secretive in their movements close to their nest trees. Approaches to, landings at, and takeoffs from nests are all done silently. Further, Red-lored Parrot pairs often wait for long periods in a tree distant from the nest tree before moving to a nest. Pairs are usually very loud during interior or intraspecific interactions, but this is usually distant from the nest and rarely helpful in determining a nest location. The routines for each pair are difficult to establish and on several occasions have led to mistakes in identifying their nest locations.

In contrast, the nests of the Red-crowned Parrot are not difficult to find, because the approach of an adult (whether a lone male approaching a nest to feed a female or both birds arriving together) is very deliberate and is announced by a series of characteristic calls. Often members of a pair do not land directly on the nest tree but close to it, with subsequent flight to the nesting tree. If the female is inside the nest, the male usually calls and the female promptly comes out. Both birds usually fly together with characteristic takeoff squawks and land nearby. This series of events is stereotyped and clearly advertises the presence and location of the nest. If the birds are disturbed by a human coming close to the nest location, they take off with loud raucous calls but land nearby and soon return to the nest (within 14–79 minutes, n = 13), if the human observer has concealed him- or herself.

The nests of the Yellow-headed Parrot are intermediate in difficulty of detection. Pairs of this species tend to vocalize for long periods near the nest tree, but they rarely approach the actual nest tree and do not move to the nest tree if they perceive the presence of an observer. In response to the arrival of the male, the female sometimes comes out of the nest promptly, but more often she takes many minutes to come out. In contrast to the Red-crowned Parrot, Yellow-headed Parrots do not give any characteristic calls when departing from the nest. Together, these characteristics make it relatively difficult to find nests of Yellow-headed Parrots.

In keeping with the relative difficulties in finding nests of the three species, the first new nests located each breeding season in the study of Enkerlin-Hoeflich (1995) were predominantly those of Red-crowned Parrots (13 of 21), whereas nests found in the second half of the breeding season were predominantly those of Red-lored Parrots (16 of 21). Although the timing of egg laying was the same in both these species, these differences reflect the much longer times it takes to find the nests of Red-lored Parrots.

Thus, the easy detectability of nests has evidently made the Red-crowned Parrot exceedingly vulnerable to illegal harvest of nestlings, and although nests of the Yellow-headed Parrot are considerably more difficult to find, the high market value of this species has likely greatly increased the motivation of poachers to overcome the problems involved in finding its nests. In contrast, the extreme difficulty in finding nests of the Red-lored Parrot and its lesser market value appear to have enabled it to survive and even thrive in spite of unregulated harvest. One might hypothesize that species such as the Red-crowned Parrot and the Yellow-headed Parrot are likely under strong selective pressures toward becoming less conspicuous around nests, but as yet any such potential changes in behavior have apparently been insufficient to prevent continuous population declines.

The amazon species of the West Indies vary greatly in their conspicuousness around nests. Many are relatively conspicuous, advertising nest locations by loud vocalizations, but two species— the Imperial Parrot and the Cayman Brac Parrot—are so extremely inconspicuous around nests that their nests are infrequently found and harvested. This has been especially true for the

Imperial Parrot. On Cayman Brac, the harvest has been more frequent due to the concerted searching efforts of poachers and absence of many nest trees that are difficult to climb. As in Mexico, harvest of nestlings of the West Indian species has been especially severe for the species that are most conspicuous, and of the island amazons perhaps only those in the Lesser Antilles have received any substantial protection from poachers by relatively frequent inaccessibility of their nests in enormous and difficult-to-climb canopy trees. However, despite such difficulties, poachers on St. Vincent have traditionally managed a substantial harvest, having become especially adept climbers.

Both species of *Rhynchopsitta* in Mexico are conspicuously noisy around nests and nests are not difficult to find, yet there has been relatively little harvest of nestlings of either species. For *R. terrisi*, the main factor preventing nestling harvest has surely been the awesome inaccessibility of essentially all nests. Nests are all in deep solution holes high in precipitous, towering cliffs, and even if climbers might occasionally get to especially low nest entrances, they can rarely get to the chicks far within. For *R. pachyrhyncha*, there has been some harvest of nestlings, but a substantial fraction of nests have been in huge dead trees that are difficult and unsafe to climb and too large to be cut down easily.

Thus both inconspicuousness and inaccessibility of nests appear to be important factors decreasing poaching rates of *Amazona* and *Rhynchopsitta* parrot nests, and although some species have apparently benefited by possessing one or the other or both of these traits, a great many others have been stressed, apparently to the point of endangerment in some cases, by lacking either trait.

DEFICITS IN BREEDING EFFORT

The Yellow-headed Parrot of Mexico and the Puerto Rican Parrot have shown a chronic tendency for the existence of many pairs that adopt nest sites but do not lay eggs (Snyder et al. 1987; Enkerlin-Hoeflich 1995). Roughly half the pairs of the Puerto Rican Parrot studied over the years have been non-egg-laying, and statistics have been worse with the Yellow-headed Parrot. Similarly, various macaws in the Amazon and in Mexico have a large proportion of non-breeders (Munn 1992; Marineros S. 1993; Iñigo-Elias

1996). As many of these species are considered endangered, it would be highly advantageous to discover the causes of the apparent reluctance to breed in many pairs, as the causes may be susceptible to reversal by conservation actions.

In both *Amazona* just mentioned, the causes of low breeding effort do not appear to lie in a scarcity of good nest sites, but research to date has not yielded a clear understanding of what other causes may be involved. Among the various hypotheses are potential dietary limitations, problems with sex ratios and homosexual pairs, and problems with abnormal age distributions in populations.

The comparative approach has not yet yielded a clear resolution among alternatives, although it may do so in the future. In most amazons under study, the pairs adopting and defending nest sites have almost always been egg-laying pairs, but it is possible in these other species that pairs with no real potential for egg laying may generally fail to form associations with nest sites, so they are simply missed by standard survey techniques. But, assuming that all species may have similar tendencies to form associations with nest holes, we have been unable to find other obvious features that could explain the apparent differences in proportions of breeding pairs in any conclusive fashion.

Nevertheless, with the Puerto Rican Parrot, a fortuitous event in 1989 has provided some intriguing and suggestive clues. This was the direct strike of the parrot range by Hurricane Hugo. Although this storm caused tremendous damage to vegetation and a loss of approximately half the parrot population, it was remarkably followed by a tremendous *increase* in the numbers of breeding pairs, which lasted for several years and then subsided back to a more usual level. Clearly a substantial number of birds that had been chronic non-breeders before the storm became breeders after the storm, but the effect did not last for more than a few years. These facts strongly suggest that the basic causes of non-breeding were not to be found in sex ratio or age distribution problems.

Instead, we suspect that the causes are much more likely to be found in some subtle dietary relationships. Many trees and shrubs of Caribbean rain forests show greatly enhanced fruiting following hurricanes, and there are also well-documented insect blooms following hurricanes that apparently underlie enhanced breeding in other avian species following hurricanes (Arendt 1992; Wunderle 1995; Wiley & Wunderle 1993). Detailed dietary studies of species such as the Puerto Rican Parrot and the Yellow-headed Parrot in comparison with other species, especially using crop-sampling techniques carried out over periods of many years, might shed light on the possibility that the species showing generally low breeding effort might suffer from nutritional limitations and might respond to dietary modifications that could be introduced as management techniques.

As an aside, we point out that despite the obvious devastating effects of Caribbean hurricanes on diverse amazon parrots, these storms may have an important positive role to play in the biology of these species, not just from a dietary standpoint but also from the standpoint of creation of nest sites through breakage and subsequent rotting of tree limbs. Breeding in the Puerto Rican Parrot was evidently sufficiently enhanced by Hurricane Hugo such that the population had recovered to nearly 90% of its former size only four years after the storm. Further, it is conceivable that some frequency of hurricanes is actually beneficial and even necessary to the ecology of this species. The absence of major hurricanes between the 1930s and 1989 could have been an important factor in the progressive decline of the species.

SUMMARY

Comparative studies of the behavior and ecology of *Amazona* and *Rhynchopsitta* parrots allow the evaluation of a variety of hypotheses concerning the determinants of important characteristics of the species. While many of the conclusions presented here are tentative and demand further research for confirmation, they offer potentials for enhancing the conservation of the species in a number of respects. We particularly emphasize the potential benefits of careful quantitative dietary studies of many species utilizing crop-sampling techniques, as dietary relationships may underlie much of the behavior of these species.

ACKNOWLEDGMENTS

Much of the information reported has resulted from a long-term program focused on parrot ecology and conservation initiated by the first author in 1990 as part of doctoral studies at Texas A&M University and continued at Monterrey Institute of Technology (ITESM), Mexico, since 1994. The "parrot team" that provided direct assistance in many years of field work was led at different times by Claudia Macías-Caballero, Tiberio Monterrubio-Rico, Miguel Angel Cruz-Nieto, S. Gabriela Ortiz-Maciel and included a large number of volunteers, students, ranch hands, indigenous and local communities, and so forth. This project would not have been possible without assistance and cooperation from a wide range of people and institutions. I particularly appreciate the help and advice of Jane Packard, who chaired my doctoral advisory committee. Also Randy Brue, Wylie Barrow, Michael Schindlinger, Tila Pérez, and Robert B. Hamilton. Among these I want to thank for participation in different stages of the field research Jim Shiflett, Martjan Lammertink, Steve Scheid, Javier Cruz, Diana Venegas, Roger Otto, Emilio Rojas, Ali Taylor, the Tutuaca Ejido, and the community of Vallecillo.

The project could never have succeeded without the financial and administrative support of Centro de Calidad Ambiental at ITESM.

Financial support was generously provided by many agencies and organizations. Wildlife Trust provided consistent economic support during these studies. CONABIO (Mexican Commission for Biodiversity Research), FMCN (Mexican Fund for Nature Conservation), CONACYT (Consejo Nacional de Ciencia y Tecnologia), the American Zoo and Aquarium Association, the Sacramento Zoo, the National Fish and Wildlife Foundation, the Arizona Game and Fish Department, and the USFWS/SEMARNAT (U.S. Fish and Wildlife Service/Secretaria de Medio Ambiente y Recursos Naturales) program in Biodiversity Conservation all were important financial contributors. Additional support has been provided by Louisiana State University and a number of private individual donors.

REFERENCES

Arendt, W.J. 1992. Impact of Hurricane Hugo on pearly-eyed thrasher reproduction in the Luquillo rain forest, Puerto Rico. *Pitirre* 5(3):13–14.

Clinton-Eitniear, J. 1986. Status of the green-cheeked amazon in Northeastern Mexico. *Watchbird* Dec/Jan:22–24.

Cruz-Nieto, M.A., E. Enkerlin-Hoeflich, and N.F.R. Snyder. 1998. "Estatus y ecología de anidación de la Cotorra Serrana Occidental (*Rhynchopsitta pachyrhyncha*) en México: efectos de las prácticas del uso del suelo y perspectivas futuras de manejo." In *Congreso de Investigación y Extensión del Sistema ITESM. Generación, transferencia y aplicación del conocimiento,* ed. ITESM, pp. 73–81. Monterrey, N.L. Mexico: Tomo I.

Enkerlin-Hoeflich, E.C. 1995. Comparative ecology and reproductive biology of three species of *Amazona* parrots in northeastern Mexico. PhD diss., Texas A&M University, College Station.

Enkerlin-Hoeflich, E.C., and K.M. Hogan. 1997. "Red-crowned Parrot, *Amazona viridigenalis.*" In *The birds of North America,* ed. F.B. Gill and A. Poole, p. 20. Philadelphia, PA: American Ornithologists' Union and Academy of Natural Sciences of Philadelphia.

Enkerlin-Hoeflich, E.C., J.M. Packard, and J.J. González-Elizondo. 1999. Safe field techniques for nest inspections and nestling crop sampling of parrots. *J Field Ornithology* 70:8–17.

Forshaw, J.M. 1990. *Parrots of the world.* Ontario, Canada: Silvio Matachione & Co.

Gálvez-Aguilera, X., J. Rivera R., F. Quiala G., and J.W. Wiley. 1998. Breeding season diet of the Cuban parrot *Amazona leucocephala* in Los Indios Ecological Reserve, Isla de Juventud, Cuba. *Papageienkunde* 2:325–334.

Gnam, R.S. 1991. Breeding biology of the Bahama parrot (*Amazona leucocephala bahamensis*). PhD thesis, the City University of New York, New York.

Hayward, G.D., and P.H. Hayward. 1993. "Boreal owl (*Aegolius funereus*)." In *The birds of North America,* No. 63, ed. A. Poole and F. Gill. Philadelphia: Academy of Natural Sciences; Washington, DC: American Ornithologists' Union.

Iñigo-Elias, E.E. 1996. Ecology and breeding biology of the Scarlet Macaw (*Ara macao*) in the Usumacinta drainage basin of Mexico and Guatemala. PhD diss., University of Florida, Gainesville.

Iñigo-Elias, E.E., and M.A. Ramos. 1997. "El comercio de los psitácidos en México." In *Uso y conservación de la vida silvestre neotropical,* ed. J.G. Robinson, K.H. Redford, and J.E. Rabinovich, pp. 445–458.. México: Fondo de Cultura Económica.

Juniper, T., and M. Parr. 1998. *Parrots: A guide to parrots of the world.* New Haven and London: Yale University Press.

Koenig, S.E. 1999. The reproductive biology of Jamaica's black-billed parrot (*Amazona agilis*) and conservation implications. PhD diss., Yale University, New Haven, CT.

Krebs, J.R. 1974. Colonial nesting and social feeding as strategies for exploiting food resources in the great blue heron (*Ardea herodias*). *Behaviour* 51:99–134.

Lanning, D.V., and J.T. Shiflett. 1981. "Status and nesting ecology of the thick-billed parrot (*Rhynchopsitta*

pachyrhyncha)." In *Conservation of new world parrots,* ed. R.F. Pasquier, pp. 393–401. St. Lucia: Smithsonian Institution Press.

Lanning, D.V., and J.T. Shiflett. 1983. Nesting ecology of thick-billed parrots. *Condor* 85:66–73.

Lawson, P.W., and D.V. Lanning. 1982. "Nesting and status of the maroon-fronted parrot (*Rhynchopsitta terrisi*)." In *Conservation of new world parrots,* ed. R.F. Pasquier, pp. 385–392. St. Lucia: Smithsonian Institution Press.

Mabb, K.T. 1997. Roosting behavior of naturalized parrots in the San Gabriel Valley, California. *Western Birds* 28:202–208.

Macías-Caballero, C.M., E. Enkerlin-Hoeflich, G. Ortíz-Maciel, A. Madero-Farias, J.J. Manzano-Loza, and M.-L. J.R. 2001. Estudio de la cotorra serrana oriental (*Rhynchopsitta terrisi*) en México: programa de conservación y manejo de ecosistemas. Reporte final presentado al FMCN. Proyecto A-1-98/93 Centro de Calidad Ambiental, ITESM, Monterrey, N.L. Mexico.

Marineros S., M. 1993. La Lapa Roja (Psittacidae: Ara macao): ecología, turismo y pautas para su manejo en la reserva biológica Carara, Costa Rica. Maestría en Manejo de Vida Silvestre. Universidad Nacional, Heredia, Costa Rica.

Munn, C.A. 1992. Macaw biology and ecotourism, or "When a bird in the bush is worth two in the hand." In *New world parrots in crisis: Solutions from conservation biology,* ed. S.R. Beissinger and N.F.R. Snyder, pp. 47–72. Washington, DC: Smithsonian Institution Press.

Rea, A.M. 1997. "The indeterminate parrot of Nuevo Leon." In *The era of Alan R. Phillips: A festschrift,* pp. 167–176. Albuquerque, NM: Horizon.

Renton, K., and A. Salinas-Melgoza. 1999. Nesting behavior of the lilac-crowned parrot. *Wilson Bull* 111:488–493.

Rojas-Suárez, F. 1994. "Biología reproductiva de la cotorra *Amazona barbadensis* (Aves: Psittaciformes) en la península de Macanao, estado Nueva Esparta." In *Biología y conservación de los psitácidos en Venezuela, Caracas,* ed. G. Morales, I. Novo, D. Bigio, A. Luy, and F. Rojas-Suárez, pp. 73–87. Caracas, Venezuela: PROVITA.

Rowley, I., and G. Chapman. 1991. The breeding biology, food, social organisation, demography and conservation of the Major Mitchell or pink cockatoo, (*Cacatua leadbeateri*), on the margin of the Western Australian wheatbelt. *Australian Journal of Zoology* 39:211–261.

Saunders, D.A. 1982. The breeding behaviour and biology of the short-billed form of the white-tailed black cockatoo *Calyptorhynchus funereus. Ibis* 124: 422–455.

Snyder, N.F.R., E.C. Enkerlin-Hoeflich, and M.A. Cruz-Nieto. 1999. "Thick-billed parrot, *Rhynchopsitta pachyrhyncha*." In *The birds of North America,* ed. F.B. Gill and A. Poole. Philadelphia: American Ornithologists' Union and Academy of Natural Sciences of Philadelphia.

Snyder, N.F.R., W.B. King, and C.B. Kepler. 1982. Biology and conservation of the Bahama parrot. *Living Bird* 19:91–114.

Snyder, N., P. McGowan, J. Gilardi, and A. Grajal, eds. 2000. *Parrots: Status survey and conservation action plan 2000–2004.* Gland, Switzerland and Cambridge, U.K.: IUCN World Conservation Union.

Snyder, N.F.R., and K. Russell. 2002. "Carolina parakeet (*Conuropsis carolinensis*)." In *The birds of North America,* No. 667, ed. A. Poole and F. Gill. Philadelphia: Birds of North America, Inc.

Snyder, N.F.R., and N.J. Schmitt. 2002. "California condor (*Gymnogyps californianus*)." In *The birds of*

North America, No. 610, ed. A. Poole and F. Gill. Philadelphia: Birds of North America, Inc.

Snyder, N.F.R., J.W. Wiley, and C.B. Kepler. 1987. *The parrots of Luquillo: Natural history and conservation of the Puerto Rican parrot.* Los Angeles: Western Foundation of Vertebrate Zoology.

Wiley, J.W., and J.M. Wunderle, Jr. 1993. The effects of hurricanes on birds, with special reference to Caribbean islands. *Bird Conservation International* 3 (4): 319–349.

Wunderle, J.M., Jr. 1995. Pre- and post-hurricane fruiting phenologies: Potential implications for Puerto Rican parrots. *Pitirre* 10 (1):38.

Yamashita, C. 1987. Field observation and comments on the indigo macaw (*Anodorhynchus leari*), a highly endangered species from northeastern Brazil. *Wilson Bull* 99:280–282.

3
Parrot Conservation, Trade, and Reintroduction

Charles A. Munn

CONSERVATION AND TRADE

Of the 345 or so species of parrots, about a third of them are threatened or declining, about three times the rate of threat found in average birds, of which about 10% are threatened. Of these threatened species of parrots, about half are endangered primarily by trade, and the other half by conversion of their habitats to agricultural lands. The species endangered by trade are invariably colorful, large, or good talkers. It is no accident that the larger wild parrots in private collections (as opposed to the ubiquitous, captive-bred Budgerigars and Cockatiels) match closely the colorful, large, talking species that are endangered by trade. For nearly all of these wild parrots kept as pets, destruction of their wild habitat is a minor or very much secondary conservation issue for these species, while regional, national, and international demand for the pet trade is the main threat to their survival in the wild. In not a single case so far in the history of the world has the keeping of captive parrots by private citizens been of significant use in a successful recovery effort for a threatened population of wild parrots.

Conversely, none of the parrots threatened by habitat destruction are popular in captivity, even though they are exactly the species that could potentially benefit from a backup population in case they disappear in the wild because of near total destruction of their wild habitat. Of course, private parrot owners feel appropriately guilty about keeping wild parrots in cages while trying to justify it by saying it is helpful to the species. They justify this keeping and breeding of colorful, large, talking wild parrots by saying, in part, that they are "saving wild Polly from having his habitat rug pulled out from under him," or words to that effect. In fact, the reason that the large, colorful, talkative species of wild parrots are in trouble is not because of shortage of habitat but because so many humans like to keep them as pets. Loving them to death, it would seem!

When a number of years ago I suggested to 200 parrot owners, breeders, and dealers that they should house backup populations of the primarily drab, small, non-talking species of parrots that are in danger of extinction because of habitat destruction, the idea was received with stony silence. No one showed interest in donating to establishing backup populations of species that have "no commercial value."

Trade in all wild parrots clearly should be illegal (as it has been for ten years now in the United States) unless the source country can prove to serious, independent "conservation inspectors" that there is no harm to wild populations and that the trade is helping add value to wild habitat and produce rural jobs related to parrot conservation. Theoretically, at least, a system of wild ranching of parrots could be devised, but so far no one has done so. Any such systems would have to be immune to the obvious and less obvious forms of cheating, including banding or chipping unsustainably trapped wild birds to launder them for sale as sustainably ranched. By outlawing all international trade in wild parrots that cannot be shown to be sustainably produced, the world may eventually see the development of independently verifiable methods of sustainable, humane ranching of wild parrots.

While talking about humane methods of ranching wild parrots, it could be argued that the only humane, conservative, and responsible way to ranch wild parrots would be by harvesting the last hatched babies from some or all nests. But before any harvest of wild babies, it would be important to raise the wild populations to carrying capacity and beyond by supplemental feeding of the wild population and by erecting nest boxes or otherwise improving natural nest cavities and wild habitat and ensuring that all hatched young are treated for parasites and fledge in good condition. One might be able to raise the carrying capacity of the wild habitat by adding balanced food supplementation and nest sites. Such measures might permit a controlled harvest of last-hatched young or even entire first clutches while providing supplemental food to the laying hens, who would in many cases re-lay. In other words, use the best techniques from traditional aviculture and, in general, livestock ranching to increase the output of the population, while not worrying about psychological or plucking problems in the wild birds, as wild birds never pluck and don't need behaviorists and psychologists.

All the simple quota-based harvest systems that are used still in some tropical countries in northeastern South America and West and Central Africa are particularly crude and inhumane, as they break up families and even catch breeding adults that leave babies to starve in wild nests. Thus, I am unalterably opposed to simple capture or export quotas of parrots. The only humane and sustainable method for parrot ranching for the pet trade would have to be the harvest of the last, starvation-bound babies in wild populations kept at carrying capacity. If these wild populations are totally protected from hunting or trapping while also given supplemental feeding and an overabundance of superb nest cavities, then there is every reason to think that their wild populations might increase to a new, higher carrying capacity. In other words, parrot producers should treat wild parrots as a rancher would treat his or her most pampered cattle. Wild parrots brought to pampered carrying capacity in a wilderness setting will add more value to the habitat than any other use of the forest—by being major tourist attractions in the wild at the same time that they are the raw material that produce valuable babies reliably every year.

So far, every example of parrot trapping in the tropics around the world BUT ONE is a classic case of the tragedy of the commons, in which roving bands of greedy trappers catch all wild birds, adults and babies, while cutting down or hacking open all nest trees and breaking up breeding families. Each trapper figures that he might as well trap and sell the last adults and babies before the next guy gets them.

The one example that I know of a trapper (a former trapper in this case) being a rational parrot rancher (to the extent that he could be given the constraints of acting outside the legal system) is one of the most skilled Hyacinth trappers of all time—Lourival Lima of the state of Piaui, Brazil. Lima and his band of followers effectively had a unique bird harvesting concession in an extensive area of roughly 1,000 square miles of wilderness in the dry forest region of northeastern Brazil. Lima never allowed any of his band of eight expert trappers to catch or hurt the adult population of breeding birds. Rather, as over decades his father (who himself was master macaw trapper) and later he himself had established a territorial system to keep other wholesalers out of his part of Brazil, he managed the Hyacinth Macaw resource rationally, like a responsible rancher. That is, he only took babies from his professional providers, and he knew that by not hurting adults, he was guaranteed a sustainable, never-ending harvest of healthy, happy wild babies. He also knew that his cliff-climbing trappers could not reach more than perhaps 50% of all wild nests of the species, and experience showed that each year, the same pairs of Hyacinths would lay eggs and hatch young in the same cliff cavities, despite the depredations by his band of pro climbers. This system ensured a steady, never-ending supply of high-quality, parent-hatched, parent-fed Hyacinth nestlings, which his team would harvest in their third month of life—when they were large and strong and would survive the harvesting very well.

Lima reports that using these methods, his team never lost a single baby Hyacinth, and his father and he sold perhaps 1,000 large Hyacinth babies between 1976 and 1994, when he stopped trading and started protecting all wildlife in his region as a paid warden, paid by funds supplied by me and by the Bird Clubs of Virginia. In this 18-year period, the Hyacinth population never showed any sign of decline.

I wish I could say that there are many examples of such informal but effective "harvest concessions" that produced incentives for rational management such as practiced by Lima. But to this day, I have never heard of or seen another rational, sustainable example of macaw or parrot harvest anywhere else on Earth. And I have heard of more than 100 or 200 examples of unsustainable, "tragedy of the commons" examples of the annihilation of parrot populations in Indonesia to Central Africa, Mexico, Central America, and South America.

If we could find ways to experiment with Lima's system in different parts of the globe, it might be possible to get it right, as Lima got it right. During the entire time that he and his father were trapping and trading thousands of macaws from that part of Brazil, the practice was illegal. Nevertheless, no one ever caught them or even made a serious attempt to catch them, and they managed their Hyacinth populations sustainably. Weird but true—an example of a successful experiment in sustainability.

The only reason that Lima started working for me as a parrot protector instead of trader is that by the mid-90s, law enforcement in Brazil was finally catching up with parrot trappers, and Lima realized that he could not continue for more than a few more years without having a nasty run-in with the law. His major buyer had gone to prison for wildlife dealing, and he realized that the jig was up and he had to look for other options. Fortunately, in my work for the Wildlife Conservation Society I long had been interested in converting Lima to the "good side of the force," as it were. I had met him in 1987 while investigating traffic in Hyacinths, and he was "the Man." By 1994, however, with law enforcement breathing down his neck, I was able to convert him. He has never gone back.

Despite the fact that he has renounced bird trapping, there is no question in my mind that he was the first and perhaps only sustainable harvester of Hyacinths in the world, if not the world's first and only documented case of a sustainable harvester of any large, commercially valuable parrot. He has a lot to teach field conservationists and writers of environmental laws. He considered that brutalizing or catching adult breeding birds was a cretinous, destructive practice, yet most armchair theorists on the topic of parrot quotas and trade still espouse standard catch and export quotas, regardless of the resulting "tragedy of the commons" race to remove from the forest ALL wild parrots of any age.

Parrot trade normally is tragic and destructive to wild populations of commercially valuable wild parrots. The only way to change this and make wild parrots a force for habitat conservation and rural development is to develop systems that grant unique, enforceable concessions of parrot habitat to individuals, clans, or organized communities so that they can ranch and pamper their own wild populations of valuable parrots. Such a system would have to include independent monitoring, as few tropical countries currently have adequate abilities to police remote parrot production areas. The details do not have to be worked out here, as they are beyond the scope of this chapter. Suffice it to say that parrot trade currently is out of control virtually everywhere on the planet except where it is either too difficult to get the birds out to markets (e.g., remote parts of the Amazon or the interior of New Guinea) or where the local cultures value wild birds more in the wild than as trade goods to be sold as pets. The only places that seem to cherish wild parrot populations in the wild and prohibit trapping are Australia, New Zealand, Gabon, and parts of Costa Rica, Peru, Ecuador, and Brazil. In the first three countries, cultural norms prohibit parrot trapping, while in the latter four cases, parrot ecotourism has become significant business and so has created a local conservation culture that diverges from the national norm.

Unfortunately, the areas that protect wild parrots and prevent all trade in large parrots are unlikely to amount to more than 10% of the remaining major tropical forest parrot habitat around the globe, but we would like to protect ALL remaining tropical forests. Therefore, we should experiment with methods for making the parrots in the rest of the world's tropical forests worth more alive and free flying in the wild than trapped to extinction decades before their forest home is in any significant danger. Sustainably ranched wild parrots might provide an option for maintaining forest cover and rural livelihoods in 20–30% of the remaining tropical forests of the world. The sooner we start systematic experiments with sustainable ranching of wild parrots, the sooner we can stop all the current wasteful, unsustainable, and inhumane quote-based trade.

The World Parrot Trust's proposal to ban parrot import into the European Union is a very useful move, as would be experiments with methods such as those pioneered by Lourival Lima in the 1970s and 1980s in Brazil.

REINTRODUCTION

It is obvious to anyone who travels to Palm Beach or Miami, Florida, to parts of San Francisco or other parts of coastal California, to Lima, Peru, or hundreds or thousands of other towns and cities around the tropics, subtropics, and milder parts of the temperate latitudes that many species of parrots have become reintroduced and are flourishing. These birds all were inadvertently "reintroduced" by release or escape of cage birds. So there is no question that parrots can be reintroduced. This truth, however, does not contradict the fact that not all of the hundreds of species of parrots will be equally easy to reintroduce. In fact, reintroduction should rarely, if ever, be a method that one should have to rely on to save wild populations of the very rarest parrots.

The reasons for this are mostly economic. Unless a wild species is down to a population of less than 100 wild birds and less than five or ten wild nests, the option of reintroducing captive-bred individuals normally will prove to be a much more expensive or riskier way of increasing wild parrot populations than simply increasing the output from existing wild nests or translocating wild birds from other locations.

A good example of a parrot species that deserves a major effort in reintroduction is the Spix's Macaw. The species went extinct in the wild in 2000 when the last wild bird perished, yet there are more than 70 birds in captivity, most of which are very inbred and for whom the studbook data have not been made available by the private owners. If the private owners of Spix's Macaw cannot organize themselves to reintroduce the Spix's Macaw to the wild, then what hope is there that any other private owners of rare parrots will ever contribute captive birds to a future reintroduction effort for a similarly endangered parrot species?

Possibly the Blue-throated Macaw qualifies for a reintroduction effort, but so far, only nonprofit, public-interest conservation organizations and their board members have shown interest in developing a technically valid reintroduction project for this species. Private owners of the species have not come forward to help.

The most successful parrot recovery effort in history is that of the Echo Parakeet, which has recovered from less than 20 birds 15 years ago to more than 200 birds in the wild now, all thanks to the generous work of a number of nonprofit conservation groups such as the Jersey Wildlife Preservation Trust and the World Parrot Trust. But none of the birds used in this successful reintroduction effort came from private bird owners or collectors. Rather, they were bred at the nonprofit Wildlife Preservation Trust or, more typically, produced by assisting the fledging of wild-laid eggs in wild nests. In fact, work with the Echo Parakeet in Mauritius, and with Scarlet and Green-winged Macaws in Manu and Tambopata, Peru, and in Costa Rica, has shown that the best way to increase the local parrot population in a wild setting is to help all wild-laid eggs survive to hatch and fledge healthy young. The methods for doing this may involve assisting eggs or babies in wild nests, or temporarily removing wild eggs or wild babies to field-based labs where they can be assisted to fledge into adjacent, appropriate habitat as soon as possible, thus minimizing their temporary captivity.

Another notably successful parrot reintroduction project was that of the Margarita Amazon in Venezuela, a project that reintroduced hundreds of birds confiscated from trappers and traders. With very few quarantine precautions and with a minimum of fuss and muss, it appears that most of these reintroduced birds flourished and became actively reproductive, thus increasing the wild population by severalfold in just a few years. Persons who are wary of disease risks caution that this case may have been handled less cautiously than is appropriate according to the best practices of modern avian veterinarians, but then it also is possible that many diseases seen in captive parrots may be a manifestation of captivity itself rather than a problem for wild birds. In other words, perhaps wild birds are largely free of clinical signs of many diseases that are present in the wild, while captive birds become ill and often die from the same diseases, with captivity itself being the culprit rather than the pathogen, per se. It is important to examine the assumptions surrounding pathogens in captivity and in the wild before planning a major release effort for captive birds.

It also is notable that, without taking any special precautions whatsoever, wild parrots have reintroduced themselves successfully in so many thousands of tropical, subtropical, and temperate locations around the globe. It would be a fertile research field for avian veterinarians to investigate which diseases are caused by or are exacerbated by captivity.

The best example of a reintroduction project gone awry may have been the attempt to reintroduce naive, lab-raised Thick-billed Parrots in southern Arizona. In this case, the project suffered from a number of problems, namely the fact that the Thick-billed Parrot is among the most difficult of parrots to reintroduce and the reintroduction area was plagued with a high density of hungry Red-tailed Hawks happy to eat reintroduced birds. The Thick-bill is among the hardest of all parrots to reintroduce because it has a very specialized feeding ecology and normally lives in tight flocks that fly each day at high speed for enormous distances. Thus, in order to blend into a wild flock and so not be singled out and attacked by hungry hawks, released Thick-bills need to be able to extract pinecone seeds at a phenomenally fast rate and then blend perfectly into a flock as it twists and turns in high-speed, marathon daily flights. The only reintroduced Thick-bills to have notable survival success after release were wild birds that were captured in forests in Mexico and quickly released in the target forest in southern Arizona. These wild birds knew how to eat efficiently and fly fast and precisely, and so were able to survive in the face of the major hawk populations in that part of the United States.

A notable advantage of using a variety of techniques to increase the productivity of wild nests and wild populations is that you will normally not need to take very elaborate, expensive precautions to prevent disease transmission, as these techniques involve either no or very little time in captivity, and even when in captivity, the birds are kept in single-species, dedicated facilities close to or in the wild habitat.

Thus, normally, reintroduction of captive-bred parrots should be avoided unless there are few or no wild birds left to work with. It will be much less expensive, much easier, and much more successful to assist wild populations to increase as fast as possible (as was the case with the Echo Parakeet). Working to help wild populations increase their reproductive success avoids all the complications and expense of elaborate quarantines for captive-raised birds. Additionally, captive-bred birds often will be naive and at high risk in the wild when compared with savvy, wild-born or wild-trained birds.

4
Sensory Capacities of Parrots

Jennifer Graham, Timothy F. Wright,
Robert J. Dooling, and Ruediger Korbel

INTRODUCTION

Parrots are gregarious and vocal creatures that communicate in ways we have yet to understand. How do parrots perceive the world? By understanding some of the unique adaptations of avian anatomy, we may better understand parrot behavior. This chapter will discuss the sensory capacities of parrots including vision, hearing, taste, smell, and touch perceptions.

VISION

The majority of birds rely heavily on visual abilities in their daily activities. Visual acuity is enhanced in avian species, approximately two to eight times higher than in mammals, as the avian eye is large in relation to the size of the head, allowing a large image to be projected on the retina.[1–5] Visual acuity is also enhanced because the retina of diurnal birds has a large number of cones compared to humans; for example, the hawk fovea contains around 300,000 cones/mm^2, while the human fovea contains around 147,000 cones/mm^2.[1] In addition, nearly every cone in the avian eye is represented by an individual axon traveling to the brain, while the eye of humans contains six to seven million cones but only one million axons in the entire optic nerve.[1]

While eyes come in different shapes depending on the species of bird, parrots have a "flat" eye. The flat eyeball is characterized by a short axis that projects a relatively smaller image on the retina, decreasing visual acuity compared to other species such as birds of prey.[1] The eyeball of birds is asymmetric, favoring binocular vision.[1]

The sclera of the eye is strengthened by ten to 18 small bones called scleral ossicles.[1–5]

Because the eyeball almost completely fills the orbit, the eye movements of the bird are generally fewer than those of mammals.[1] However, birds can move their heads and necks extensively, and this compensates for the small eye movements.[1] Movement of the orbits is independent between both eyes in parrots, in contrast to mammals.[1]

A feature of the avian eye is that the sphincter and dilator muscles of the pupil contain mainly striated fibers, compared to the mammalian counterpart that contains only smooth muscle.[1–5] Because of this anatomic feature, the pupillary opening is under voluntary control in parrots. Rapid dilation and constriction of the pupillary opening is often observed in aggressive or excited parrots.[6] While pupillary light reflexes do occur in birds, complete decussation of the optic nerve axons prevents true consensual pupillary light reflex.[2, 3] The iris is the colored part of the eye that contains chromatophores that can create varying iris colors based on age, gender, and species of the parrot.[1–3]

Unlike the mammalian counterpart, the avian retina is devoid of blood vessels, which decreases scattering of light and shadows.[5] The pecten is a unique vascular structure found only in the avian eye in association with the retina. The function of the pecten is likely to provide nutrition to the eye, as retinal vessels are lacking.[1, 5, 7]

Parrots often turn their head or body sideways when presented with a new toy or object. Behavioral studies in many birds have shown that they prefer the use of a lateral and monocular field to observe distant objects.[5, 8–12] Based on monocular data in pigeons, visual resolution is higher in the lateral field than frontal field, thus explaining this preference.[5, 13]

The lens of the avian eye is softer than that of mammalian species.[1] Unlike the yellow-tinted mammalian lens that filters out wavelengths of light below 400 nm, the clear avian lens transmits wavelengths below 400 nm.[1] Colored oil droplets on the ends of the cones provide protection against the effects of ultraviolet (UV) light.[5, 14] Birds are able to see UV light below 400 nm due to the combined effects of cone oil droplets and visual pigments.[4, 5, 15] While trichromatic color vision in humans is based on three colors (blue, green, and red), the tetrachromatic, or pentachromatic in some avian species, system of birds includes UV, fluorescent, blue, green, and red.[4, 16–24] UV perception of parrots likely plays an important role in behavior. Many parrots' feathers reflect UV and studies have shown that UV reflection of feathers affects mate choice (see Plates 1 and 2 in color section).[4, 16, 25–29] While some parrots are not visibly sexually dimorphic to the human eye, UV reflection from plumage and skin varies between sexes of some birds.[4] Some types of fruits and berries, such as kaki, green grapes, and figs, reflect UV light and ripeness of the food may be determined by this characteristic.[4, 30] Certain flower patterns, insects, and urine and feces of rodents also reflect UV light that can be detected by birds.[4, 30–32] Additionally, highly UV-reflective areas within the oral cavity play an important role in triggering reflexes to feed young birds that demonstrate their oral cavity to their parents. Birds may use UV receptors in combination with color receptors for navigation by detecting sun-based color gradients.[33–35] Fluorescence, which occurs when short wavelength light is absorbed and re-emitted at a longer wavelength, occurs on parrot feathers and may be an important avian signaller.[25, 36]

Birds are able to detect a spatial frequency of around 160 frames/second or hertz (Hz), compared to 50–60 Hz in humans.[37–39] Because most artificial lights produce noncontinuous light at a frequency of around 100–120 Hz, a stroboscopic effect not detectable to humans results and may be detrimental to birds.[4, 39–41] In addition, artificial lights and sunlight passing through windows do not provide full-spectrum light. While studies are currently under way to examine the effects of artificial lights on birds, current recommendations have been made to provide full-spectrum light and high frequency sources that emit continuous light.[37] Suggestions have also been made to consider light source and presence of full-spectrum light when performing ethological studies.[17, 37, 42, 43] Because video or computer monitors have refresh rates of around 50–95 Hz, welfare issues may arise when performing video playback experiments in birds.[39, 44–46]

Familiarity with the unique anatomic and physiologic variations of the avian eye compared to that of mammals is important when assessing behavior alterations in parrots. Behavior changes, such as reluctance to fly or step onto an extended hand, abnormal head posture, inappetence, and others, can certainly result from ocular abnormalities. In addition, permanent ocular problems, such as blindness resulting from cataract formation, are a common occurrence in parrots and can be managed in such a way as to maintain quality of life. Provision of full-spectrum lighting, normal light cycles, and continuous-emitting light sources should be considered when addressing behavioral problems in birds.

HEARING

Birds rely on their hearing ability for detecting predators and prey, orienting in the environment, and communicating with conspecifics. The songs and calls produced by birds are among the most complex auditory signals known,[47] and this complexity has generated much interest in how birds hear sounds.[48] In the case of parrots, many of these vocalizations appear to be learned through experience,[49] which has led to further interest in the connections between perception, learning, and vocal production.

The anatomy of the avian ear presents some marked contrasts to the more familiar mammalian ear. These differences include the absence of an external ear; a single middle ear bone, the columella, in place of the three bones found in mammals; and the much shorter sensory auditory epithelium in the inner ear. In Budgerigars, for instance, the sensory surface of the inner ear, the basilar papilla, is about 3–4 mm in length (compared to around 30 mm in humans). The columellar middle ear and the short auditory sensory epithelium in birds probably both exert limitations on the range of hearing in birds compared to mammals.[50] Another interesting difference between birds and mammals is in the organization of sensory hair cells on the auditory epithelium. Mammals typically have one row of inner hair cells and three rows of outer hair cells across the width of the auditory epithelium, while birds show more rows of hair cells and considerable variation in the structure and orientation of these hair cells.[51] The functional consequence of these differences remains obscure. But, in striking contrast to mammalian hair cells, avian hair cells are known to be capable of regenerating after damage caused by exposure to excessive noise or ototoxic drugs.[52, 53] Here the functional consequences are enormous. Birds regain their hearing when their hair cells regenerate. Many forms of human deafness are related to defects in or loss of hair cell function,[54] and thus the discovery of hair cell regeneration in birds has spurred a renewed interest in avian ear anatomy.

The anatomical complexity of the bird ear is not fully understood and has led to much interest in how well birds are able to detect, discriminate, and learn complex sounds. We are fortunate to know a great deal about the hearing in one parrot species, the Budgerigar, because of its small size and tractability in the laboratory for behavioral studies of hearing. Less is known of the hearing abilities in other parrot species, but what is known suggests that many abilities of the Budgerigar are shared across species. The behavioral methods used for studying hearing involve operant conditioning or training the bird to respond to a sound—or the change in a sound—by pecking a switch in order to obtain food.[55] These methods have been highly successful and have been used in a wide range of studies examining how parrots and other birds detect sounds, discriminate among similar sounds, and classify sounds into perceptual categories.

One of the most basic measures of hearing abilities is the audiogram. The audiogram is a plot of the least detectable amount of sound energy a bird can hear in the quiet at different frequencies over its range of hearing. Figure 4.1 shows audiograms for three parrots—the Budgerigar, the Cockatiel, and the Orange-fronted Conure. These audiograms show that these parrots, like many

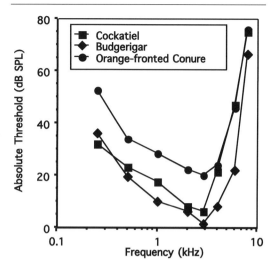

Figure 4.1. Hearing thresholds under quiet conditions for three species of parrot. Figure redrawn from Wright et al. (2003).

bird species, hear best at frequencies between about 1 and 5 kHz and less well at frequencies below about 500 Hz and above 10 kHz. The lowest threshold approaches 0 dB in the Budgerigar, 5 dB in the Cockatiel, and 20 dB in the Orange-fronted Conure.[56, 57]

In all three species these lowest thresholds in the quiet occur at frequencies between 2 and 4 kHz. This is also the frequency range in which most of the acoustic energy is found in their most common type of vocalizations, the contact call.[57, 58] Contact calls are probably designed for distance communication under more noisy conditions than found in the laboratory. Interestingly, when hearing thresholds are measured in the presence of a masking noise, Budgerigars, Cockatiels, and Orange-fronted Conures also show the best signal-to-noise ratios in this same frequency region. These signal-to-noise ratios (called critical ratios) are shown in Figure 4.2. These critical ratio functions show the level (in decibels) above the background noise that a sound must be in order to be heard. Most birds show a pattern like the Cockatiel; that is, critical ratios increase monotonically at roughly 3 dB for every octave increase in frequency. The Budgerigar and Orange-fronted Conure, by contrast, show a 5–10 dB increase in sensitivity between 2 and 4 kHz relative to the typical avian critical

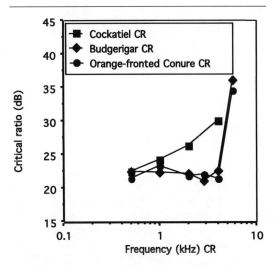

Figure 4.2. Hearing thresholds under noisy conditions for three species of parrot. Thresholds are given as the critical ratio between signal level and the masking noise at the threshold of detection. Figure redrawn from Wright et al. (2003).

is borne out, while in other areas the abilities of birds are very similar to those of mammals and other terrestrial animals. For example, studies of frequency discrimination in the Budgerigar and the Orange-fronted Conure have shown that, like most birds, they are able to discriminate among tones that differ by about 1% of their frequency.[57, 60] This threshold is roughly in the range of humans and other animals that have been tested. In contrast, these parrots are worse than humans at discriminating differences in the intensity of two tones; humans can discriminate a 1 dB difference in the intensity of pure tones, while birds, including Budgerigars and Orange-fronted Conures, typically require a difference of 2–5 dB.[57, 61] One can imagine that in discriminating vocalizations in the real world, frequency cues might be far more reliable than intensity cues due to degradation of signals during transmission through the environment, so perhaps this is one reason that intensity discrimination abilities are less well developed.

The detection abilities measured using pure tone stimuli may not be perfect predictors of the ability of parrots to distinguish among complex species-specific calls. Several studies have examined the ability of parrots to discriminate among and classify their contact calls. One study compared the abilities of Budgerigars and Zebra Finches to detect the presence of contact calls in a noisy background, and compared these threshold levels to those found when birds were asked to discriminate among the same calls in the presence of noise.[62] Thresholds were 2–5 dB lower for detection than for discrimination among the same calls, suggesting that discrimination is a more difficult task requiring more of the information in the calls to be clearly perceived.

A second study compared the ability of Budgerigars, Zebra Finches, and Canaries to discriminate among a set of stimuli including four contact calls from each species.[63] All three species had more difficulty discriminating between calls from the same species than between calls from different species. Furthermore, all three species could discriminate more easily between calls from their own species than between two calls from a different species. These results suggest that discrimination is more difficult when calls are acoustically more similar (i.e., from the same species) but that different species may have spe-

ratio function.[56, 57] While the function of this increased sensitivity in these species is uncertain, it is intriguing to note that it corresponds well to the frequency range of maximum energy in their contact calls and may help in discriminating among different calls within large noisy flocks.

Birds in general, with the exception of nocturnal predators such as the Barn Owl, are not very good at localizing sound. Because of their small heads and closely spaced ears, the time difference or intensity difference between sounds arriving at the two ears of a bird is negligible. One parrot, the Budgerigar, has been tested in the laboratory and minimum audible angles are in the range of 22–52 degrees for pure tones and 24 degrees for broadband sounds such as noises and vocalizations.[59]

Hearing is much more than the detection or localization of sounds. In order to communicate, an animal also must be able to discriminate among different sounds with potentially very different meanings. The complex temporal and frequency structure of many bird vocalizations has long prompted suspicions that birds may have particularly good abilities to detect small differences in frequency, amplitude, and temporal characteristics of sound. In some cases this prediction cial hearing abilities that aid in the perception of their own calls. Such specializations may arise either through innate differences in auditory capabilities or through learned preferences developed through selective exposure to conspecific sounds as nestlings or fledglings.

A third study examined the ability of the Orange-fronted Conure to form perceptual categories for different individuals based on the acoustic properties of their calls (T. Wright, K. Cortopassi, J. Bradbury, and R. Dooling, unpublished data). Subjects listened to a repeating background of ten calls from a single individual interspersed with calls from different individuals. Subjects quickly learned to avoid responding to the differences between different renditions of the contact call by a single individual and to respond to the differences among calls of different individuals. Their ability to learn this distinction rapidly suggests that they are able to form perceptual categories for the calls of different individuals that allow them to focus on those acoustic features that reliably differ between different individuals. Such perceptual abilities may be critical for acoustic recognition of a variety of social levels in parrots, including individuals, pairs, flocks, roosts, and geographic regions.

TASTE AND SMELL

Taste buds lie on the tongue base in most of the avian species studied such as the chicken, pigeon, swift, raptor, and songbird.[1, 64, 65] In parrots, taste buds are found along the choanal opening on the roof of the oropharynx in association with salivary glands.[1, 65] Compared to mammals, birds have a poor sense of taste; while humans have around 9,000 taste buds, parrots are estimated to have 300–400.[66, 67] Parrots have a higher number of taste buds than most other avian species, such as the chicken with 250–350 and the pigeon with only 37–75.[64, 66, 67] Despite the low number of taste buds found in birds, many studies have shown that flavors can affect food choice and quantity consumed.[66, 68–76] While it has been stated that most birds easily detect salts and acids but sweet substances are not effective stimuli, the response to different flavors varies widely among birds.[1, 76] Some parrots and Budgerigars, as well as other birds, have been shown to prefer sugar solutions over water.[67] Studies in captive Cockatiels examined threshold

and preference for water, sodium chloride, potassium chloride, sucrose, glucose, fructose, sodium phosphate buffer, and citric acid buffer solutions.[66, 76] In the Cockatiel studies, all tested compounds added to the water resulted in decreased consumption of the test solution and increased consumption of pure water. No test compound was preferred by the Cockatiels.[66, 76] While future study is needed to determine the significance of taste preference in parrots, there is no question that taste plays a role in food acceptance and avoidance.

The receptors of the nasal cavity that detect odor are generally located on the caudal nasal conchae.[1] Receptor nerve fibers run from the conchae olfactory epithelium to an area within the brain called the olfactory bulb, which is relatively small in the parrot compared to other avian species.[1] Interestingly, the avian orders with relatively small olfactory bulbs have high olfactory thresholds.[77, 78] Compared to mammals such as man, dogs, and rats, birds have proven to have comparable olfactory capacities in conditioning studies.[77, 79–83] Although research into psittacine olfactory abilities is scarce, various avian species use olfactory cues for food location, orientation and navigation, returning to nest sites, reproduction and parenting, and selection of nest material.[81, 84–89]

TOUCH

There are many types of sensory receptors, including those for touch, heat, and pain, located within the parrot beak and skin that give the bird more information about its environment. The different types of touch receptors, or mechanoreceptors, in birds are Herbst corpuscles, Merkel cell receptors, Grandry corpuscles, and Ruffini endings.[90] Herbst corpuscles, which are vibration-sensitive, are the most numerous skin receptors and are found in the beak, leg, and skin.[90, 91] Because they lie in close association with feather follicles and muscles associated with the follicles, Herbst corpuscles relay feather position in relation to the body. Merkel cells are found mainly in the beak of non-aquatic birds, while Grandry corpuscles are present in aquatic birds; both are numerous in the bill tip organ that is important for food prehension.[90, 91] While Ruffini's corpuscles can be found in joint capsules of birds, Ruffini endings have only been identified in the bill of geese and the beak of the Japanese quail.[90, 92–94] Mechanoreceptors are involved with behavioral responses, including the initiation of a feeding response in baby birds upon beak manipulation and the ability of parrots to manipulate food with their beak and feet.[90] The sensitive mechanoreceptors in the feet of parrots may allow them to feel earthquakes that are undetectable to owners.[90, 95] Disorders of the plumage may be detected by mechanoreceptors and stimulate preening behavior.[90, 96] Flight control and patterns may be regulated by mechanoreceptors detecting vibrations caused by air stream turbulence.[90, 97, 98]

Avian thermoreceptors may be free nerve endings and are present in the skin, especially the beak and tongue.[90, 99] Thermoreceptors in the skin assist with body thermoregulation and those in the beak may be used for regulating incubation temperatures in some birds.[100] Pain receptors, or nociceptors, respond to mechanical and thermal stimuli and are present in the beak and skin.[90, 101, 102] Research indicates that birds respond to pain by either a reflex/escape response or by immobility; these responses may be mediated by different types of pain receptors.[103] In addition, beak amputation studies show that birds may experience chronic pain.[103]

CONCLUSION

Parrots experience the world in ways both similar and different to mammals. It is apparent that vision, hearing and vocalization, taste, olfaction, and touch perception play vital roles in the daily life of the parrot. Many of the normal and abnormal behaviors of parrots can be better understood by examining how birds perceive the environment around them. Further research in the area of sensory perception of parrots will expand our knowledge and likely enable us to improve the lives of these magnificent creatures.

REFERENCES

1. King, A., and J. McLelland, 1984. "Special sense organs." In *Birds, their structure and function*, ed. A. King and J. McLelland, pp. 284–314. Philadelphia: Balliere-Tindall.
2. Williams, D. 1994. "Ophthalmology." In *Avian medicine: Principles and application*, ed. B.W. Ritchie, G.J. Harrison, and L.R. Harrison, pp. 673–694. Lake Worth, FL: Wingers Publishing.
3. Kern, T.J. 1997. "Disorders of the special senses." In *Avian medicine and surgery*, ed. R.B. Altman, S.L. Clubb, G.M. Dorrestein, and K. Quesenberry, pp. 563–589. Philadelphia: WB Saunders.
4. Korbel, R.T. 2000. "Avian ophthalmology: A clinically oriented approach." Proceedings of the Association of Avian Veterinarians, pp. 439–456.
5. Gunturkun, O. 2000. "Sensory physiology: Vision." In *Sturkie's avian physiology*, ed. G.C. Whittow, pp. 1–19. San Diego: Academic Press.
6. Blanchard, S. 1999. *The companion parrot handbook*. Oakland: PBIC, Inc., p. 162.
7. Korbel, R.T., B. Nell, P.T. Redig, I. Walde, and S. Reese. 2000. "Video fluorescein angiography in the eyes of various raptors and mammals." Proceedings of the Association of Avian Veterinarians, pp. 89–95.
8. Blough, P.M. 1971. The visual acuity of the pigeon for distant targets. *Journal of the Experimental Analysis of Behavior* 15:57–67.
9. Bischof, H.J. 1988. The visual field and visually guided behavior in the zebra finch (*Taeniopygia guttata*). *Journal of Comparative Physiology* 163:329–337.
10. Fox, R., Lehmkuhle S.W., and D.H. Westendorf. 1976. Falcon visual acuity. *Science* 192:263–265.
11. Friedman, M.B. 1975. "How birds use their eyes." In *Neural and endocrine aspects of behaviour in birds*, ed. P. Wright, P. Cryl, and D.M. Volwes, pp. 182–204. Amsterdam: Elsevier.
12. Reymond, L. 1985. Spatial visual acuity of the eagle Aquila audax: A behavioral, optical, and anatomic investigation. *Vision Res* 25:1477–1491.
13. Gunturkun, O., and U. Hahmann. 1994. Cerebral asymmetries and visual acuity in pigeons. *Behav Brain Res* 60171–175.
14. Emmerton, J. 1983. "Vision." In *Physiology and behavior of the pigeon*, ed. M. Abs, pp. 245–266. London: Academic Press.
15. Chen, D.M., and T.H. Goldsmith. 1986. Four spectral classes of cone in the retinas of birds. *J Comp Physiol* 159:473–479.
16. Burkhardt, D. 1989. UV vision: a bird's eye view of feathers. *Journal of Comparative Physiology* A164:787–196.
17. Cuthill, I., J.C. Partridge, and A.T. Bennett. 2000. "Avian UV vision and sexual selection." In *Animal signals. Signalling and signal design in animal communication,* ed. Y. Epsmark, T. Amundsen, and G. Rosenqvist, pp. 87–106. Trondheim, Norway: Royal Norwegian Society of Sciences and Letters, The Foundation Tapir Publishers.
18. Cuthill, I., J.C. Partridge, A.T. Bennett, S.C. Church, and N.S. Hart. 2000. Ultraviolet vision in birds. *Adv Study Behav* 29:159–214.

19. Bennett, A.T., I. Cuthill, and K. Norris. 1994. Sexual selection and the mismeasure of color. *Am Nat* 144:848–860.

20. Osorio, D., M. Vorobyev, and C.D. Jones. 1999. Colour vision of domestic chicks. *J Exp Biol* 202:2951–2959.

21. Osorio, D., C.D. Jones, and M. Vorobyev. 1999. Accurate memory for colour but not pattern contrast in chicks. *Curr Biol* 9:199–202.

22. Vorobyev, M., D. Osorio, A.T. Bennett, N.J. Marshall, and I. Cuthill. 1998. Tetrachromacy, oil droplets and bird plumage colors. *J Comp Physiol* A183:621–633.

23. Bowmaker, J.K., L.A. Heath, S.E. Wilkie, and D.M. Hunt. 1997. Visual pigments and oil droplets from six classes of photoreceptors in the retinas of birds. *Vis Res* 37:2183–2194.

24. Wilkie, S.E., P.M. Vissers, D. Das, W.J. DeGrip, J.K. Bowmaker, and D.M. Hunt. 1998. The molecular basis for UV vision in birds: Special characteristics, cDNA sequence and retinal localisation of the UV-sensitive pigment of the budgerigar (*Melopsittacus undulatus*). *Biochem J* 330:541–547.

25. Pearn, S.M., T.D. Andrew, A.T. Bennett, and I. Cuthill. 2001. Ultraviolet selection, fluorescence and mate choice in a parrot, the budgerigar *Melopsittacus undulatus*. *Proc R Soc Lond* 268:2273–2279.

26. Burkhardt, D., and E. Finger. 1991. Black, white, and UV: How birds see birds. *Naturwissenschaften* 78:279–280.

27. Cuthill, I., A.T. Bennett, J.C. Partridge, and E. Maier. 1999. Plumage reflectance and the objective assessment of avian sexual dichromatism. *Am Nat* 160:183–200.

28. Finger, E., and D. Burkhardt. 1994. Biological aspects of bird colouration and avian colour vision including ultraviolet range. *Vis Res* 34:1509–1514.

29. Finger, E., D. Burkhardt, and J. Dyck. 1992. Avian plumage colors: Origin of UV reflection in a black parrot. *Naturwissenschaften* 79:187–188.

30. Burkhardt, D. 1982. Birds, berries, and UV. A note on some consequences of UV vision in birds. *Naturwissenschaften* 69(4):153–157.

31. Viitala, J., E. Korplmakl, P. Palokangas, and M. Kolvula. 1994. Attraction of kestrels to vole scent marks visible in ultraviolet light. *Nature* 373:425–427.

32. Chittka, L., A. Shmida, N. Troje, and R. Menzel. 1994. Ultraviolet as a component of flower reflections, and the color perception of Hymenoptera. *Vis Res* 34(11):1489–1508.

33. Bradbury, J.W., and S.L. Vehrencamp. 1998. "Light signal reception." In *Principles of animal communication*, ed. A.D. Sinauer, pp. 239–278. Sunderland, MA: Sinauer Associates, Inc.

34. Bennett, A.T., and I. Cuthill. 1994. Ultraviolet vision in birds: What is its function? *Vis Res* 34:1471–1478.

35. Coemans, M.A., J.J. vos Hzn, and J.F.W. Nuboer. 1994. The relation between celestial colour gradients and the position of the sun, with regard to the sun compass. *Vis Res* 34:1461–1470.

36. Arnold, K.E., I.P. Owens, and N.J. Marshall. 2002. Fluorescent signaling in parrots. *Science* 295:92.

37. Korbel, R.T., and U. Gropp. "Ultraviolet perception in birds." Proceedings of the Association of Avian Veterinarians, pp. 77–81.

38. Brundett, G.W. 1974. Human sensitivity to flicker. *Lighting Res Technol* 6:127–143.

39. Maddocks, S.A., A.R. Goldsmith, and I. Cuthill. 2001. The influence of flicker rate on plasma corticosterone levels of European starlings, *Sturnus vulgaris*. *Gen Comp Endocrinol* 124 (3):315–320.

40. Boshouwers, F.M.G., and E. Nicaise. 1992. Artificial light sources and their influence on physical activity and energy expenditure of laying hens. *Brit Poultry Sci* 34:11–19.

41. Nuboer, J.F.W. 1993. "Visual ecology in poultry houses." Proceedings of the Fourth Symposium of Poultry Welfare, Edinburgh, Scotland, pp. 39–44.

42. D'Eath, R.B., and M.S. Dawkins. 1996. Laying hens do not discriminate between video images of conspecifics. *Anim Behav* 52:903–912.

43. Hunt, S., I. Cuthill, J.P. Swaddle, and A.T. Bennett. 1997. *Ultraviolet vision and band-colour preferences in female zebra finches, Taeniopygia guttata*. *Anim Behav* 54:1383–1392.

44. D'Eath, R.B. 1998. Can video images imitate real stimuli in animal behaviour experiments? *Biol Rev* 73:267–292.

45. Fleishman, L.J., and J.A. Endler. 2000. Some comments on visual perception and the use of video playback in animal behaviour studies. *Acta Ethol* 3:15–27.

46. Cuthill, I., N.S. Hart, J.C. Partridge, A.T. Bennett, S. Hunt, and S.C. Church. 2000. Avian colour vision and avian video playback experiments. *Acta Ethol* 3:29–37.

47. Catchpole, C.K., and P.J.B. Slater. 1995. *Bird song: Biological themes and variations*. Cambridge: Cambridge Univ. Press.

48. Dooling, R.J., B. Lohr, and M.L. Dent. 2000. "Hearing in birds and reptiles." In *Comparative hearing in birds and reptiles*, ed. R.J. Dooling,

R.R. Fay, and A.N. Popper, pp. 308–359. New York: Springer-Verlag.

49. Farabaugh, S.M., and R.J. Dooling. 1996. "Acoustic communication in parrots: Laboratory and field studies of Budgerigars, *Melopsittacus undulatus.*" In *Ecology and evolution of acoustic communication in birds*, ed. D.E. Kroodsma and E.H. Miller, pp. 97–117. Ithaca, NY: Cornell University Press.

50. Saunders, J.C., R.K. Duncan, D.E. Doan, and Y.L. Werner. 2000. "The middle ear of reptiles and birds." In *Comparative earing: Birds and reptiles*, ed. R.J. Dooling, A.N. Popper, and R.R. Fay, pp. 13–69. New York: Springer-Verlag.

51. Gleich, O., and G.A. Manley. 2000. "The hearing organ of birds and Crocodilia." In *Comparative hearing: Birds and reptiles*, ed. R.J. Dooling, A.N. Popper, and R.R. Fay, pp. 70–138. New York: Springer-Verlag.

52. Ryals, B.M., and E.W. Rubel. 1988. Hair cell regeneration after acoustic trauma in adult Coturnix quail. *Science* 240:1774–1776.

53. Corwin, J.T., and D.A. Cotanche. 1988. Regeneration of sensory hair cells after acoustic trauma. *Science* 240:1772–1774.

54. Steel, K.P., and C.J. Kros. 2001. A genetic approach to understanding auditory function. *Nature Genet* 22:143–149.

55. Park, T.J., K. Okanoya, and R.J. Dooling. 1985. Operant conditioning of small birds for acoustic discrimination. *J Ethol* 3:5–9.

56. Okanoya, K., and R.J. Dooling. 1987. Hearing in passerine and psittacine birds: A comparative study of absolute and masked thresholds. *J Comp Psychol* 101 (1):7–15.

57. Wright, T.F., K.A. Cortopassi, J.W. Bradbury, and R.J. Dooling. In press. Hearing and vocalizations in the orange-fronted conure, *Aratinga canicularis. J Comp Psychol.*

58. Farabaugh, S.M., M.L. Dent, and R.J. Dooling. 1998. Hearing and vocalizations of wild-caught Australian budgerigars (*Melopsittacus undulatus*). *J Comp Psychol* 112:74–81.

59. Park, T.J., and R.J. Dooling. 1991. Sound localization in small birds: Absolute localization in azimuth. *J Comp Psychol* 105:125–133.

60. Dent, M.L., R.J. Dooling, and A.S. Pierce. 2000. Frequency discrimination in budgerigars (*Melopsittacus undulatus*): Effects of tone duration and tonal context. *J Acoust Soc Am* 107(5): 2657–2664.

61. Dooling, R.J., and J.C. Saunders. 1975. Auditory intensity discrimination in the parakeet (*Melopsittacus undulatus*). *J Acoust Soc Am* 58: 1308–1310.

62. Lohr, B., T.F. Wright, and R.J. Dooling. In press. Detection and discrimination of natural calls in masking noise by birds: Estimating the active space of a signal. *Anim Behav.*

63. Dooling, R.J., S.D. Brown, G.M. Klump, and K. Okanoya. 1992. Auditory perception of conspecific and heterospecific vocalizations in birds: Evidence for special processes. *J Comp Psychol* 106:20–28.

64. El Boushy, A.R., A.F.B. Van der Poel, J.C.J. Verhaart, and D.A. Kennedy. 1989. Sensory involvement control feed intake in poultry. *Feedstuffs* 61 (25):16–41.

65. Nalavade, M.N., and A.T. Varute. 1977. Histochemical studies on the mucins of the vertebrate tongues. XI. Histochemical analysis of mucosubstances in the lingual glands and taste buds of some birds. *Acta Histochem* 60 (1): 18–31.

66. Matson, K.D., J.R. Millam, and K.C. Klasing. 2000. Taste threshold determination and side-preference in captive cockatiels (*Nymphicus hollandicus*). 2000. *Applied Animal Behaviour Science* 69:313–326.

67. Kare, M.R., and J.R. Mason. 1986. "The chemical senses in birds." In *Avian physiology*, ed. P.D. Sturkie, pp. 59–73. New York: Springer-Verlag.

68. Bartholomew, G.A., and T.J. Cade. 1958. Effects of sodium chloride on the water consumption of house sparrows. *Physiol Zool* 31:304–310.

69. Cummings, J.L., J.R. Mason, D.L. Otis, J.E. Davis, and T.J. Ohashi. 1994. Evaluation of methiocarb, ziram, and methyl anthranilate as bird repellants applied to dendrobium orchids. *Wildl Soc Bull* 22:633–638.

70. Hainsworth, F.R., and L.L. Wolf. 1976. Nectar characteristics and food selection by hummingbirds. *Oecologia* 25:101–113.

71. Harriman, A.E., and M.R. Kare. 1966. Aversion to saline solutions in starlings, purple grackles, and herring gulls. *Physiol Zool* 39:123–126.

72. Harriman, A.E., and J.S. Milner. 1969. Preference for sucrose solutions by Japanese quail (*Coturnix coturnix japonica*) in two-bottle drinking tests. *Am Midland Natural* 81:575–578.

73. Harriman, A.E., and E.G. Fry. 1990. Solution acceptance by common ravens (*Corvus corax*) given two-bottle preference tests. *Psychol Rep* 67:19–26.

74. Kare, M.R., and H.L. Pick. 1960. The influence of the sense of taste on feed and fluid consumption. *Poult Sci* 39:697–706.

75. Kare, M.R., R. Black, and E.G. Allison. 1957. The sense of taste in the fowl. *Poult Sci* 36: 129–138.

76. Matson, K.D., J.R. Millam, and K.C. Klasing. 2001. Thresholds for sweet, salt, and sour taste stimuli in cockatiels (*Nymphicus hollandicus*). *Zoo Biology* 20:1–13.

77. Mason, J.R., and L. Clark. 2000. "The chemical senses in birds." In *Sturkie's avian physiology*, ed. G.C. Whittow, pp. 39–56. San Diego: Academic Press.

78. Clark, L., and P.S. Shah. 1993. Chemical bird repellants: Possible use in cyanide ponds. *J Wildl Manage* 57:657–664.

79. Davis, R.G. 1973. Olfactory psychophysical parameters in man, rat, dog, and pigeon. *J Comp Physiol Psychol* 85:221–232.

80. Clark, L., and J.R. Mason. 1987. Olfactory discrimination of plant volatiles by the European starling. *Anim Behav* 35:227–235.

81. Clark, L., and C.A. Smeraski. 1990. Seasonal shifts in odor acuity by starlings. *J Exp Zool* 177:673–680.

82. Clark, L. 1991. Odor detection thresholds in tree swallows and cedar waxwings. *Auk* 108:177–180.

83. Clark, L., K.V. Avilova, and N.J. Bean. 1993. Odor thresholds in passerines. *Comp Biochem Physiol* 104:305–312.

84. Houston, D.C. 1987. Scavenging efficiency of turkey vultures in tropical forests. *Condor* 88:318–323.

85. Clark, L., and P.S. Shah. 1992. "Information content of prey odor fumes: What do foraging Leach's storm petrels know?" In *Chemical signals in vertebrates*, ed. R.L. Doty and D. Muller-Schwarze, pp. 421–428. New York: Plenum Press.

86. Wallraff, H.G., J. Kiepenheuer, and A. Streng. 1993. Further experiments on olfactory navigation and non-olfactory pilotage by homing pigeons. *Behav Ecol Sociobiol* 32:387–390.

87. Harriman, A.E., and R.H. Berger. 1986. Olfactory acuity in the common raven (*Corvus corax*). *Physiol Behav* 36:257–262.

88. Cohen, J. 1981. Olfaction and parental behavior in Ring Doves. *Biochem Sys Ecol* 9:351–354.

89. Clark, L., and J.R. Mason. 1988. Effect of biologically active plants used as nest material and the derived benefit to starling nestlings. *Oecologia* 77:174–180.

90. Necker, R. 2000. "The somatosensory system." In *Sturkie's avian physiology*, ed. G.C. Whittow, pp. 57–69. San Diego: Academic Press.

91. Gottschaldt, K.M. 1985. "Structure and function of avian somatosensory receptors." In *Form and function in birds*, ed. A. King and J. McLelland, pp. 375–461. London: Academic Press.

92. Halata, Z., and B.L. Munger. 1980. The ultra-structure of Ruffini and Herbst corpuscles in the articular capsule of domestic pigeon. *Anat Rec* 198:681–692.

93. Halata, Z., and M. Grim. 1993. Sensory nerve endings in the beak skin of Japanese quail. *Anat Embryol* 187:131–138.

94. Gottschaldt, K.M., H. Fruhstorfer, W. Schmidt, and I. Kraft. 1982. Thermosensitivity and its possible fine-structural basis in mechanoreceptors in the beak skin of geese. *J Comp Neurol* 205:219–245.

95. Shen, J.X., and Z.M. Xu. 1994. Response characteristics of Herbst corpuscles in the interosseous region of the pigeon's hind limb. *J Comp Physiol* 175:667–674.

96. Delius, J.D. 1988. Preening and associated comfort behaviour in birds. *Ann NY Acad Sci* 525:40–55.

97. Gewecke, M., and M. Woike. 1978. Breast feathers as an air-current sense organ for the control of flight behaviour in a songbird (*Carduelis spinus*). *Z Tierpsychol* 47:293–298.

98. Bilo, D., and A. Bilo. 1978. Wind stimuli control vestibular and optokinetic reflexes in the pigeon. *Naturwissenschaften* 65:161–162.

99. Hensel, H. 1973. "Cutaneous thermoreceptors." In *Handbook of sensory physiology: Somatosensory system*, ed. A. Iggo, pp. 79–110. Berlin/Heidelberg/New York: Springer-Verlag.

100. Frith, H.J. 1959. Incubator birds. *Sci Am* 201:52–58.

101. Necker, R., and B. Reiner. 1980. Temperature-sensitive mechanoreceptors, thermoreceptors, and heat nociceptors in the feathered skin of pigeons. *J Comp Physiol* 135:201–207.

102. Gentle, M.J. 1989. Cutaneous sensory afferents recorded from the nervus intramandibularis of *Gallus gallus var. domesticus*. *J Comp Physiol* 164:763–774.

103. Gentle, M.J. 1992. *Pain in birds. Anim Welfare,* 1:235–247.

5
Social Behavior of Psittacine Birds

Lynne M. Seibert

Due to the popularity of keeping psittacine birds as pets, a better understanding of their social behavior, in both natural and captive environments, is crucial in order to provide for their social and physical needs. Many psittacine species do not have an extensive history of domestication. Understanding and addressing their social needs will improve the welfare of captive psittacine birds, behavior problems may be more effectively managed, and captive breeding programs can benefit when social behaviors are better understood. Social behavior varies among the different psittacine species. Solitary behavior is the exception (Kakapo, *Strigops habroptilus*), with most species showing complex social organization.

FLOCK FORMATION

Flock formation is important for predator detection and avoidance, access to mates, defense of territories, and foraging efficiency (Wilson 1975). Psittacine birds often form flocks, a behavior that is promoted by unstable food resources (irregularly distributed sources that are unpredictable through time) and indefensible areas. Feeding together in organized flocks may be advantageous to the individual, who is able to benefit from the collective knowledge of the group. By following the flock, an individual has a better chance of locating adequate amounts of food when resources are unpredictable. Small foraging groups are better able than individual birds to exclude competitors from feeding sites (Wilson 1975). There is some evidence that smaller birds with more limited fasting ability are more likely to flock than larger birds (Gill 1995).

Indefensible areas also promote flocking behavior in birds. There is increased security in a large group, with individuals nearest the center of the flock having the least chance of becoming the victim of a predator. Flocking improves the efficiency of predator detection, allowing the individual more time for other activities. Alarm calling is common among flocks and serves to alert other members of the group to possible danger. Birds may also participate in cooperative mobbing behavior against intruders (Gill 1995).

Flocks range in size and species composition, with mixed-species flocks observed in native habitats. Nuclear species form the main elements of the organization, while additional species that join the flock opportunistically are referred to as "followers." The formation of multi-species flocks appears to provide additional advantages for group members. There may be less conspecific competition for similar food and nesting sites. One theory that explains the variety of distinctive plumage coloration in psittacine birds proposes that the coloration promotes recognition of conspecifics for breeding purposes when different species are living in close proximity (Butcher & Rohwer 1989).

DOMINANCE RELATIONSHIPS

The importance and meaning of dominance interactions in psittacine social groups was reviewed by Seibert (2003). Stability of social groups requires both mutual recognition of members and a system for allocation of limited group resources. A dominance relationship exists when predictable dominance-subordinance responses occur between members of a stable social group, based on the outcome of prior interactions between the individuals. Once relationships are established, there is consistency in social interactions, resulting in fewer, or less intense, aggressive assertions of dominance (Bernstein 1981). Dominance relationships function to reduce the occurrence of competitive conflicts between members of a social group.

Agonistic behaviors consist of both aggressive and submissive actions within the context of a social interaction (Wilson 1975). Agonistic encounters are observed more frequently when relationships are unclear, such as the introduction of new individuals. Dominance relationships also appear to require periodic reinforcement, even in the absence of incentive, to prevent extinction (Bernstein 1981).

Subordinate individuals respond to aggressive behaviors performed by higher-ranking individuals with appeasement or submissive signals. Submissive postures allow avoidance of combat. Patterns of communication that function to terminate aggression are labeled submissive (Bernstein 1981).

BENEFITS OF RANK

The advantages of occupying positions of higher status in the flock have not been determined for most psittacine species. Higher-ranking individuals may have greater access to feeding or roosting sites, lower visibility to predators, or more mating opportunities. Aggressive encounters in a group of Orange-fronted Parakeets were most frequent during feeding, followed by bathing or seeking roosting places (Hardy 1965). However, no aggression occurred in the context of foraging in a captive flock of Cockatiels, but higher-ranking males did appear to have greater access to mates and preferred nest boxes (Seibert & Crowell-Davis 2001). Female domestic gallinaceous hens were found to select mates with larger than average combs, or higher-ranking males if information about social dominance was available (Graves et al. 1985). Female Speckled Parrotlets also appeared to pursue higher-ranking partners, but males showed no preference for higher-ranking females (Garnetzke-Stollmann & Franck 1991).

GENDER EFFECTS ON AGGRESSIVENESS

In most avian species studied, males show higher frequencies of aggressive behaviors than females (Jackson 1991; Nol et al. 1996; Seibert &

Crowell-Davis 2001; Wilson 1992; Wingfield et al. 1987; Woolfenden & Fitzpatrick 1977). However, Sandell and Smith (1997) found that female European Starlings became more aggressive than males during the breeding season. Tarvin and Woolfenden (1997) reported similar findings in female Blue Jays during the breeding season. Further studies are needed to explore the causes of gender differences in aggressiveness.

Seibert and Crowell-Davis (2001), studying a captive flock of Cockatiels, found that females were significantly more likely to direct aggression against other females than against males in the flock. There was not a significant difference for the male Cockatiels in the gender of their opponents. Female competition for access to mates has been suggested as an explanation for these gender differences in female aggressiveness (Sandell & Smith 1997; Tarvin & Woolfenden 1997).

INDICATORS OF DOMINANCE

Reliable indicators of dominance status have not been determined for most psittacine species. Some postulated indicators of dominance relationships are the frequency of threats and attacks and access to resources. Rushen (1984) proposed that social dominance within established flocks of domestic chickens could be determined using observations of agonistic encounters within the entire flock, rather than paired contests. Seibert and Crowell-Davis (2001) measured dominance relationships by recording the outcomes of all agonistic encounters during focal sampling of each flock member. Power (1966) recorded displacement at feeding and roosting sites to determine relative social status in a breeding flock of Orange-chinned Parakeets.

Studies of other bird populations have shown that social status is directly related to size, age, and gender (Gill 1995). However, Hardy (1965) found no correlation between dominance rank and physical attributes in the group of parrots he studied. Instead, he noted a direct correlation between pair bonding and dominance rank. Other researchers have found that pair bonding increases the social status of psittacine birds within a group (Levinson 1980).

MEASURING DOMINANCE

The agonistic display behaviors of White-fronted Amazon Parrots were classified as low, medium, or high intensity (Levinson 1980). Threat behaviors (aggressive components of agonistic behavior) are composed of one or more components that differ in valence (intimidatory effectiveness) (Hardy 1965). The displays are partially stereotyped, such that components appear in a characteristic order, but the display may be terminated at any point in the series when intimidation has been accomplished.

In species for which dominance interactions have been recorded, the following behaviors were recorded as aggressive (Garnetzke-Stollmann & Franck 1991; Hardy 1965; Levinson 1980; Power 1966; Seibert & Crowell-Davis 2001).

Turn threat: the aggressing bird abruptly turned toward opponent with head and neck extended

Beak gape: aggressing bird directed open beak toward opponent

Peck threat: aggressor pecked at opponent but did not make contact

Beak spar: short bouts in which birds' beaks made contact

Peck: aggressor's beak closed on some part of recipient

Wing flapping: perched aggressor flapped wings while facing opponent

Sidle approach: perched aggressor approached with side of the body directed toward opponent

Slow advance: perched aggressor walked directly toward opponent

Rushing: perched aggressor ran at opponent

Flight approach: aggressor flew directly toward opponent

Hardy (1965) and Power (1966) also reported stationary threat behaviors including plumage appression, or sleeking of the body feathers, and malar fluffing, fluffing of feathers in the malar region, which causes the bird's head to appear larger and draws attention to the beak.

Submissive behaviors, also referred to as appeasement behaviors, appear to be less ritualized. Submissive behaviors performed in response to aggressive displays consist of crouching, fluffing feathers, head wagging, foot lifting, or avoidance (Hardy 1965).

Variations in threat display complexity of different psittacine species may be explained by the games-theory approach. Games theory predicts that as the risk of physical injury increases,

species evolve less dangerous strategies for resolving disputes, such as more complex ritualized postural displays. Serpell (1982) studied nine different taxa of *Trichoglossus* parrots that differed in their beak size and the complexity of threat displays. The findings of this study suggest that an interspecific difference in beak length, which is directly related to the risk of injury from the bites of conspecifics, influences the nature of threat displays. With increasing beak size, displays became more complex, and there was a reduced inclination to attack a mirror-image opponent (Serpell 1982).

GENDER EFFECTS ON DOMINANCE RELATIONSHIPS

Several studies have found that male birds tend to occupy higher social positions than female birds (Seibert & Crowell-Davis 2001; Tarvin & Woolfenden 1997; Weinhold 1998; Woolfenden & Fitzpatrick 1977).

Aggressiveness, or the tendency to initiate agonistic interactions, may or may not be correlated with dominance status. Cloutier et al. (1995) found that subordinate hens were less likely to engage in aggressive behaviors than dominant hens. Graves et al. (1985) also found that aggressiveness was correlated with dominance rank in White Leghorn cocks. Higher-ranking Cockatiels had significantly higher rates of aggression than lower-ranking flock members (Seibert & Crowell-Davis 2001).

AFFILIATIVE RELATIONSHIPS

Affiliative behaviors in birds consist of allopreening, allofeeding, maintenance of close proximity, pair bonding, and reproductive behaviors. Garnetzke-Stollmann and Franck (1991) described affiliative interactions in a group of captive parrots (*Forpus conspicillatus*) that included perching in close contact, allopreening, and solicitation of allopreening.

Spatial organization of flock members is not random. Members maintain relationships with other flock members that can be measured based on spatial patterns and proximity. Sparks (1964) found that the members of a flock of Red Avadavats (*Amandava amandava*) were not randomly dispersed. Grigor *et al.* (1995) found that spatial associations in domestic chickens were influenced by the social relationships within the flock. Seibert and Crowell-Davis (2001) also found the spacing in a flock of Cockatiels to be non-random and indicative of preferred associations. Preferred spatial associations coincided with mating groups, but in addition, males and females in the flock sometimes had same-gender preferred associates. Other researchers have found that mated pairs of birds maintain close spatial associations (Silcox & Evans 1982; Trillmich 1976; Wechsler 1989).

ALLOPREENING

Allopreening, which occurs when an individual uses its beak to groom another bird, is cited as the most important mechanism for maintenance of the pair bond (Gill 1995). In a review of the allopreening behavior of different psittacine species, Harrison (1994) reported that allopreening was confined to the head and neck region in amazon parrots, lovebirds, and the genus _Melopsittacus_. Allopreening involved the head, wings, and tail in _Aratinga, Brotogeris, Ara_, and _Cacatua_ species.

Since allopreening behavior has been associated with the formation of pair bonds, a predilection for cross-gender allopreening has been supported in various avian species (Gaston 1977; Harrison 1965; Spruijt et al. 1992). Seibert and Crowell-Davis (2001) found that males allopreened females significantly more than they allopreened other males. However, isosexual allopreening does occur and should be viewed as evidence of a social bond. Garnetzke-Stollmann and Franck (1991) observed that preferred associations, allopreening, and support in agonistic interactions were significantly more common among siblings than among unrelated birds in a flock of Speckled Parrotlets.

ALLOFEEDING

Allofeeding is closely associated with copulation in birds (Skeate 1984). The female solicits feeding by crouching, lowering her head, ruffling her feathers, and vocalizing. The male displays head bobbing, grasps the female's beak at a right angle, and regurgitates food to the female. Allofeeding occurs year-round in some amazon parrots, conures, lovebirds, and Grey-cheeked Parakeets (Harrison 1994).

PAIR BONDING

Pair bonding has been defined as a mutually beneficial relationship between sexually mature female and male birds, serving primarily for the cooperative rearing of young (Doane & Qualkinbush 1994; Wilson 1975). Pairs are characterized by allofeeding, pair participation in agonistic encounters, and close spatial associations (Garnetzke-Stollmann & Franck 1991; Levinson 1980; Trillmich 1976). Many psittacine species are thought to maintain pair bonds throughout the year.

Advent of the breeding season can alter the social hierarchy. Power (1966) found that single birds were more successful in an aggressive encounter if their mate was nearby, even if the mate did not appear to be actively participating. Levinson (1980) reported pair participation in agonistic encounters in White-fronted Amazon Parrots (_Amazona albifrons_), a species that maintained pair bonds throughout the year.

According to Butterfield (1970), perching in close proximity can be interpreted as evidence of pair bond formation. Arrowood (1988) observed close spatial associations among bonded pairs of Canary-winged Parakeets (_Brotogeris v. versicolorus_). Mates maintained very close proximity, usually touching. In addition, once pairing was achieved, individual mates no longer displayed affiliative behaviors toward any other flock members, as long as the mate was present in the flock, and agonistic displays did not occur between pair-bonded individuals.

MATING PAIRS AND GROUPS

The social behavior of most psittacine species has not been studied in natural habitats, and captive populations have commonly been housed in pairs for breeding. The assumption that psittacine birds maintain exclusive pair bonds is not accurate for all species. Extra-pair matings have been observed in Speckled Parrotlets, Budgerigars, and Cockatiels (Baltz & Clark 1997; Garnetzke-Stollmann & Franck 1991; Seibert & Crowell-Davis 2001). Allopreening occurs less frequently between the male and the secondary female. Extra-pair courtship activities tend to occur while the primary female partner is incubating eggs and unable to observe the activity (Baltz & Clark 1997).

While some psittacine males will actually assist in incubating the eggs (Cockatiels, macaws, conures, and some cockatoo species), all male psittacine birds appear to assist in the rearing of young. Male birds feed the hen as she incubates, guard the nest entrance, and feed the hatchlings. Many psittacine offspring have relatively long infancies, with weaning taking up to a year in some species, increasing the requirement for parental care (Doane & Qualkinbush 1994).

Successful nesting behavior has been described for endangered Puerto Rican Parrots (*Amazona vittata*) in a field setting. Successful mating pairs, or those producing fledged chicks, followed distinct patterns of nesting activities (Wilson et al. 1995). Females increased nest attendance during egg laying and incubation, while males rarely entered the nest at this stage. Allofeeding of the hen occurred close to the nest. During early chick rearing, male attentiveness increased, while females began to spend more time away from the nest. Regular allofeeding of the young by the male was essential for proper growth. Knowledge of the typical patterns of nest attendance can be used to detect problems in captive breeding programs.

CONCLUSION

An understanding of the social behaviors of psittacine birds has implications for the prevention and treatment of various undesirable behaviors of pet birds. Problems may occur in birds not provided with appropriate socialization opportunities, or as the birds reach sexual maturity, with reports of behaviors that seem to indicate bonding with a human caregiver. Undesirable behaviors include attempts to preen, allofeed (regurgitate), and copulate with the person; masturbation; aggressive attempts to drive away other members of the family; and defense of the cage as a nesting site (Harrison & Davis 1986). In addition to sexual behaviors, abnormal behaviors indicative of stress or anxiety can occur including feather picking, barbering, and self-mutilation; screaming, aggression and biting; and phobias. The importance of flock social interactions to various species and the effects of isolation or pair housing on welfare are pertinent issues. Spatial and social relationships have important implications for the management of psittacine species, including providing the appropriate amount of space for the flock, optimizing feeding locations, determining stocking density, and identifying mating pairs.

REFERENCES

Arrowood, P.C. 1988. Duetting, pair bonding, and agonistic display in parakeet pairs. *Behaviour* 106: 129–157.

Baltz, A.P., and A.B. Clark. 1997. Extra-pair courtship behaviour of male budgerigars and the effect of an audience. *Animal Behavior* 53:1017–1024.

Bernstein, I.S. 1981. Dominance: The baby and the bath water. *Behavioral and Brain Sciences* 4:419–457.

Butcher, G.S., and S. Rohwer. 1989. The evolution of conspicuous and distinctive coloration for communication in birds. *Current Ornithology* 6:51–108.

Butterfield, P.A. 1970. "The pair bond of the zebra finch." In *Social behavior in birds and mammals: Essays on the social ethology of animals*, ed. J.H. Crook, pp. 249–278. New York: Academic Press.

Cloutier, S., J.P. Beaugrand, and P.C. Laguë. 1995. The effect of prior victory or defeat in the same site as that of subsequent encounter on the determination of dyadic dominance in the domestic hen. *Behav Proc* 34:293–298.

Doane, B.M., and T. Qualkinbush. 1994. *My parrot, my friend: An owner's guide to parrot behavior*. New York: Macmillan.

Garnetzke-Stollmann, K., and D. Franck. 1991. Socialisation tactics of the speckled parrotlet (*Forpus conspicillatus*). *Behaviour* 119:1–29.

Gaston, A.J. 1977. Social behaviour within groups of jungle babblers (*Turdoides striatus*). *Animal Behavior* 25:828–848.

Gill, F.B. 1995. *Ornithology*, 2nd ed. New York: WH Freeman and Company.

Graves, H.B., C.P. Hable, and T.H. Jenkins. 1985. Sexual selection in Gallus: Effects of morphology and dominance on female spatial behavior. *Behav Proc* 11:189–197.

Grigor, P.N., B.O. Hughes, and M.C. Appleby. 1995. Social inhibition of movement in domestic hens. *Animal Behavior* 49:1381–1388.

Hardy, J.W. 1965. Flock social behavior of the orange-fronted parakeet. *Condor* 67:140–156.

Harrison, C.J.O. 1965. Allopreening as agonistic behaviour. *Behaviour* 24:161–209.

Harrison, G.J. 1994. "Perspective on parrot behavior." In *Avian medicine: Principles and application*, ed. B.W. Ritchie, G.J. Harrison, and L.R. Harrison, pp. 96–108. Lake Worth, FL: Wingers Publishing.

Harrison, G.J., and C. Davis. 1986. "Captive behavior and its modification." In *Clinical avian medicine and surgery*, ed. G.J. Harrison, pp. 20–28. Philadelphia: WB Saunders Company.

Jackson, W.M. 1991. Why do winners keep winning? *Behav Ecol Sociobiol* 28:271–276.

Levinson, S.T. 1980. The social behavior of the white-fronted Amazon (*Amazona albifrons*). In *Conservation of new world parrots: Proceedings of the ICBP Parrot Working Group Meeting*, ed. R.F. Pasquier, pp. 403–417. Washington, DC: Smithsonian Institution Press.

Nol, E., K. Cheng, and C. Nichols. 1996. Heritability and phenotypic correlations of behaviour and dominance rank of Japanese quail. *Anim Behav* 52:813–820.

Power, D.M. 1966. Agonistic behavior and vocalizations of orange-chinned parakeets in captivity. *Condor* 68:562–581.

Rushen, J. 1984. How peck orders in chickens are measured: A critical review. *Appl Anim Ethol* 11:255–264.

Sandell, M.I., and Smith, H.G. 1997. Female aggression in the European starling during the breeding season. *Anim Behav* 53:13–23.

Seibert L.M. 2003. "Social dominance: The peck order revealed." Proc Assoc Avian Vet, Pittsburgh, PA, pp. 187–188.

Seibert, L.M., and Crowell-Davis, S.L. 2001. Gender effects on aggression, dominance rank, and affiliative behaviors in a flock of captive adult cockatiels (*Nymphicus hollandicus*). *Appl Anim Behav Sci* 71 (2):155–170.

Serpell, J.A. 1982. Factors influencing fighting and threat in the parrot genus *Trichoglossus*. *Animal Behaviour* 30:1244–1251.

Silcox, A.P., and Evans, S.M. 1982. Factors affecting the formation and maintenance of pair bonds in the zebra finch, *Taeniopygia guttata*. *Anim Behav* 30:1237–1243.

Skeate, S.T. 1984. Courtship and reproductive behaviour of captive white-fronted Amazon parrots (*Amazona albifrons*). *Bird Behaviour* 5:103–109.

Sparks, J.H. 1964. Flock structure of the red avadavat with particular reference to clumping and allopreening. *Anim Behav* 12:125–136.

Spruijt, B.M., VanHooff, J.A., and Gispen, W.H. 1992. Ethology and neurobiology of grooming behavior. *Physiol Rev* 72:825–852.

Tarvin, K.A., and Woolfenden, G.E. 1997. Patterns of dominance and aggressive behavior in blue jays at a feeder. *Condor* 99:434–444.

Trillmich, F. 1976. Spatial proximity and mate-specific behaviour in a flock of budgerigars. *Z Tierpsychol* 41:307–331.

Wechsler, B. 1989. Measuring pair relationships in jackdaws. *Ethology* 80:307–317.

Weinhold, J. 1998. Analysis of the social behavior of a community of blue-fronted Amazons (*Amazona aestiva*) kept in an aviary. *Amazona Quarterly* 14:11–13.

Wilson, E.O. 1975. *Sociobiology*. Cambridge: Belknap Press.

Wilson, J.D. 1992. Correlates of agonistic display by great tit Parus major. *Behaviour* 121:168–214.

Wilson, K.A., Field, R., and Wilson, M.H. 1995. Successful nesting behavior of Puerto Rican parrots. *Wilson Bulletin* 107 (3):518–529.

Wingfield, J.C., Ball, G.F., Dufty, A.M., Hegner, R.E., and Ramenofsky, M. 1987. Testosterone and aggression in birds. *Amer Scientist* 75:602–608.

Woolfenden, G.E., and Fitzpatrick, J.W. 1977. Dominance in the Florida scrub jay. *Condor* 79:1–12.

6

Captive Parrot Nutrition: Interactions with Anatomy, Physiology, and Behavior

Kevin David Matson and Elizabeth A. Koutsos

OVERVIEW OF PSITTACINE NUTRITION

The selection or formulation of appropriate diets that meet the nutrient requirements of psittacine birds is based upon several factors. First, the wild-type foraging habits and behaviors of a particular parrot species provide important information regarding the animal's evolutionary adaptations to feeds and feeding. Second, an understanding of an animal's digestive anatomy and physiology, which often reflects its wild-type feeding habits, assists nutritionists in determining the nutrient and food requirements of that species. Third, optimal diet formulation is enabled by experimental data concerning the specific nutrient requirements of a particular species, based on data collected in either that species or in a closely related species. This factor is especially important, since knowledge of an animal's wild-type foraging strategies and its digestive anatomy and physiology only provide estimates of nutritional needs, while experimental data tests hypotheses and firmly establishes nutritional needs for a particular animal. This chapter explores topics in parrot nutrition including wild-type feeding strategies, digestive anatomy, and physiology with a special focus on avian gustation, calculated and experimentally determined nutrient requirements, and behavioral and immunological impacts of an improper diet.

WILD-TYPE DIETS

In the wild, the majority of parrots and other members of the order Psittaciformes consume plant-based (folivorous) diets. Folivorous psit-

tacines range from nectarivorous (nectar-/pollen-eating) to granivorous (seed-eating), while consumption of several plant-based feedstuffs (omnivory) is most common. A condensed listing of wild-type feeding strategy and common diet ingredients can be found in Table 6-1, and more detailed information concerning a wider range of species is available (Koutsos et al. 2001a).

DIGESTIVE ANATOMY AND PHYSIOLOGY

A bird's digestive anatomy, including the beak and oral cavity, esophagus, crop, proventriculus, gizzard, small and large intestine, ceca (generally absent in parrots), and cloaca, determines its ability to acquire, digest, and absorb nutrients, and often reflects its wild-type diet. For example, beak shape and size is generally correlated to wild-type diets (Klasing 1998). Granivorous birds often have ridged beaks that enhance seed-cracking abilities (Homberger & Brush 1986), and large granivores (particularly parrots) generally have a cartilaginous connection between the skull and beak to absorb the shock of cracking large seeds. Compared to granivores, frugivorous birds tend to have wider beaks and oral cavities. The remainder of the gastrointestinal tract, including the crop, proventriculus, gizzard, and intestines, is generally similar in psittacine birds, although the gizzards of frugivorous birds tend to have reduced musculature as compared to granivores or omnivores, reflecting the reduced need for particle grinding (Klasing 1998). Finally,

Table 6.1. Feeding strategies and common diet ingredients of some wild Psittaciformes

Species name	Strategy	Common diet ingredients	References
Blue and Gold macaw (*A. ararauna*)	Florivore	Seeds, fruits, nuts	(Abramson et al. 1995)
Red-faced parrot (*H. pyrrhops*)	Florivore	Flowers, berries, shoots, seeds, seed pods	(Toyne & Flanagan 1997)
Scaly-headed parrot (*P. maximiliani*)	Florivore	Seeds (70%), flowers (20%), grain (8%), fruit pulp (2%)	(Galetti 1993)
Blue-throated macaw (*A. glaucogularis*)	Frugivore	Palm fruit, nuts, milk	(Abramson et al. 1995)
Buffon's macaw (*A. ambigua*)	Frugivore	Fruits, flowers	(Abramson et al. 1995)
Green-winged macaw (*A. chloroptera*)	Frugivore	Fruits (*Hymenaea*), palm nuts, seeds	(Abramson et al. 1995)
Orange-winged amazon (*A. amazonica*)	Frugivore	Fruit (85% from palm fruit)	(Bonadie & Bacon 2000)
Red-bellied macaw (*A. manilata*)	Frugivore	Fruit (96% from palm fruit), flowers, seed pods	(Bonadie & Bacon 2000)
Vulturine parrot (*P. fulgidus*)	Frugivore	One or two of the 38 extant species of figs (*Ficus* spp.)	(Mack & Wright 1998)
Red-fronted macaw (*A. rubrogenys*)	Frugivore-Granivore	Fruits, seeds	(Pitter & Christiansen 1995)
Regents parrot (*P. anthopeplus*)	Frugivore-Granivore	Fruits, seeds	(Long & Mawson 1994)
Scarlet macaw (*A. macao*)	Frugivore-Granivore	Fruits, nuts, bark, leaves and shoots	(Abramson et al. 1995)
Budgerigar (*M. undulatus*)	Granivore	Seeds	(Wyndham 1980)
Cockatiel (*N. hollandicus*)	Granivore	Seeds (prefers soft, young over mature, hard seeds)	(Jones 1987)
Ground parrot (*P. wallicus*)	Granivore	Seeds, some insect larvae	(Mcfarland 1991)
Hyacinth macaw (*A. hyacinthinus*)	Granivore	Palm nuts (50% lipid content)	(Abramson et al. 1995)
Lear's macaw (*A. leari*)	Granivore	1° palm nuts, fruit	(Abramson et al. 1995)
Red-fronted macaw (*A. rubrogenys*)	Granivore	Nuts, seeds, fruit	(Abramson et al. 1995)
Spix's macaw (*C. spixii*)	Granivore	Palm nuts	(Abramson et al. 1995)
Hooded parrot (*P. dissimilis*)	Omnivore	1° seeds (1° sesame), flowers, invertebrates,	(Garnett & Crowley 1995)
Red-tailed amazon (*A. brasiliensis*)	Omnivore	Seeds, fruits, flowers, leaves, nectar and insects	(Martuscelli 1995)

larger birds generally have longer GI tracts, which results in increased time of retention of diet ingredients as compared to that of smaller birds.

GUSTATION IN PSITTACINES

Gustation, or the act of tasting food particles, occurs in the structures of the oral cavity. In the case of birds, these structures include the salivary glands, the tongue and its associated taste buds, and the beak. One important function of the structures associated with the oral cavity is the perception of the chemical qualities of potential food. Because these qualities transmit information about the suitability of potential food, it is important to understand how parrots sense their chemical environment.

Chemosensory Perception

The importance of chemosensory perception (i.e., gustation and olfaction) in birds has typically been downplayed with the emphasis, instead, being placed on sight and hearing. Nonetheless, olfaction and gustation are employed by birds in a variety of nutritive pursuits. For example, the Procellariiform "tubenose" seabirds use scent to locate food sources when navigating vast pelagic environments (Malakoff 1999; Nevitt 1999b; Nevitt 1999a), while Red-winged Blackbirds (*Agelaius phoeniceus*) reject dilute solutions of arthropod defensive secretions on the basis of taste (Yang & Kare 1968). In addition to toxin avoidance, foodstuffs are also evaluated by taste in order to detect nutrient levels (Herness & Gilbertson 1999). This phenomenon has been extensively researched in nectarivores such as hummingbirds and sunbirds (Martinez del Rio 1990; Martinez del Rio et al. 1992; Downs & Perrin 1996). Further, plasticity in the transduction pathways of gustatory chemoreceptors may result in a connection between the nutritional status of birds and their taste responses, thereby allowing for "specific appetites" for certain minerals (Herness & Gilbertson 1999).

While the avian sense of taste has received little attention, is has been demonstrated that taste buds are present in the oral cavity of birds on the floor of the pharynx and the base of the tongue (El Boushy et al. 1989). The number of avian taste buds appears to be extremely low compared to mammals. Humans (with about 9,000) have around 25 times more taste buds than parrots, which are reported to have 300–400 (Kare & Mason 1986). Fibers stemming from the glossopharyngeal nerve innervate the taste buds (El Boushy et al. 1989). Most of the additional studies of the microanatomy and physiology of taste buds have been limited to mammals, and little is known about what generalities about these structures can be made across taxa.

Testing Taste in Birds

The gustatory abilities of birds have been tested in several species by a variety of methods. The methods typically involve comparisons of consumption variables (e.g., number of sips or pecks or volume consumed) that are measured simultaneously for pure water compared to an aqueous solution of the test chemical, offered in separate bottles. Most commonly, two-choice taste-preference tests are conducted. However, concerns about arbitrary side preferences or biases have resulted in some investigators varying the number of bottles (from two to six), the relative position of each bottle (usually changing on an hourly or daily basis), and the location of bottles within each cage (Bartholomew & Cade 1958; Harriman & Fry 1990; Jackson et al. 1998). In addition to numerous studies testing the sugar preferences of nectarivores and frugivores, many wild and domestic species have been tested to determine whether consumption patterns change following the addition of taste stimuli: domestic chickens (*Gallus domesticus* [Kare et al. 1957; Kare & Pick 1960; Fuerst & Kare 1962; Gentle 1972]), Rock Doves (*Columba livia* [Duncan 1960; Crocker et al. 1993]), common crows (*Corvus corax* [Harriman & Fry 1990]), Japanese Quail (*Coturnix coturnix japonica* [Brindley 1965; Harriman & Milner 1969]), Bobwhite Quail (*Colinus virginianus* [Brindley 1965; Brindley & Prior 1968]), Laughing Gulls (*Larus atricilla* [Harriman 1967]), Herring Gulls (*Larus argentatus smithsonianus*), European Starlings (*Sturnus vulgaris*), Common Grackles (*Quiscalus quiscula* [Harriman & Kare 1966]), and House Finches (*Carpodacus mexicanus* [Bartholomew & Cade 1958]). This group of studies suggests that birds respond differently to a range of taste stimuli and the response depends on the species, the compound, and the concentrations being tested.

Taste Thresholds of Cockatiels

To better understand the role of taste in food choice of parrots, a series of tests were conducted using captive Cockatiels, *Nymphicus hollandicus*, as a model (Matson et al. 2000; Matson et al. 2001). Two-choice taste-preference tests were designed to determine thresholds of taste for various taste stimuli in the sweet, salt, bitter, and sour categories. Taste threshold was defined as the lowest concentration at which the consumed volume of a solution of test compound was significantly different from the consumed volume of pure water.

Results of this work are summarized in Table 6-2. In general, these results show that the birds' gustatory acuity differs according to taste category (i.e., salt, sweet, bitter, or sour). A 4,000-fold difference in concentration was found between

Table 6.2.   Taste thresholds of Cockatiels, *Nymphicus hollandicus*

Taste category	Chemical stimulus	Test range	Taste threshold
Salt	Sodium chloride	20.0–180.0 mmol*L^{-1}	160.0 mmol*L^{-1}
	Potassium chloride	100.0–250.0	160.0
Sweet	Fructose	160.0–490.0 mmol*L^{-1}	400.0 mmol*L^{-1}
	Glucose	160.0–200.0	160.0
	Sucrose	80.0–560.0	360.0
Bitter	Quinine	0.001–0.5 mmol*L^{-1}	0.1 mmol*L^{-1}
	Gramine	0.001–1.0	1.0
	Tannic acid	0.001–1.0	0.5
	Watte tannins	0.001–10.0	10.0
Sour	Citrate buffer (0.05 mol*L^{-1})	pH 5.0–5.5	pH 5.5
	Phosphate buffer (0.05 mol*L^{-1})	pH 4.9–7.7	None determined

Source: Matson et al. 2000; Matson et al. 2001; Matson, unpublished data.

the highest (sweet, using fructose) and lowest (bitter, using quinine) thresholds. Further, for all test substances, the Cockatiels either significantly increased intake of pure water or significantly decreased intake of the test solution—no solutions were preferable to water.

Cockatiels demonstrated the greatest gustatory acuity for bitter flavors. Thresholds for these compounds ranged from 0.1–10 mmol*L^{-1}, with the lowest threshold for quinine (0.1 mmol*L^{-1})—a commonly used bitter tasting alkaloid (K. Matson, unpublished data). The quinine threshold of Cockatiels is similar to the threshold of most humans (0.09 mmol*L^{-1} in distilled water [Schall 1990]), but lower than the thresholds of mammalian florivores (e.g., browser threshold, 3.0 mmol*L^{-1}; grazer threshold, 0.67 mmol*L^{-1} [Glendinning 1994]).

Both chloride salts that were tested were detected at the same threshold (160.0 mmol*L^{-1}) (Matson et al. 2001). As the normal range for circulating sodium concentrations in captive parrots is 130.0–157.0 mmol*L^{-1}, the threshold levels represent a marginally hypertonic concentration (Lane 1996; Polo et al. 1998). Rejection of hypertonic salt solutions is common in birds. For example, Laughing Gulls, Herring Gulls, and European Starlings show an aversion to solutions of sodium chloride in the range of 150.0–200.0 mmol*L^{-1} (Harriman & Kare 1966; Harriman 1967). One possible explanation for salt rejection is that hormones responsible for regulating water and salt balance also regulate the amiloride-

sensitive sodium channel, a sodium gustatory transduction mechanism (Herness & Gilbertson 1999).

Some reports indicate that parrots prefer solutions of sugar to pure water, while others hypothesize that granivores, such as Cockatiels, should react neutrally or negatively to sugar consumption (El Boushy et al. 1989; Kare & Mason 1986, respectively). No significant preferences were found when two monosaccharides (glucose and fructose) and one disaccharide (sucrose) were tested independently (Matson et al. 2000; Matson et al. 2001). Threshold concentrations were, however, higher on average than those found for bitter and salt compounds.

Sour taste is mostly based upon acidity or free protons (H^+). Therefore, two buffer systems were used so that the concentration of free protons could be manipulated—a 0.05 mol*L^{-1} buffer of sodium citrate and citric acid and a 0.05 mol*L^{-1} buffer of mono- and dibasic sodium phosphate. For these stimuli, the pH (rather than simple concentration) was varied and the pH was used as well for reporting taste thresholds. Despite the ability of protons to trigger many classes of ion channels that serve as gustatory transduction mechanisms, only citrate buffer resulted in the determination of a threshold (Matson et al. 2000; Matson et al. 2001). Thus, taste trials in Cockatiels, as well as in chickens, correspond to neurological studies demonstrating greater responses to organic acids (i.e., citrate buffer) than inorganic acids (i.e., phosphate buffer [Fuerst & Kare 1962]).

Implications

Given the wide range of Cockatiel taste thresholds, it is important to consider the effects of gustation on diet formulation and dietary changes in captive psittacines. Food palatability is the product of the food's chemical qualities and the bird's taste abilities. Despite the fact that the gustatory acuity of Cockatiels and other birds is generally equal to or less than humans, certain chemicals— particularly bitter ones—are rejected by birds on the basis of taste and these should be avoided when formulating diets. Various levels of bitter-tasting tannins are present in many grains crops and if these grains are used in seed mixes or formulated diets, food intake may be reduced. Other tastes, such as salt and sweet, are associated with nutrients required by all birds, and thus, the acceptance or rejection response to these taste stimuli may vary with nutritional status. Finally, tastes and specific appetites may sometimes drive consumption. Therefore, it is possible that because the Cockatiels used in the taste preference trials just described were all offered a salt and energy sufficient diet ad libitum (0.18% Na, 0.27% Cl, crude protein minimum 11%; five primary ingredients: ground corn, ground wheat, peanut meal, soy oil, and soy meal; Maintenance Crumbles, Roudybush, Inc., Cameron Park, California), the thresholds as measured may have been affected. If the birds had been fed a deficient diet, preferences for solutions containing the deficient nutrient might be expected.

THEORETICAL AND CALCULATED NUTRIENT REQUIREMENTS

Knowledge of an animal's wild-type diet, gastrointestinal anatomy and physiology, and gustatory capacity in combination with experimental data obtained in that species or related species can be used to determine specific nutrient requirements. It is important to keep in mind, however, that nutrient requirements are generally based upon meeting the nutrient needs of the majority of a population. Inevitably, there are animals whose individual nutrient needs are different from the majority of the population. Therefore, even when feeding individual animals a diet believed to be nutritionally adequate, it is important to be observant for signs of deficiency or toxicity, in addition to behavioral changes indicating nutritional problems.

Water

Water is often overlooked as a nutrient, but must be supplied to maintain cellular homeostasis, food digestion processes, waste excretion, and numerous metabolic reactions. Water requirements will vary with size of the animal (in general, smaller animals need less water) and environmental temperature (warmer temperatures tend to increase water requirements). Under thermo-neutral conditions, the daily water requirement of adult parrots is calculated to be ~2.4% of body weight (MacMillen & Baudinette 1993).

Energy

Energy can be supplied in the diet by lipid, protein, or carbohydrate, and functions to support basal metabolism, thermoregulation, and activity. A bird's energy requirement will change with environmental temperature (colder temperatures increase energy needs), activity level (higher activity levels also increase energy needs), and physiological state (maintenance animals require less energy than breeding or growing animals). Estimates of the daily metabolizable energy requirements for adult psittacine birds range from 154.6 kcal/$kg^{0.75}$ (indoor cage) to 226.1 kcal/$kg^{0.75}$ (outdoor aviary, cold weather) (see Koutsos et al. 2001a).

Protein/Amino Acids

Birds require 12 essential amino acids: phenylalanine, valine, tryptophan, methionine, arginine, threonine, hisitidine, isoleucine, lysine, leucine, glycine, and proline. Additionally, a source of nitrogen (e.g., protein) must also be present in the diet. Like energy requirements, the physiological state of an animal has a dramatic effect on its protein and amino acid requirements. In general, requirements are highest in growing chicks and females laying large clutches of eggs, while requirements are generally lowest for adult animals at maintenance. For example, the African Grey Parrot (*Psittacus erithacus*) requires 10–15% protein for maintenance (Kamphues et al. 1997), but higher requirements would be predicted for growing chicks and egg-laying females. Similarly, 11% crude protein is sufficient to support Cockatiels (*Nymphicus hollandicus)* at maintenance (Koutsos et al. 2001b), but growing Cockatiel chicks require 20% crude protein (Roudybush & Grau 1986).

In addition to physiological state, dietary feeding strategy impacts the protein requirement of animals. For example, frugivorous species of birds have lower rates of obligatory nitrogen losses as compared to granivorous species (Pryor 1999). Therefore, these specialist feeders are expected to have lower protein requirements than granivores or omnivores, and this hypothesis has been confirmed in the Rainbow Lorikeet (*Trichoglossus haemotodus*), which required less than 3% crude protein when provided a high-quality protein source (egg white) (Frankel & Avram 2001).

Lipids

Birds, like other animals, require essential fatty acids to provide membrane integrity, intracellular signaling molecules, and hormones. However, little research has been conducted to quantify the fatty acid requirements of psittacines. Therefore, nutritionists generally use poultry guidelines as a reference (NRC 1994); domesticated poultry require approximately 1% linoleic acid and 4–5% total lipid in poultry diets is not uncommon.

Vitamins

Presumably, parrots and other psittacines require the same vitamins as do other birds. However, little research has been conducted to quantify these requirements. In general, research has focused on the fat-soluble vitamins (A, D, E, and K); due to their chemical nature, these vitamins can be difficult to excrete, resulting in enhanced susceptibility to toxicity. Research in Cockatiels has demonstrated that diets containing 2,000–10,000 IU vitamin A/kg were sufficient to support animals at maintenance, and 4,000 IU vitamin A/kg diet was sufficient to support chick growth to fledging (Koutsos & Klasing 2002). Interestingly, in the same trial, adult birds fed 100,000 IU vitamin A/kg diet developed vitamin A toxicity within 3 months, while birds fed 0 IU vitamin A/kg diet did not develop a vitamin A deficiency during the two-year experimental period. However, 0 IU vitamin A/kg diet did not support normal growth and development of Cockatiel chicks. These results demonstrate that adult Cockatiels are more susceptible to vitamin A toxicity than to vitamin A deficiency, and that growing chicks require a dietary vitamin A source. Additionally, Cockatiel chicks fed 2.4 mg ß-carotene/kg diet and no vita-

min A grew normally and exhibited no signs of vitamin A deficiency. This observation supports the use of pro-vitamin A carotenoids in psittacine diets, perhaps as a means to avoid vitamin A toxicity. However, the exact rate of ß-carotene conversion to vitamin A in psittacines has not yet been determined.

Minerals

Because of the requirements for eggshell formation and skeletal calcification, as well as variable levels of calcium in different diet ingredients, the primary mineral of concern to avian nutritionists is calcium. The calcium requirement for psittacines has not been experimentally determined, so the established chicken requirement of 0.1% of the diet (NRC 1994) is commonly used. This is of particular importance when diets composed entirely of seed are fed, since seeds generally contain less than 0.1% calcium. Additionally, higher calcium requirements are expected during periods of eggshell formation and laying; egg-laying chickens are commonly fed 3–4% calcium. African Grey Parrots are commonly diagnosed with hypocalcemia (Rosskopf et al. 1985), although whether the calcium requirements or deficiency pathologies of this species are similar across parrot species remains to be determined. As with calcium, the requirements of psittacines for other essential minerals have not been examined, and poultry guidelines are often the only data available concerning avian mineral requirements.

EFFECTS OF NUTRIENT DEFICIENCIES/ EXCESSES

Nutrient deficiency and excess can induce numerous pathologies, which can include defects in reproduction, embryogenesis, and the growth and development of chicks; increased susceptibility to disease; undesired behavioral changes; poor health; and ultimately, death. A deficiency or toxicity of an individual nutrient will likely result in a unique combination of signs and symptoms, although the underlying etiology of these pathologies is often very similar.

Immune Function Effects

The immune response can be dramatically altered by the nutritional status of an animal (see review by Koutsos & Klasing 2001). These effects are most pronounced when deficiencies or toxicities occur during development, and a chronic deficiency of virtually any required nutrient during the period of immune system development (primarily during in ovo development, but also in post-hatch chicks) negatively impacts immunocompetence. In general, those required nutrients that function in regulating cell differentiation (e.g., vitamins A and D) are particularly detrimental to the development of immunocompetence. Similarly, post-hatch nutritional status can affect all facets of the immune system, and nutrient deficiency or excess may lead to increased disease susceptibility and may enhance the virulence or pathogenicity of certain organisms. Finally, many nutrients, specifically fatty acids and antioxidants, may modulate the immune response depending on their rate of dietary inclusion. For example, vitamin E has been shown to have anti-inflammatory properties at moderate dietary levels, while high dietary levels are associated with dampened immune responsiveness (e.g., broiler chickens [Leshchinsky & Klasing 2001]). However, the optimal levels of these nutrients for psittacine birds have not been determined, therefore excessive supplementation should be avoided until further research has been completed.

Behavioral Effects

Nutritional deficiency and excess can impact animal behavior in a variety of ways. First, a severe nutrient deficiency can change the behavior of an animal in terms of activity level. In rats, for example, deficiencies of protein, vitamin D, vitamin A, thiamin, riboflavin, or magnesium cause reductions in activity (Hughes & Wood-Gush 1973). Calcium-deficient chicks have increased movement and pecking behaviors, while sodium-deficient chickens have increased pecking frequency (Hughes & Wood-Gush 1973). Second, some nutrient deficiencies result in a "specific appetite" for that particular nutrient. This term refers to the ability of an animal to identify the proportion of a particular nutrient in a feedstuff, and to adjust the consumption of that feedstuff relative to its nutrient needs (Murphy 1994). For example, a specific appetite for calcium has been demonstrated in egg-laying female pheasants, in which increased consumption of a calcium-containing supplement (limestone) occurred when birds were fed calcium-deficient diets. While less research has been completed in birds as compared

to mammals, specific appetites for calcium (Hughes & Wood-Gush 1971a; Ranft & Hennig 1993), sodium (Hughes & Wood-Gush 1971b), amino acids (Newman & Sands 1983; Noble et al. 1993), protein (Ranft & Hennig 1993), energy (Ranft & Hennig 1993), and thiamin (Hughes & Wood-Gush 1971b) have been identified in birds. Third, undernourishment during post-hatch development may have severe consequences on the development of behavior and motor coordination, since cerebellum development (which plays a major role in the development of motor coordination in birds and mammals) is more affected by undernutrition than other parts of the brain. In mammals, undernourished infants have reduced locomotor activity, which is not reversed by refeeding (Altman et al. 1971). Finally, novel behavior effects resulting from nutritional deficiency or excess have recently been reported. Cockatiels fed deficient (0 IU vitamin A/kg diet), excessive (10,000 IU vitamin A/kg diet), or toxic (100,000 IU vitamin A/kg diet) levels of vitamin A had altered vocalization patterns compared to animals maintained on adequate vitamin A diets (2,000 IU/kg diet) (Koutsos et al. 2001c). Specifically, the total number of vocalizations (Figure 6.1), average length of vocalizations (reduced by

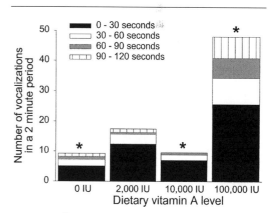

* Statistically significant difference compared to 2,000 IU vitamin A (P<0.05).

Figure 6.1. Effect of dietary vitamin A level on the number of vocalizations over a two-minute period made by adult female Cockatiels (*Nymphicus hollandicus*) at maintenance. Birds had consumed assigned diets for three months prior to vocalization analysis. Data from Koutsos et al. 2001c.

high or low vitamin A), peak frequency (Hz) of vocalizations (reduced by high or low vitamin A), and peak amplitude (dB) and total power (dB) (reduced by deficient diets) were significantly affected by dietary vitamin A level.

In addition to the effects of nutrient deficiency and excess, other types of behavioral responses to diet and nutrition have been demonstrated. First, specific preferences for food types have been demonstrated in cockatoos (Rowley et al. 1989). In general, when offered a choice of seed size, smaller birds preferred smaller seeds and larger birds preferred larger seeds, although individual preference was quite variable. Additionally, the novelty of a food item may play a role in the animal's response, since animals tend to ingest smaller amounts of a novel food as compared to consumption of a familiar food (Forbes 1998). Second, "nutritional enrichment" provides a mechanism for altered behavior patterns in response to diet choice and/or presentation. For example, providing sources of foraging enrichment altered parrot behavior (Coulton et al. 1997). Specifically, birds spent more time with the enrichment tool, altered the time spent on other perches, and increased allopreening events. In addition, birds chose to work for food by participating in the foraging enrichment apparatus, although identical food was freely available. A willingness to "work" for food has been observed in a variety of species. When starlings (*Sturnus vulgaris*) were offered a choice between freely available mealworms and hidden mealworms (requiring searching and foraging behaviors), they preferentially foraged for and ate hidden mealworms (Inglis & Ferguson 1986). Only when birds were nutritionally deprived for long periods of time did they choose freely available mealworms. Similar results have been seen in pigeons (Neuringer 1969) and in domestic fowl (Duncan & Hughes 1972). Finally, aversion to a novel food will occur if the food contains excessive toxins, has a major nutrient imbalance (e.g. amino acid imbalance), and/or causes nausea or discomfort (Forbes 1998).

CONCLUSIONS

Determining the nutrient requirements of an animal requires knowledge of its wild-type feeding strategy, gastrointestinal anatomy and physiology, and calculated and theoretical nutrient requirements. Once nutrient requirements have been established, diets may be selected to meet those nutrient needs, although several considerations should be made at this time. First, the bird's evolutionary adaptations may direct the choice of feedstuffs (e.g., incorporating large seeds in the case of a large parrot or liquid diet in the case of a nectarivore). Second, knowledge of specific appetites can allow for effective supplementation of diets (e.g., providing a supplemental calcium source to egg-laying birds). Third, knowledge of gustatory preferences and aversions can facilitate diet formulation by maximizing palatability and feed acceptance. Fourth, providing enrichment through nutrition (e.g., providing foraging opportunities) may enhance the animal's feeding experience and reduce stereotypic behaviors. Finally, it is critical to observe an animal subjected to dietary changes in order to evaluate its response to the new diet and, if necessary, to respond appropriately to changes in the animal's condition, health, and behavior.

REFERENCES

Abramson, J, B.L. Speer, and J.B. Thomson. 1995. *The large macaws*. Fort Bragg, CA: Raintree.

Altman, J., K. Sudarshan, G.D. Das, N. McCormick, and D. Barnes. 1971. The influence of nutrition on neural and behavioral development. 3. Development of some motor, particularly locomotor patterns during infancy. *Dev Psychobiol* 4 (2):97–114.

Bartholomew, G.A., and T.J. Cade. 1958. Effects of sodium chloride on the water consumption of house finches. *Phys Zool* 31:304–310.

Bonadie, W.A., and P.R. Bacon. 2000. Year-round utilisation of fragmented palm swamp forest by red-bellied macaws (*Ara manilata*) and orange-winged parrots (*Amazona amazonica*) in the Nariva Swamp (Trinidad). *Biol Cons* 95:1–5.

Brindley, L.D. 1965. Taste discrimination in bobwhite and Japanese quail. *Anim Behav* 16:304–307.

Brindley, L.D., and S. Prior. 1968. Effects of age on taste discrimination in the bobwhite quail. *Anim Behav* 16 (2):304–307.

Coulton, L.E., N.K. Waran, and R.J. Young. 1997. Effects of foraging enrichment on the behaviour of parrots. *Anim Welfare* 6 (4):357–363.

Crocker, D.R., S.M. Perry, M. Wilson, J.D. Bishop, and C.B. Scanlon. 1993. Repellency of cinnamic acid derivatives to captive rock doves. *J Wildl Manag* 57 (1):113–122.

Downs, C.T., and M.R. Perrin. 1996. Sugar preferences of some southern African nectarivorous birds. *Ibis* 138 (3):455–459.

Duncan, C.J. 1960. Preference tests and the sense of taste in the feral pigeon (*Columba livia* Var Gmelin). *Anim Behav* 8:54–60.

Duncan, I.J.H., and B.O. Hughes. 1972. Free and operant feeding in domestic fowls. *Anim Behav* 20:775–777.

El Boushy, A.R., A.F.B. Van der Poel, J.C.J. Verhaart, and D.A. Kennedy. 1989. Sensory involvement controls feed intake in poultry. *Feedstuffs* 61 (25): 16–41.

Forbes, J.M. 1998. Dietary awareness. *Appl Anim Behav Sci* 57 (3–4):287–297.

Frankel, T.L., and D.S. Avram. 2001. Protein requirements of rainbow lorikeets, *Trichoglossus haematodus. Aust J Zool* 49:435–443.

Fuerst, W.F., and M.R. Kare. 1962. The influence of pH on fluid tolerance and preferences. *Poult Sci* 41: 71–77.

Galetti, M. 1993. Diet of the scaly-headed parrot (*Pionus maximiliani*) in a semideciduous forest in Southeastern Brazil. *Biotropica* 25:419–425.

Garnett, S., and G. Crowley. 1995. Feeding ecology of hooded parrots *Psephotus dissimilis* during the early wet season. *Emu* 95:54–61.

Gentle, M.J. 1972. Taste preference in the chicken (*Gallus domesticus L.*). *Br Poult Sci* 13 (2):141–155.

Glendinning, J.I. 1994. Is the bitter rejection response always adaptive? *Physiol Behav* 56 (6):1217–1227.

Harriman, A.E. 1967. Laughing gulls offered saline in preference and survival tests. *Physiol Zool* 40:273–279.

Harriman, A.E., and E.G. Fry. 1990. Solution acceptance by common ravens (*Corvus corax*) given two-bottle preference tests. *Psychol Rep* 67 (1):19–26.

Harriman, A.E., and M.R. Kare. 1966. Aversion to saline solutions in starlings, purple grackles, and herring gulls. *Physiol Zool* 39:123–126.

Harriman, A.E., and J.S. Milner. 1969. Preference for sucrose solutions by Japanese quail (*Coturnix coturnix japonica*) in two-bottle drinking tests. *Am Midland Natur* 81:575–578.

Herness, M.S., and T.A. Gilbertson. 1999. Cellular mechanisms of taste transduction. *Annu Rev Physiol* 61:873–900.

Homberger, D.G., and A.H. Brush. 1986. Functional-morphological and biochemical correlations of the keratinized structures in the African gray parrot, *Psittacus erithacus* (Aves). *Zoomorphology (Berl)* 106:103–114.

Hughes, B.O., and D.G.M. Wood-Gush. 1971a. A specific appetite for calcium in domestic chickens. *Anim Behav* 19:490–499.

Hughes, B.O., and D.G.M. Wood-Gush. 1971b. Investigations into specific appetites for sodium and thiamine in domestic fowls. *Physiol Behav* 6 (4):331–339.

Hughes, B.O., and D.G.M. Wood-Gush. 1973. An increase in activity of domestic fowls produced by nutritional deficiency. *Anim Behav* 21:10–17.

Inglis, I.R., and N.J.K. Ferguson. 1986. Starlings search for food rather than eat freely-available identical food. *Anim Behav* 34 (2):614–617.

Jackson, S., S.W. Nicolson, and C.N. Lotz. 1998. Sugar preferences and "side bias" in cape sugarbirds and lesser double-collared sunbirds. *Auk* 115 (1):156–165.

Jones, D. 1987. Feeding ecology of the cockatiel, *Nymphicus hollandicus*, in a grain-growing area. *Aust Wild Res* 14:105–115.

Kamphues, J., W. Otte, and P. Wolf. 1997. "Effects of increasing protein intake on various parameters of nitrogen metabolism in grey parrots (*Psittacus erithacus erithacus*)." In *First International Symposium on Pet Bird Nutrition,* ed. J. Kamphues, P. Wolf, and N. Rabehl, p. 118. Hannover, Germany: Institut fur Tierernahrung.

Kare, M.R., R. Black, and E.G. Allison. 1957. The sense of taste in the fowl. *Poult Sci* 36:129–138.

Kare, M.R., and J.R. Mason. 1986. "The chemical senses in birds." In *Avian physiology,* ed. P.D. Sturkie and C.A. Benzo, pp. 59–73. New York: Springer-Verlag.

Kare, M.R., and H.L. Pick. 1960. The influence of the sense of taste on feed and fluid consumption. *Poult Sci* 39:697–706.

Klasing, K.C. (1998). *Comparative avian nutrition.* New York: CAB International.

Koutsos, E.A., and K.C. Klasing. 2001. "Interactions between the immune system, nutrition, and productivity of animals." In *Recent advances in animal nutrition,* ed. P.C. Garnsworthy & J. Wiseman. Nottingham: Nottingham University Press.

Koutsos, E.A., and K.C. Klasing. 2002. "Vitamin A nutrition of cockatiels." In *Proc. Comparative Nutrition Society,* pp. 210–211. Silver Spring, MD: Comparative Nutrition Society.

Koutsos, E.A., K.D. Matson, and K.C. Klasing. 2001a. Nutrition of birds in the order Psittaciformes: A review. *J Avian Med Surg* 15:237–275.

Koutsos, E.A., H.N. Pham, J.R. Millam, and K.C. Klasing. 2001b. "Vocalizations of cockatiels (*Nymphicus hollandicus*) are affected by dietary vitamin A concentration." 35th International Congress of the ISAE, Davis, CA.

Koutsos, E.A., J. Smith, L. Woods, and K.C. Klasing. 2001c. Adult cockatiels (*Nymphicus hollandicus*) undergo metabolic adaptation to high protein diets. *J Nutr* 131:2014–2020.

Lane, R.A. 1996. "Avian hematology: Basic cell identification, white blood cell count determinations, and
clinical pathology." In *Diseases of cage and aviary
birds,* ed. W.J. Rosskopf and R.W. Woerpel, pp.
739–772. Baltimore: Williams and Wilkins.

Leshchinsky, T.V., and K.C. Klasing. 2001. Relationship between the level of dietary vitamin E and
the immune response of broiler chickens. *Poult Sci*
80 (11):1590–1599.

Long, J.L., and P.R. Mawson. 1994. Diet of regent parrots (*Polytelis anthopeplus*) in the south-west of
Western Australia. *Western Austr Natur* 19:293–299.

Mack, A.L., and D.D. Wright. 1998. The vulturine parrot, *Psittrichas fulgidus,* a threatened New Guinea
endemic: Notes on its biology and conservation.
Bird Cons Int 8:185–194.

MacMillen, R.E., and R.V. Baudinette. 1993. Water
economy of granivorous birds: Australian parrots.
Functional Ecol 7 (6):704–712.

Malakoff, D. 1999. Following the scent of avian olfaction. *Science* 286 (5440):704–705.

Martinez del Rio, C. 1990. Sugar preferences in hummingbirds: The influence of subtle chemical differences on food choice. *Condor* 92 (4):1022–1030.

Martinez del Rio, C., H.G. Baker, and I. Baker. 1992.
Ecological and evolutionary implications of digestive processes: Bird preferences and the sugar constituents of floral nectar and fruit pulp. *Experientia*
48 (6):544–551.

Martuscelli, P. 1995. Ecology and conservation of the
red-tailed amazon *Amazona brasiliensis* in southeastern Brazil. *Bird Cons Int* 5:405–420.

Matson, K.D., J.R. Millam, and K.C. Klasing. 2000.
Taste threshold determination and side-preference in
captive cockatiels (*Nymphicus hollandicus*). *Appl
Anim Behav Sci* 69 (4):313–326.

Matson, K.D., J.R. Millam, and K.C. Klasing. 2001.
Thresholds for sweet, salt, and sour taste stimuli in
cockatiels (*Nymphicus hollandicus*). *Zoo Biol* 20
(1):1–13.

Mcfarland, D.C. 1991. The biology of the ground par-
rot, *Pezoporus wallicus,* in Queensland [Australia]:
I. Microhabitat use, activity cycle and diet. *Wildlife
Res* 18:168–184.

Murphy, M.E. 1994. Dietary complementation by wild
birds: Considerations for field studies. *J Biosci
(Bangalore)* 19 (4):355–368.

Neuringer, A.J. 1969. Animals respond for food in the
presence of free food. *Science* 166 (903):399–401.

Nevitt, G. 1999a. Foraging by seabirds on an olfactory
landscape. *American Scientist* 87 (1):46–53.

Nevitt, G. 1999b. Olfactory foraging in Antarctic
seabirds: A species-specific attraction to krill odors.
Marine Ecology Progress Series 177:235–241.

Newman, R.K., and D.C. Sands. 1983. Dietary selection for lysine by the chicks. *Physiology and
Behaviour* 31:13–20.

Noble, D.O., M.L. Picard, E.A. Dunnington, G. Uzu,
A.S. Larsen, and P.B. Siegel. 1993. Food intake adjustments of chicks: Short term reactions of genetic
stocks to deficiencies in lysine, methionine or tryptophan. *Br Poult Sci* 34 (4):725–735.

NRC, ed. 1994. *Nutrient requirements of poultry.*
Washington, D.C.: National Academy Press.

Pitter, E., and M.B. Christiansen. 1995. Ecology, status
and conservation of the red-fronted macaw *Ara
rubrogenys. Bird Cons Int* 5:61–78.

Polo, F.J., V.I. Peinado, G. Viscor, and J. Palomeque.
1998. Hematologic and plasma chemistry values in
captive psittacine birds. *Avian Dis* 42 (3):523–535.

Pryor, G.S. 1999. Comparative protein requirements
and digestive strategies of three species of parrots
with distinct dietary specializations. *Am Zool* 39
(5):93A.

Ranft, U., and A. Hennig (1993). "New experimental
results on nutrient selection of laying hens." In
*Endocrine and nutritional control of basic biologi-
cal functions,* ed. H. Lehnert, pp. 167–172. Seattle:
Hogrefe & Huber.

Rosskopf, W.J., R.W. Woerpel, and R.A. Lane. 1985.
"The hypocalcemia syndrome in African greys: An
updated clinical viewpoint with current recommendations for treatment." Proc Assoc Avian Vet:
129–131.

Roudybush, T.E., and C.R. Grau. 1986. Food and water
interrelations and the protein requirement for growth
of an altricial bird, the cockatiel (*Nymphicus hollandicus*). *J Nutr* 116:552–559.

Rowley, I., E. Russell, and M. Palmer. 1989. The food
preference of cockatoos: An aviary experiment.
Austr Wildl Res 16 (1):19–32.

Schall, J.J. 1990. Aversion of whiptail lizards
Cnemidophorus to a model alkaloid. *Herpetologica*
46 (1):34–38.

Toyne, E.P., and J.N.M. Flanagan. 1997. Observations
on the breeding, diet and behaviour of the red-faced
parrot *Hapalopsittaca pyrrhops* in southern
Ecuador. *Bull Br Ornithologists' Club* 117:257–263.

Wyndham, E. 1980. Environment and food of the
budgerigar *Melopsittacus undulatus. Aust J Ecol*
5:47–61.

Yang, R.S.H., and M.R. Kare. 1968. Taste response of
a bird to constituents of arthropod defense secretions. *Ann Entomol Soc America* 61:781–782.

7
Comfort Behavior and Sleep

Laurie Bergman and Ulrike S. Reinisch

Although many people are attracted to parrots as pets by their playful antics and vocal mimicry, when looking at the time budgets of most parrot species in the wild one sees that these birds spend the most time each day engaged in relatively quiet and sedate activities. Sleep and rest occupy the major part of a 24-hour day. The activities that take up the greatest portions of their waking day are foraging and grooming. Grooming and other comfort behaviors are major behavioral activities for parrots of all species.

There are two basic ways to look at sleep: studying the patterns of brain waves during the different phases of sleep and looking at sleep as part of an animal's daily activity pattern. Electroencephalographic (EEG) studies, recording brain activity, electromyographic (EMG) studies, recording muscular activity, and electrooculographic studies, recording eye movements, have been performed in several species of birds, including two psittacine species, Half-moon Conures (*Aratinga canicularis*) and Budgerigars (*Melopsittacus undulatus*) (Ayala-Guerrero et al. 1987, 1989). As in mammals, birds have been found to have two phases of sleep. The first, slow wave sleep (SWS) is characterized by slow, high-voltage brain waves. This type of sleep appears to be the most important sleep stage, the one that may have restorative functions. The second, called paradoxical sleep (PS) or REM (rapid eye movement) sleep, shows low-voltage brain waves, similar to those seen during wakefulness. These low-voltage brain waves are often accompanied by movement of the eyes. In people, dreaming occurs during PS. PS may be involved in brain development and learning (Carlson 2001).

In the psittacines studied, PS was always preceded by SWS. These birds were found to have spent shorter overall percentages of their total sleep time in PS than mammals or most other avian species. However, this may represent changes in the birds' sleep patterns due to being kept in constant light for the studies, not an actual difference in psittacine PS as compared to other birds (Ayala-Guerrero et al. 1987, 1989).

Missing from the sleep of all avian species studied are sleep spindles, bursts of activity that are thought to represent a mechanism that decreases the individual's sensitivity to sensory input. Sleep spindles arise from the neocortex, a structure that is not well developed in the avian brain (Ookawa 1972; Ayala-Guerrero et al. 1987).

Unihemispheric sleep was observed in the Half-moon Conures studied. Unihemispheric sleep is a means of maintaining predator detection where only one hemisphere of the brain is asleep at a time. EEGs of the conures showed times of low-voltage fast waves in one cerebral hemisphere and large amplitude slow waves in the other hemisphere (Ayala-Guerrero et al. 1987). It is believed that while flying, especially on migratory flights over waters, birds engage in unihemispheric sleep. Unihemispheric sleep has been observed in most orders of birds and in marine mammals (Rattenburg et al. 2000).

Sleep is the single behavior that occupies the greatest proportion of a parrot's day (Rowley 1990; Snyder 1987; Wirminghaus et al. 2001). Even when kept under constant illumination, the Half-moon Conure was found to spend almost 57% of a 24-hour period in some state of sleep (drowsiness, SWS, or PS). Budgerigars in similar conditions slept for an average of 38% of a 24-hour day. These studies also showed sustained periods of slow wave sleep and an increase in paradoxical sleep between 7:00 P.M. and 7:00 A.M. This implies that this sleep pattern is due to endogenous circadian rhythms, not simply due to entrainment by external stimuli (Ayala-Guerrero et al. 1987, 1989).

As a social species, a parrot flock usually sleeps and rests as a group. In general, a flock's waking day begins with sunrise or before, with the first light of the day, and ends with sunset. Parrot flocks usually sleep in a roosting area that is distinct from the feeding area where they have spent the day. In the case of breeding pairs with a nest the roosting area is near or at the nest site. Non-breeding birds may roost in trees that are convenient to the area where they have been feeding. As dusk approaches birds will return to their roosting area or a nearby convenient area. During the middle of the day parrots will also have a period of quiet time during which they may sleep or drowse (Rowley 1990; Snyder 1987; Wirminghaus et al. 2001). During this rest period the birds may experience short periods of SWS and PS (Ayala-Guerrero et al. 1987).

A parrot typically sleeps while perching upright or lowered in a somewhat horizontal position with its body touching the perch. As the parrot becomes drowsy it will fluff its feathers and blinking and eye movements will decrease. Once the bird is asleep its eyes are closed. In REM sleep the eyes remain closed and the head may droop as neck muscle tone decreases. At the end of a period of PS the birds often suddenly raise their heads but do not awaken, returning to SWS. In prolonged sleep parrots turn their heads 180 degrees and tuck their heads under their scapular feathers. Parrots may sleep with both feet on the perch or with one foot raised (Ayala-Guerrero et al. 1987; Rowley 1990).

Although sleep is recognized as an essential behavior in both humans and animals and is the subject of much research, little is actually known about the functions of sleep. It is believed that SWS provides a restorative period for the brain and PS is involved in memory and learning. Laboratory animals subjected to prolonged sleep deprivation eventually died (Carlson 2001). It has been estimated that as much as 50% of the adult human population of America is sleep deprived (Maas 1999). This may also be true for our psittacine pets and may contribute to some behavior problems. As most species of parrots are from tropical or semi-tropical regions, their days normally have roughly 12 hours of light and 12 hours of dark (Forshaw 1989). Despite the laboratory findings that parakeets kept in constant light continued to do the bulk of their sleeping between 7:00 P.M. and 7:00 A.M. (Ayala-Guerrero et al. 1987, 1989), it appears that many pet parrots are not given the opportunity to sleep as they would in the wild. Pet parrots are often kept in cages located in the main living areas of homes, where they are exposed not only to durations of "daylight" that extend beyond 12 hours/day but also to noises and visual stimulation from televisions, radios, and people moving about the house. Pet parrots should be provided with a quiet, dark sleeping area, ideally separate from their daytime living area (e.g., a separate small sleep cage), and close to 12 hours of "nighttime" to sleep.

In addition to sleep, parrots spend a great deal of time engaged in grooming: preening and other body maintenance behaviors. Collectively these behaviors are often called comfort behaviors. Not only do these behaviors normally occur when the bird is comfortable and at ease but the behaviors themselves appear to be comforting and soothing to the birds. It is probably due to this aspect of these behaviors that they often appear as displacement behaviors when parrots are under stress or behaviorally conflicted. This can lead to these behaviors becoming liberated from their normal contexts and appearing as "problem behaviors" ranging from minor annoyances to owners to self-injurious behaviors such as feather picking and self-mutilation.

Grooming occupies the largest amount of a wild parrot's waking hours after foraging (Rowley 1990; Snyder 1987). Preening serves several functions, starting with maintenance of feathers. Maintaining feathers in good condition is not only crucial for flight but also for thermoregulation, waterproofing, camouflage, and communication (Cech et al. 2001). Other grooming behaviors that have been noted in parrots include scratching with the feet, cleaning feet and legs with the beak, stretching, yawning, and beak rubbing and grinding (Lefebvre 1982; Rowley 1990; Wirminghaus et al. 2000).

Despite their widespread geographic distribution, parrots of different species tend to have similar grooming behaviors (Lefebvre 1982; Rowley 1990; Wirminghaus et al. 2000). Based on a study of grooming behavior in Budgerigars, grooming tends to proceed from head-to-toe as has also been found to be the case in several species of mammals. Also in common with other species studied, Budgerigars moved from grooming one region of the body to the next based mainly on adjacency and clustered their grooming in distinct anatomical regions (e.g., head, wings and trunk, lower region, and preen gland) (Lefebvre 1982). Individual feathers are preened by grasping the feather in the beak and pulling it between the upper and lower beak while nibbling at the feather. This serves to reattach disconnected barbules (Rowley 1990).

Long and short grooming bouts were noted in the Budgerigars studied. Bouts were defined as a sequence of grooming acts that was uninterrupted by non-grooming behavior for less that 30 seconds. Short bouts contained seven or fewer acts/bout, whereas the number of acts/bout in a long bout could be over 100. Short bouts seemed to occur mainly in response to an irritating stimulus. Short bouts of grooming often included behaviors such as shaking, stretching, and scratching, whereas preening took place almost exclusively in long bouts (Lefebvre 1982).

The other types of grooming behaviors that have been described in parrots are also well preserved between the species. Scratching with feet is an important grooming behavior. Because of these birds' flexibility they are able to reach most areas on the head that are inaccessible to preening with their feet. Stretching has also been described in parrots, often occurring after a period of rest before beginning another activity, including as the opening sequences of a grooming bout. Yawning, also called jaw or beak stretching, commonly occurs. There are also a variety of stretches that involve the wings, including arching the wings over the back and stretching a wing and ipsilateral leg downward at the same time. This stretch is accompanied by tail fanning. This procedure is then repeated with the other wing and leg. This often occurs before flight. Other grooming behaviors include chewing at inedible objects and beak grinding, both of which serve to keep the beak in good condition by wearing down any overgrowth and sharpening the cutting edge of the mandible. Beak grinding produces a soft, audible grinding sound (Lefebvre 1982; Rowley 1990).

In addition to self-directed grooming, when given the opportunity, parrots also engage in allogrooming. Allogrooming serves a variety of functions. It allows for grooming of areas, specifically the head, which are inaccessible by the individual being groomed. It also is an important social behavior. Allopreening is often reciprocal and usually, but not always, takes place between a bonded pair or parents and offspring. However, allopreening does occur between non-related, non-bonded individuals in a flock. Allopreening is usually solicited by one bird lowering its head to present its neck to be preened. The preening bird then moves on to groom the neck, head, and face of the other bird. The birds will often switch roles after a bout of allopreening. In Budgerigars, the proportion of allopreening given versus received was almost the same (Lefebvre 1982; Rowley 1990). The importance of allopreening can be seen in the amount of time devoted to it. Galahs have been reported to engage in allopreening sessions that last as long as five minutes (Rowley 1990). In Budgerigars allopreening occupied almost the same proportion of long grooming bouts as preening of the wings (Lefebvre 1982).

Parrot flocks will groom for a brief period in the morning before flying from their nighttime roosting area to forage for the day. After feeding and filling their crops the flock will rest in a convenient tree (near the foraging area or, if they are feeding young, in the roosting/nesting area). The birds will groom while digesting their morning meal. This pattern is repeated with grooming after an afternoon meal and upon arriving at the roosting area at dusk (Rowley 1990; Snyder 1987).

As was noted earlier, comfort behaviors can become problematic, either of their own right or as signs of underlying stress. Shortly after one of the authors adopted a rescued parrot that had been housed in a dark basement, she noticed small piles of black powder in the bird's cage in the morning. These piles were the result of the bird continually grinding his beak through the night. In this case, the bird did not do any permanent damage to himself and, as he became more relaxed and less fearful in his new home, the beak grinding stopped. Pet parrots may substitute petting from their owners for allogrooming, which may contribute to problems with aggression, vocalizations, and misplaced sexual behavior, due to "pair bonding" with the owner. These and other behavior problems related to comfort behaviors, such as feather picking and self-mutilation, are discussed in chapters 18, 21, and 23.

REFERENCES

Ayala-Guerrero, F., M.C. Perez, and A. Calderon. 1987. Sleep patterns in the bird *Aratinga canicularis*. *Physiology and Behavior* 43 (5):585–589.

Ayala-Guerrero, F. 1989. Sleep patterns in the parakeet *Melopsittacus undulates*. *Physiology and Behavior* 46 (5):787–791.

Carlson, N.R. 2001. *Physiology of behavior.* Boston: Allyn and Bacon.

Cech, R., J.B. Dunning Jr., and C. Elphick. 2001. "Behavior." In *The Sibley guide to bird life and behavior*, ed. Chris Elphick, John B. Dunning, Jr., and David Allen Sibley, pp. 51–79. New York; Alfred A. Knopf.

Forshaw, J.M. 1989. *Parrots of the world,* 3rd (rev.) ed. London: Blandford.

Lefebvre, L. 1982. The organization of grooming in budgerigars. *Behavioural Processes* 7:93–106.

Maas, J. 1999. *Power sleep: The revolutionary program that prepares your mind for peak performance.* New York: Harper Collins.

Ookawa, T. 1972. Avian wakefulness and sleep on the basis of recent electroencephalographic observations. *Poultry Science* 51:1565–1574.

Rattenburg, W.C. et al. 2000. Behavioral, neurophysiological and evolutionary perspectives on unihemispheric sleep. *Neuroscience and Biobehavioral Reviews* 24 (8):817–842.

Rowley, I. 1990. *Behavioral ecology of the galah, Eolophus roseicapillus: In the wheatbelt of Western Australia.* Chipping Norton, NSW: Surrey Beatty.

Snyder, N.F.R. 1987. *The parrots of Luquillo: Natural history and conservation of the Puerto Rican parrot.* Los Angeles: Western Foundation of Vertebrate Zoology.

Wirminghaus, J.O., C.T. Downs, C.T. Symes, E. Dempster, and M.R. Perrin. 2000. Vocalizations and behaviours of the cape parrot *Poicephalus robustus* (Psittaciformes:Psittacidae). *Durban Museum Novitates* 25:12–17.

Wirminghaus, J.O., C.T. Downs, M.R. Perrin, C.T. Symes. 2001. Abundance and activity patterns of the cape parrot (*Poicephalus robustus*) in two afromontane forests in South Africa. *African Zoology* 36 (1):71–77.

8

Parrot Reproductive Behavior, or Who Associates, Who Mates, and Who Cares?

Tracey R. Spoon

INTRODUCTION

Thorough knowledge of parrot breeding biology requires information about the composition of breeding groups, the process by which individuals form breeding relationships, nest-site establishment, parental care patterns, and factors that influence breeding success. A comprehensive understanding also requires an evaluation and appreciation of the variation both between and within species regarding these aspects of psittacine reproductive behavior. On the surface, parrots appear to represent a fairly uniform group with respect to reproductive biology, but recent evidence suggests more variability and complexity than initially believed. Researching parrot reproductive biology not only has a basic scientific importance but has practical implications as well. Given the poor conservation status of a significant number of parrot species (Collar & Juniper 1992; Bennett & Owens 1997), an in-depth understanding of the reproductive systems of psittacines becomes crucial to protecting and restoring declining populations. Management practices both in the wild and in captivity would benefit from additional rigorous scientific studies of the reproductive behavior of psittacines (e.g., Monterrubio et al. 2002; Manning et al. 2004). For example, recent studies indicate that supplemental feeding of breeding female Kakapos, an extremely endangered psittacine with a rare lek-type mating system (see later), appears to result in an undesirable male bias in offspring sex ratios (Clout et al. 2002; Sutherland 2002).

With these issues in the forefront, I will begin this review of psittacine reproductive behavior with a few caveats about methodology. Next, this chapter will review the mating systems of parrots with a particular eye toward discerning variation within species and discrepancies between the social and genetic aspects of mating patterns. Finally, I will turn to behaviors used by parrots during mate assessment, courtship, and breeding and follow with a consideration of psittacine parental care. I give preference to studies conducted on wild populations or semi-natural captive groups that allow individuals to express variation in behavior. Compared to captive breeding situations with individuals housed in pairs, large captive populations of mixed sex and age likely offer a more complete picture of the process by which individuals form breeding relationships and the degree of variation that exists in the species. Such studies likely provide the most valid and reliable scientific information. On a practical note, management practices in the wild and in captivity that preserve the behavioral variation in a species and fulfill the behavioral needs of individuals will likely have the most success in breeding productivity and long-term conservation goals (Derrickson & Snyder 1992).

The following discussion of psittacine mating patterns and reproductive behavior requires a few methodological qualifications. First, assessments of psittacine mating systems are often based on observations of the number of parrots attending a nest or the social associations between individuals within a larger flock. For example, based on observations of two individuals attending a nest or duos of birds associating within a larger flock, researchers usually assert that a particular species exhibits monogamy, a mating system in which each breeding unit consists of one male and one female. However, in order to definitively state that a species truly exhibits a particular mating system, the members of breeding units must be individually identifiable either through naturally occurring physical differences or marks placed by observers—a formidable task for many parrot species. Due to the inherent difficulty of tracking birds beyond the immediate vicinity of the nest site, a member of an assumed monogamous pair may attend more than one nest, or more than one male or female may attend a single nest unbeknownst to an observer who cannot identify individuals. For instance, in a study of Glossy Black Cockatoos (*Calyptorhynchus lathami*), a species identified as strongly monogamous, occasionally a male approached and fed an incubating female only to be chased off by a different male who also fed the female and then accompanied her back to the nest (Garnett et al. 1999). Determining the social and mating relationships in such cases requires long-term studies on known individuals.

A second difficulty in studying the reproductive behavior of parrots rests on the fact that many species display sexual monomorphism (Forshaw 1981, 1989; Alderton 1991); in other words, males and females cannot be readily distinguished based on physical characteristics. In many cases, individuals are assigned a sex based on behavioral differences in nest attendance and sexual behavior. Because sex identification then relies on behavioral differences, this methodology may obscure rather than reveal important behavioral variability within the sexes both between and within species.

MATING SYSTEMS

Although a moderate degree of variation exists among parrot species, most psittacines appear to exhibit social monogamy, meaning that the predominant breeding unit consists of one male and one female (Forshaw 1981, 1989; Higgins 1999). Social monogamy differs from genetic monogamy in that socially monogamous pairmates may associate primarily with each other and may jointly establish a nest but may copulate and cre-

ate offspring with an individual other than their social mate (Dunn & Lifjeld 1994). Because of difficulties observing parrots in the wild and testing genetic parentage, most studies have focused on the social aspects of mating systems. For example, detailed studies on identifiable individuals in the wild have revealed that White-tailed Black Cockatoos (*Calyptorhynchus funereus*, Saunders 1982), Puerto Rican Amazons (*Amazona vittata*, Snyder et al. 1987), Galahs (*Eolophus roseicapillus*, Rowley 1990), Major Mitchell's Cockatoos (*Cacatua leadbeateri*, Rowley & Chapman 1991), Green-rumped Parrotlets (*Forpus passerinus*, Waltman & Beissinger 1992), Monk Parakeets (*Myiopsitta monachus*, Eberhard 1998), and Burrowing Parrots (*Cyanoliseus patagonus*, Masello et al. 2002) predominantly or exclusively exhibit social monogamy. Additional studies in the wild on Crimson Rosellas (*Platycercus elegans*, Krebs 1998), Glossy Black Cockatoos (Garnett et al. 1999), and several species of amazon parrots (Yellow-headed, *Amazona oratrix*; Red-crowned, *A. viridigenalis*; Red-lored, *A. autumnalis* [Enkerlin-Hoeflich 1995]; Lilaccrowned, *A. finschi* [Renton & Salinas-Melgoza 1999]; Black-billed, *A. agilis,* and Yellow-billed, *A. collaria* [Koenig 2001]) strongly suggest a socially monogamous mating system, although the identification of individuals and sex in these studies typically or occasionally relied on observations of nest attendance, association patterns, and behavioral patterns rather than an independent assessment of identification and sex. Likewise, in several studies on captive groups that allowed individuals to express variability in mating patterns, several species of lovebirds (*Agapornis* species, Dilger 1960; Stamm 1962), Orange-fronted Conures (*Aratinga canicularis*, Hardy 1963), Budgerigars (*Melopsittacus undulatus*, Brockway 1964; Trillmich 1976), White-fronted Amazons (*Amazona albifrons*, Levinson 1980), Rainbow and Scaly-breasted Lorikeets (*Trichoglossus haematodus* and *T. chlorolepidotus*, Serpell 1981), Canary-winged Parakeets (*Brotogeris versicolorus*, Arrowood 1987), Spectacled Parrotlets (*Forpus conspicillatus*, Garnetzke-Stollman & Franck 1991), and Cockatiels (*Nymphicus hollandicus*, Spoon et al. 2004) predominately formed socially monogamous breeding groups. These monogamous pair relationships seem particularly strong as evidenced by the close association between mates who perform most of their daily activities together throughout the year (e.g., Rainbow and Scaly-breasted Lorikeets [Serpell 1981]; Canary-winged Parakeets [Arrowood 1987]; Galahs [Rowley 1990]; Spectacled Parrotlets [Garnetzke-Stollman & Franck 1991, Wanker et al. 1996 cited in Wanker et al. 1998]; Cockatiels [Spoon et al. 2004]; Brown-headed Parrots, *Poicephalus cryptoxanthus* [Taylor & Perrin 2004]). Galah mates, for example, return to their nest site together every evening to roost (Rowley 1990).

Despite this tendency toward monogamy, several typically monogamous species exhibit variation in breeding group composition. For example, polygamous groups have been observed in Masked Lovebirds (*Agapornis personata*, Stamm 1962), Spectacled Parrotlets (Garnetzke-Stollman & Franck 1991), Yellow-headed Amazons (Enkerlin-Hoeflich 1995), Monk Parakeets (Eberhard 1998), and Cockatiels (Seibert & Crowell-Davis 2001). The role of these "extra" birds in breeding remains little understood. Normally the accessory bird in trios of Yellow-headed Amazons only flew with the breeding pair, but in one trio the accessory bird participated minimally in nesting and was once observed feeding the female (Enkerlin-Hoeflich 1995). In a captive group of Cockatiels, both males of a polygamous trio cared for the female's young although she was only observed to copulate with one of them, and a male who associated and copulated with two females subsequently cared for the young of both in two separate nest boxes (Seibert & Crowell-Davis 2001). As noted previously, instances of two birds feeding one nesting female have been recorded in Glossy Black Cockatoos (Garnett et al. 1999). In two Monk Parakeet trios consisting of one female and two males, both males participated in nest building and feeding the female. Interestingly, a complete copulation bout between the two males was observed near the nest in which the female was incubating (Eberhard 1998). In a Monk Parakeet trio of two females and one male, all three participated in nest building but only one female incubated the eggs (Eberhard 1998). Not only do polygamous trios occasionally occur in Monk Parakeets, but the species may exhibit some degree of cooperative or communal breeding among pairs with incipient helping-at-the-nest as well

(Eberhard 1998). Evidence also suggests that Golden Conures (*Aratinga guarouba*) may possess a communal breeding system in which groups of several males and females or possibly groups of pairs utilize the same nest cavity with multiple females contributing eggs and multiple male and female attendants subsequently caring for the young; single pairs may also breed alone (Oren & Novaes 1986; Forshaw 1989). This cooperative or communal pattern is quite different from the more general pattern in which monogamous pairs aggregate with conspecifics during feeding and roosting and then defend the nest site from other pairs during breeding (Rowley & Chapman 1991; Wanker et al. 1998).

In addition to variation in the composition of breeding units, the degree of permanency of pair relationships also varies between individuals and species. Long-term studies on White-tailed Black Cockatoos (Saunders 1982), Puerto Rican Amazons (Snyder et al. 1987), Galahs (Rowley 1990), and Major Mitchell's Cockatoos (Rowley & Chapman 1991) indicate that mates often remain together until the death of one member. In these studies, very few of the former mates of individuals known to have changed mates were observed again, suggesting that the mate change occurred because the former mate died and left the remaining member without a mate. However, these results also indicate that occasionally individuals of these species switch mates despite the fact that their former mate remains alive. In several additional studies, observations indicate that individuals usually retain their mates between breeding seasons (e.g., Green-rumped Parrotlets, Waltman & Beissinger 1992; Yellow-headed and Red-crowned Amazons, Enkerlin-Hoeflich 1995; Monk Parakeets, Eberhard 1998; Burrowing Parrots, Masello et al. 2002). In contrast, captive Cockatiels (Spoon 2002) and Canary-winged Parakeets (Arrowood 1987) were not as devoted to their mates; when several previously confined pairs were housed together or additional birds were added to the flock, several paired Cockatiels and Canary-winged Parakeets, respectively, switched mates. Similarly, in one study of captive Masked Lovebirds, mate change frequently occurred (Stamm 1962), yet Dilger (1960) claimed that lovebird mates usually remain together until death, based on his study of several lovebird species. Spectacled Parrotlet pairs remained stable even after changes in group composition (Garnetzke-Stollman & Franck 1991). Based on these studies it is difficult to tell whether captivity increases the frequency of mate change or merely renders it more easily observed.

As mentioned previously, social monogamy does not necessarily mean genetic monogamy. Galahs (Rowley 1990) and Budgerigars (Brockway 1964; Baltz & Clark 1997), for example, will engage in sexual behavior and copulate outside the pair relationship, but often restrict these extrapair interactions to times when their mates are in the nest cavity or otherwise unable to observe the infidelity. Paired Cockatiels appear to use extrapair sexual behavior and copulation to assess potential mates and form new pair relationships, apparently in response to a low degree of compatibility with their current mate (Spoon 2002). Among captive Spectacled Parrotlets, Garnetzke-Stollman and Franck (1991) observed extrapair copulations only under one very specific circumstance—the secondary female of a polygamous trio copulated repeatedly with the male of a neighboring pair while his female incubated a clutch. Interestingly, this extra-pair relationship involved only sexual behavior with no affiliative behavior or courtship feeding (Garnetzke-Stollman & Franck 1991). Very few studies have actually assessed the genetic mating systems of parrots. In a captive group of Golden Conures, the eggs of one female were fertilized by two males, but no information was available on the social relationships between the female and males or on which individuals cared for the eggs or young (Oren & Novaes 1986). In contrast, a detailed study of wild Burrowing Parrots discovered no instances of extra-pair paternity, suggesting that these parrots exhibit genetic as well as social monogamy (although the study did identify one case of apparent intraspecific brood parasitism) (Masello et al. 2002).

Despite the apparent predominance of social monogamy among parrots, some species exhibit mating systems vastly different from social monogamy. The Kakapo (*Strigops habroptilus*) and Vasa Parrot (*Coracopsis vasa*), for instance, display mating systems that differ dramatically from the socially monogamous systems just described. The highly endangered Kakapo of New Zealand appears to possess a lek-type breeding system in which males establish courts called track-and-bowl systems used to attract females for copulation (Merton et al. 1984; Powlesland et al. 1992). During mating periods, which occur only once every two to five years, females travel to the male's court, which appears to be used solely for mating and not for feeding or nesting by the female. Otherwise, Kakapos live solitarily, and females alone assume all parental responsibilities (Powlesland et al. 1992). The Greater Vasa Parrot exhibits a strongly polygynandrous mating system in which both males and females copulate with several individuals (Ekstrom 2002). Male and female Vasa Parrots do not form pair relationships or pair bonds typical of most parrots, and females generally lay clutches sired by multiple males.

PAIR RELATIONSHIPS

Although the parrot family exhibits greater diversity regarding mating systems than previously believed, the most complete information on reproductive behavior exists primarily for socially monogamous species. For these species, the relationship between pairmates not only forms the basis of the breeding unit, but because these relationships often last year-round for multiple years, they also form the basis of parrot social organization. In some species, establishing a pair relationship may prove vital to social rank within the flock. For instance, Spectacled Parrotlet pairmates hold the same rank within the flock, and monogamous pairs hold the highest ranks (Garnetzke-Stollman & Franck 1991). Similarly, Orange-fronted Conure pairmates appear to help each other establish a higher rank, and when a pair member is removed, the remaining member often loses status (Hardy 1963). Major Mitchell's Cockatoos offer further evidence of the importance of pair relationships in parrot reproductive and social behavior—reproductively immature birds may form pair bonds up to a year prior to actually breeding (Rowley & Chapman 1991). Thus, understanding these pair relationships is crucial to understanding parrot reproductive behavior.

Affiliative interactions such as close proximity, allopreening, and reduced aggression typically characterize associations between psittacine pairmates. The predominant pattern appears to be for mates to follow each other closely and maintain significantly closer proximity to each other than to non-mates. As a result, mates remain together almost constantly and perform many of their daily activities together (e.g., Budgerigars [Brockway 1964; Trillmich 1976]; Rainbow and Scaly-breasted Lorikeets [Serpell 1981]; Canary-winged Parakeets [Arrowood 1987]; Galahs [Rowley 1990]; Spectacled Parrotlets [Garnetzke-Stollman & Franck 1991]; Major Mitchell's Cockatoos [Rowley & Chapman 1991]; Cockatiels [Spoon et al. 2004]). Between mates of several lovebird species, maintenance behaviors hold a strong mimetic value such that a bird often joins its mate in performing particular behaviors such as preening (Dilger 1960). Similarly, Cockatiel pairmates not only maintain significantly closer proximity to their mates but also exhibit greater behavioral synchrony, meaning that mates often perform the same behaviors simultaneously (Spoon et al. 2004). Indeed, Cockatiel pairs that exhibit greater affiliative behavior and synchrony and less aggression enjoy greater reproductive success and display less extra-pair sexual behavior (Spoon 2002; Spoon et al., in press). This strong preference to associate with a mate extends to the auditory realm as well; in controlled choice studies, Spectacled Parrotlets prefer the contact calls of their mates over non-mates (Garnetzke-Stollman & Franck 1991). While in close proximity, members of a pair often engage in bouts of allopreening in which they preen as well as solicit preening from their partners. In most socially monogamous parrot species, allopreening occurs primarily with a mate rather than non-mate (e.g., lovebirds, Dilger 1960; Orange-fronted Conures, Hardy 1963; Rainbow and Scaly-breasted Lorikeets, Serpell 1981; Galahs, Rowley 1990; Green-rumped Parrotlets, Waltman & Beissinger 1992) and in some studies has been observed only between established mates (e.g., White-tailed Black Cockatoos, Saunders 1974; Budgerigars, Trillmich 1976; Canary-winged Parakeets, Arrowood 1987; Spectacled Parrotlets, Garnetzke-Stollman & Franck 1991; Cockatiels, Spoon et al. 2004). Bill touching, another affiliative behavior of Budgerigars, also occurs predominantly between mates (Trillmich 1976). In addition to increased affiliative behaviors, Budgerigars (Trillmich 1976) and Cockatiels (Spoon et al. 2004) display reduced aggression toward mates compared to non-mates.

Moreover in many parrot species, mates display these various affiliative behaviors during non-breeding periods, indicating the year-round nature of these relationships (e.g., Orange-fronted Conures [Hardy 1963]; Cockatiels [Zann 1965; Spoon et al. 2004]; Puerto Rican Amazons [Snyder et al. 1987]; Galahs [Rowley 1990]). As an additional indication of the specificity of these pair relationships, paired Spectacled Parrotlets (Garnetzke-Stollman & Franck 1991) and Budgerigars (Trillmich 1976), for example, tend not to display affiliative behaviors toward their extra-pair sexual partners.

Many psittacine species also display cooperative or coordinated pair behaviors especially during agonistic interactions with non-mate conspecifics. For example, Orange-chinned Parakeet (*Brotogeris jugularis*, Power 1966), Canary-winged Parakeet (Arrowood 1987), Puerto Rican Amazon (Snyder et al. 1987), and Yellow-naped Amazon (*Amazona auropalliata*, Wright & Dorin 2001) mates perform coordinated duets during agonistic or territorial encounters with non-mates. Likewise, in several different *Trichoglossus* (lorikeet) species, Serpell (1981) recorded eight distinct types of cooperative displays with both vocal and visual elements performed by mates, again often during agonistic interactions with conspecifics. Hardy (1963) also described highly coordinated vocalizations given by Orange-fronted Conure mates while approaching their nest site.

Although pair relationships form a critical part of most parrot social groups and many affiliative and sexual behaviors characterize those relationships, the process of pair formation appears subtle and remains poorly understood. For example, Arrowood (1987) and Hardy (1963) could identify no specific or obvious behavioral methods used to attract a mate or form pairs in Canary-winged Parakeets and Orange-fronted Conures, respectively. In Spectacled Parrotlets, young first establish close sibling relationships and then often form a series of non-exclusive relationships with potential mates until exclusive pair formation occurs (Garnetzke-Stollman & Franck 1991; Wanker et al. 1996). Similarly, in Cockatiels, a male often approaches and sings to one or more selected females until the female permits sexual or affiliative behavior (Zann 1965; T. Spoon, personal observation). Interestingly, in the one case of pair formation in Cockatiels that Zann (1965) observed, pairing appeared complete once the female allowed the male to allopreen her; in contrast, in the several instances of pair formation that I observed in Cockatiels, copulation often occurred prior to allopreening and seemed to consistently indicate the occurrence of pair formation (Spoon 2002). Furthermore, pair formation often occurs outside of an immediate breeding context (e.g., Budgerigars, Trillmich 1976; Cockatiels, Spoon et al. 2004). In some cases, specific behaviors do appear to be associated with pair formation; for example, head shaking by male Budgerigars (Brockway 1964) and head bowing by male Puerto Rican Amazons (Snyder et al. 1987) seem to be associated primarily with pair formation. An intriguing series of studies on Budgerigars revealed that males learn to imitate the contact calls of females with whom they are paired (Hile et al. 2000) and that the ability to do so plays an important role in mate choice and pair formation (Hile 2002; Striedter et al. 2003). A few studies have contributed vital information to understanding pair formation in parrots by examining the characteristics that individuals use to select a mate. Some degree of mate choice in Budgerigars depends on ultraviolet fluorescent properties of the plumage; both males and females prefer partners in which the fluorescent characteristics of the feathers remain visible (Pearn et al. 2001; Arnold et al. 2002). Determining whether Budgerigars use natural variation in fluorescence to select among potential mates would offer important insight into the process of mate choice in parrots. Likewise, male and female Burrowing Parrots may prefer mates with larger abdominal red feather patches, which appear to signal individual quality (Masello & Quillfeldt 2003). In a free-choice test, female but not male Spectacled Parrotlets preferred potential mates of high rank (Garnetzke-Stollman & Franck 1991). In this species, pairmates hold the same rank within the flock and selecting a high-ranking mate may confer significant advantages. Cockatiels allowed to self-select a mate experience a reproductive advantage over pairs formed randomly by investigators (Yamamoto et al. 1989); several non-psittacine species display a similar pattern (Klint & Enquist 1981; Bluhm 1985; Lupo et al. 1990; Bottoni et al. 1993; Ryan & Altmann 2001).

COURTSHIP AND COPULATION

In addition to affiliative and cooperative behaviors, courtship and pre-copulatory displays represent an important component of parrot reproductive behavior. The documented courtship displays of many socially monogamous psittacines contain several common elements. For example, male displays of several species in the Cacatuinae subfamily involve at least partially raised crests, switch sidling or strutting back and forth along a perch, head bowing, and flaring the wings or holding the carpal joints slightly away from the body (e.g., Cockatiels [Zann 1965; Spoon 2002]; White-tailed Black Cockatoos [Saunders 1974; Forshaw 1981]; Red-tailed Black Cockatoos [*Calyptorhynchus banksii,* Forshaw 1981]). Forms of repetitive strutting are also observed in such diverse species as Orange-fronted Conures (Hardy 1963), Budgerigars (Brockway 1964), Black-billed Amazons (Cruz & Gruber 1980), Monk Parakeets (Eberhard 1998), and several lovebird species (Dilger 1960). Likewise, males of various species such as Orange-fronted Conures (Hardy 1963), Budgerigars (Brockway 1964), Thick-billed Parrots (*Rhynchopsitta pachyrhyncha,* Lanning & Shiflett 1983), White-fronted Amazons (Skeate 1984), Puerto Rican Amazons (Snyder et al. 1987), Green-rumped Parrotlets (Waltman & Beissinger 1992), and several lovebird species (Dilger 1960) perform some type of head bobbing and/or head bowing display. Puerto Rican Amazon (Snyder et al. 1987) and Green-rumped Parrotlet males (Waltman & Beissinger 1992) also perform rapid wing flicking as part of their courtship displays. As in many bird species, vocalizations also comprise an important aspect of parrot courtship behavior (e.g., Orange-fronted Conures [Hardy 1963]; Budgerigars [Brockway 1964]; Cockatiels [Zann 1965; Spoon 2002]; White-tailed Black Cockatoos [Saunders 1974]; King Parrots, *Alisterus scapularis* [Forshaw 1981]). However, unlike passerines, most parrots do not produce vocalizations regarded as song. Males of a few parrot species produce courtship vocalizations that may be considered song in that the vocalizations consist of melodious, recognizable syllables (e.g., warbling in Budgerigars [Brockway 1964]; courtship song in Orange-fronted Conures [Hardy 1963] and Cockatiels [Zann 1965; Spoon 2002]). Warbling by male Budgerigars not only correlates with sperm production but also stimulates female ovarian activity and thus represents an integral component of reproductive behavior in this species (Brockway 1965). Interestingly, female Budgerigars occasionally warble but at a substantially lower rate and complexity than males (Farabaugh et al. 1992). Administering testosterone to adult male and female Budgerigars appears to lower the threshold for male-typical courtship behaviors including vocalizations (Brockway 1968; Nespor et al. 1996). Jackson (1963) also describes a yodeling song produced by female Kakas (*Nestor meridionalis*), and Ekstrom (2002) reports singing by female Greater Vasa Parrots in the context of allofeeding (see later).

Because the courtship activities of the lek-breeding Kakapo illustrate the diversity that exists within psittacines, they deserve special notice. During breeding periods, males actively maintain their courts known as track-and-bowl systems by excavating up to several shallow depressions or bowls and cleaning the trails that connect them (Merton et al. 1984). From their courts, males of this flightless, nocturnal species produce courtship vocalizations including booming, which can be heard up to several kilometers away. Indeed, males often locate their bowls at the base of natural sound reflectors. As mentioned previously, the track-and-bowl systems appear to be used exclusively for courtship and mating and not feeding or nesting. In fact, a male's track-and-bowl system usually occurs several kilometers from his home range (Merton et al. 1984).

Observers typically have recorded only males performing courtship behaviors in most parrot species. However, in a few species, observers have noted females displaying as well. For example, female Cockatiels often join their male partners in switch sidling, especially in instances that lead to female copulation solicitation (Zann 1965; T. Spoon, personal observation). In King Parrots, both males and females erect their head feathers but sleek the remaining body feathers, contract their pupils, and call (Forshaw 1981), and in Puerto Rican Amazons males and females engage in a mutual bowing display during pair formation (Snyder et al. 1987). Either member of Green-rumped Parrotlet pairs may initiate courtship behavior, which often occurs in conjunction with nest prospecting and normally consists of head bowing combined with tail fanning alternating

between mates (Waltman & Beissinger 1992). Female Budgerigars usually remain motionless (or may leave or respond aggressively) to male pre-copulatory courtship but occasionally respond with nudging or pumping, behavioral components typical of male courtship, prior to soliciting copulation (Brockway 1964).

Courtship feeding or allofeeding occurs between pairmates in numerous parrot species. In the following discussion, I use the terms "allofeeding" and "courtship feeding" interchangeably to refer to regurgitation of food by one individual for another *excluding* the provisioning of a mate during incubation or brooding and the feeding of chicks. Yet, courtship feeding and provisioning an incubating female appear interrelated—courtship feeding occurs primarily in species in which the male provides food for the female while she alone incubates. For example, species such as White-tailed Black Cockatoos (Saunders 1982), Puerto Rican Amazons (Snyder et al. 1987), Green-rumped Parrotlets (Waltman & Beissinger 1992), Monk Parakeets (Eberhard 1998), Orange-fronted Conures (Hardy 1963), Rainbow and Scaly-breasted Lorikeets (Serpell 1981; Forshaw & Cooper 1981), and Budgerigars (Brockway 1964) exhibit courtship feeding and a parental care system in which the female alone incubates while the male provisions her; in contrast, species such as Gang-gang Cockatoos (*Callocephalon fimbriatum*, Forshaw 1981), Galahs (Rowley 1990), and Cockatiels (Spoon 2002) rarely if ever engage in allofeeding and exhibit a parental care system in which both members of the pair share incubation duties and the male does not provision the female.

Most authors prefer the term "courtship feeding" because the behavior often occurs in association with courtship displays and copulation. Moreover, some courtship displays such as head bobbing and bill clasping appear to be ritualized forms of courtship feeding (Dilger 1960; Brockway 1964; Waltman & Beissinger 1992). Allofeeding or an apparently ritualized form occurs in a courtship context in Budgerigars (Brockway 1964), King Parrots (Forshaw 1981), Green-rumped Parrotlets (Waltman & Beissinger 1992), and several lovebird species (Dilger 1960). In species such as Spectacled Parrotlets (Garnetzke-Stollman & Franck 1991), Green-rumped Parrotlets (Waltman & Beissinger 1992),

Puerto Rican Amazons (Snyder et al. 1987), White-tailed Black Cockatoos (Saunders 1982), and Monk Parakeets (Eberhard 1998), allofeeding only occurs during, or at least increases in frequency at the beginning of, the breeding cycle. In Puerto Rican Amazons, for example, courtship feeding occurs in close association with copulation, although the success rate of copulation remains similar whether or not courtship feeding occurs (Snyder et al. 1987). However, in some species allofeeding occurs throughout the year or even if restricted to the breeding season may not be directly associated with copulation. Allofeeding occurs year-round in Orange-fronted Conures (Hardy 1963), White-fronted Amazons (Skeate 1984), and several lovebird species (Dilger 1960; Stamm 1962) although in lovebirds the frequency increases with the onset of breeding (Dilger 1960). In most psittacines, only the male allofeeds the female; however, female Spectacled Parrotlets (Garnetzke-Stollman & Franck 1991) and Puerto Rican Amazons (Snyder et al. 1987) rarely but occasionally feed their mates, and Madagascar (*Agapornis cana*) and Abyssinian Lovebird (*A. taranta*) females frequently feed their mates (Dilger 1960).

Some form of courtship behavior typically precedes copulation, another important component in the reproductive lives of parrots. Copulation in parrots tends to be a lengthy affair compared to other birds whose copulations generally last only a few seconds (Birkhead & Møller 1992). The following examples illustrate the extended duration of copulation in a variety of socially monogamous psittacines: mean of 30 seconds but up to 1.5 minutes in Budgerigars (Brockway 1964), approximately one minute in Black-billed Amazons (Koenig 2001) and White-tailed Black Cockatoos (Saunders 1974), approximately 1.5 minutes in Orange-fronted Conures (Hardy 1963) and Galahs (Rowley 1990), 1.5–2 minutes in Cockatiels (Zann 1965; T. Spoon, personal observation), approximately 1–3.5 minutes in Green-rumped Parrotlets (Waltman & Beissinger 1992), a few seconds to more than six minutes in lovebirds (Dilger 1960; Stamm 1962), and a mean of slightly more than 4.5 minutes with multiple mounts in Monk Parakeets (Eberhard 1998). The most remarkable copulation sequence belongs to the polygynandrous Greater Vasa Parrot, in which copulation may exceed 1.5 hours and begins with

the male mounting the female but ends with the birds perched side by side while their cloacae remain locked together (Wilkinson & Birkhead 1995). During the breeding season, the cloacae of Vasa Parrot males and, to a lesser extent, females become greatly enlarged, and during copulation, the male's cloacal protrusion appears to completely enter the female's opening. While the two remain interlocked, the male makes vigorous copulatory movements and may allofeed the female several times (Wilkinson & Birkhead 1995). In addition to the duration of copulation, another difference between parrots and most birds is that male parrots mount by stepping onto rather than flying onto the back of the female (Dilger 1960; Hardy 1963; Brockway 1964; Eberhard 1998; T. Spoon, personal observation). Male Thick-billed (Lanning & Shiflett 1983) and amazon parrots (*Amazona* species, Snyder et al. 1987) usually do not even fully mount the female during copulation but place one foot on the female's back while the other foot grasps the perch. An interesting twist occurs in Peach-faced Lovebirds and the white eye-ringed group of lovebirds in which pseudofemale copulation solicitation by males sometimes results in female mounting; the sexually dichromatic lovebird species, on the other hand, do not appear to display this behavioral reversal (Dilger 1960). The degree to which parrots limit copulation to the breeding season varies among species. Green-rumped Parrotlets (Waltman & Beissinger 1992), Budgerigars (Trillmich 1976), Galahs (Rowley 1990), and Vasa Parrots (Wilkinson & Birkhead 1995) tend to limit copulation primarily or entirely to around the time of nest prospecting and egg laying. In contrast, Cockatiel mates copulate throughout year (Zann 1965) and often multiple times a day, although the frequency tends to be highest during pair formation and breeding (Spoon et al. 2004).

NESTING

Although the majority of parrot species nest in tree cavities, psittacines exhibit a moderate degree of variability in nest sites. Most psittacines are secondary cavity nesters, meaning that they utilize existing cavities in trees as nest sites (Forshaw 1981, 1989). Some species modify the cavity by adding layers of nesting material; for example, Palm Cockatoos (*Probosciger aterrimus*) may create a layer of twigs two to three meters deep in the bottom of a cavity (Forshaw 1981), and Galahs line their nests with green leaves, the only cockatoo species known to use green material (Rowley 1990). Members of the genus *Agapornis* display a great deal of diversity in nest construction inside their nesting hollows, ranging from a simple pad in Madagascar and Abyssinian Lovebirds to a well-formed cup in Peach-faced Lovebirds to a roofed nest chamber with tunnel in Masked Lovebirds (Dilger 1960). Additionally, many parrot species, while cavity nesters, use chambers in termite or ant mounds (Red-Faced Lovebirds, *Agapornis pullaria* [Dilger 1960]; Orange-fronted Conures [Hardy 1963]; Golden-shouldered Parrots, *Psephotus chrysopterygius* [Forshaw 1981]; Canary-winged Parakeets [Paranhos & Marcondes-Machado 2000]) or cliff faces rather than trees (Maroon-fronted Parrots, *Rhynchopsitta pachyrhynchus terrisi* [Lawson & Lanning 1980]; Burrowing Parrots [Masello et al. 2001]). Rock Parakeets (*Neophema petrophila*) nest in crevices in rocks or under rock overhangs (Forshaw 1981). The use of alternative nesting niches such as chambers in termitaria, ant mounds, and cliffs may have evolved in response to increased predation pressures corresponding to the evolutionary radiation of mammalian predators (Brightsmith 2005). Several species exhibit the flexibility to nest in a variety of cavities; Paradise Parakeets (*Psephotus pulcherrimus*) may use chambers in termitaria or in banks along watercourses (Forshaw 1981), Bahama Amazons (*Amazona leucocephala bahamensis*) typically nest in tree cavities but will use limestone karst cavities in the ground on islands lacking suitable cavity-containing trees (Snyder et al. 1987), Puerto Rican and Hispaniolan Amazons (*A. ventralis*) may nest in either tree or cliff cavities (Snyder et al. 1987), and Galahs nest primarily in tree cavities but will nest in concrete pipes and crevices in rock and cliff faces (Rowley 1990). On the other hand, Ground Parrots (*Pezoporus wallicus*), Night Parrots (*Geopsittacus occidentalis*), and Kakapos do not nest in formal cavities but use shallow excavations or hollows located under overhanging vegetation or near the base of a shrub or tree (Forshaw 1981; Powlesland et al. 1992). Similarly, Keas (*Nestor notabilis*) nest in burrows normally excavated under boulders (Diamond & Bond 1999). Monk Parakeets are unusual among parrots in

that each breeding pair uses sticks to construct an enclosed nest chamber, which is often integrated with other such chambers into a large compound nest (Navarro et al. 1992; Eberhard 1998). Interestingly, both breeder and non-breeder Monk Parakeets participate in building the large, compound structure that they actively maintain year-round and use for roosting during non-breeding periods as well as nesting during the breeding season (Navarro et al. 1992; Eberhard 1998). However, twig theft commonly occurs between pairs, suggesting a lack of true cooperation in nest construction (Eberhard 1998).

Spacing between conspecific nests also varies greatly between species, ranging from colonial situations with little distance between nests to widely dispersed distributions with kilometers between nests. Species such as Maroon-fronted Parrots (Lawson & Lanning 1980; Snyder et al. 1987), Monk Parakeets (Eberhard 1998), Burrowing Parrots (Masello et al. 2002), and Peach-faced and the white-eye ringed group of lovebirds (Dilger 1960) nest colonially with little distance and often minimal aggression between breeding pairs. In contrast, Major Mitchell's Cockatoos maintain an average distance of almost three kilometers between nests (Rowley & Chapman 1991) due to intense aggression by breeding pairs toward conspecifics (Saunders et al. 1985). High levels of intraspecific aggression around nesting trees by Blue-and-yellow Macaws (*Ara ararauna*) may prevent the use of many apparently suitable nesting cavities and limit the density of breeding pairs (Renton 2004). In between these extremes, many species appear to exhibit an intermediate pattern in which nests appear somewhat clumped but not as much so as colonially breeding species (e.g., Thick-billed Parrots, Lanning & Shiflett 1983; Galahs, Rowley 1990; several *Amazona* species, reviewed in Snyder et al. 1987 and Enkerlin-Hoeflich 1995). The degree of clumping and aggression between breeding pairs may relate, in part, to the availability of suitable nesting sites. Bahama Parrots nesting in a region with superabundant nest sites in the form of solution holes in the ground exhibit little territorial aggression and close nest spacing compared to heightened territorial aggression exhibited by the same species in an area with few potential nest sites (Snyder et al. 1987). Some species such as Galahs maintain an interest in their nest sites throughout the year, and pairs return to them to roost every evening (Rowley 1990). During the non-breeding season, Puerto Rican Amazon pairs roost near their nests only intermittently and defend the territory somewhat but much less vigorously than during the breeding season (Snyder et al. 1987). Defense of nest sites by Imperial (*Amazona imperialis*) and Hispaniolan Amazon pairs has been observed during non-breeding times (Snyder et al. 1987). In contrast, White-tailed Black Cockatoos, Red-tailed Black Cockatoos, and Corellas (*Cacatua tenuirostris*) inhabit their nesting areas only during breeding (Saunders 1982; Saunders et al. 1982).

Following nest-site selection and preparation, egg laying, incubation, and chick rearing commence. "Parrot encyclopedias" such as Forshaw (1981, 1989), Alderton (1991), Collar (1997), and Higgins (1999) provide species information, when available, on age at first breeding, breeding season, clutch size, incubation, and fledging. Masello and Quillfeldt (2002) also provide a useful summary of various breeding parameters for psittacines reported in the literature. Due to space constraints, I will discuss general trends and notable variability in these reproductive parameters and refer readers to these sources for species-specific information. In general, parrots exhibit delayed sexual maturity; many of the large-bodied species of cockatoos, for example, do not reach sexual maturity until approximately four to five years of age (Forshaw 1981), while Budgerigars may pair and breed in captivity as young as five months of age (Kavanau 1987). Natural populations of parrots exhibit a remarkable range in clutch size from one in some large cockatoos (Red-tailed Black [Smith & Saunders 1986]; Glossy [Garnett et al. 1999]; Palm [Murphy et al. 2003]) to an average of six (range 1–11) in Monk Parakeets (Navarro et al. 1992) and seven (range 5–10) in Green-rumped Parrotlets (Waltman & Beissinger 1992). In species with variable clutch size, the female's nutritional status may affect clutch size; Green-rumped Parrotlet females fed more often by their mates during egg laying subsequently produced larger clutches (Waltman & Beissinger 1992). Among Australian psittacines, average clutch size decreases, egg weight increases, and incubation duration increases as species body weight increases (Saunders et al. 1984). A similar trend regarding clutch size and

body weight occurs among *Amazona* species (Enkerlin-Hoeflich 1995). This trend does not apply universally across all parrot taxa, however; Double-eyed Fig Parrots (*Opopsitta diophthalma*), for example, have both a small body weight and small clutch size (average two eggs) (Forshaw 1981). Thus, in species of large-bodied parrots such as Palm Cockatoos, the convergence of late sexual maturity, small clutch size, failure to breed every year, extremely low nesting success (81% of active nests failed to produce fledglings in one population of Palm Cockatoos), and strong competition for limited nesting sites result in populations highly sensitive to environmental perturbations (Murphy et al. 2003).

PARENTAL CARE

In most parrot species, the female incubates alone while the male provides regurgitated food to her (Forshaw 1981, 1989). In these species, the female usually leaves the nest only to receive food. For example, incubating female Glossy Black Cockatoos normally leave the nest only in the evening when the male returns from foraging to feed her (Garnett et al. 1999). Similarly, female White-tailed Black Cockatoos remain in the nest during incubation except to receive food from the male in the morning and evening (Saunders 1982). Female Green-rumped Parrotlets spend on average about 85% of their time during the day in the nest, and males feed the incubating females almost once per hour during this time (Waltman & Beissinger 1992). An interesting provisioning pattern emerges among amazon parrots—in general, males of mainland species feed their mates only twice per day, whereas males of island species feed their mates multiple times each day (Enkerlin-Hoeflich 1995; Renton & Salinas-Melgoza 1999). This pattern may relate to differential predation pressure, but again, exceptions exist to this general trend. Yellow-billed Amazons on the island of Jamaica display the twice-daily feeding pattern (Koenig 2001). Even the polygynandrous Vasa Parrot conforms to the pattern of female-only incubation coupled with male provisioning but with an interesting twist—females typically receive food from several males and each male provisions several females at widely separated nests (Ekstrom 2002). Furthermore, in keeping with the association between food and sex, female Vasa Parrots generally perform ritualized or false copulation (in the sense that it does not involve cloacal contact or the prolonged joining described previously) with each of the provisioning males.

However, the parrot family contains several notable exceptions to this pattern of female incubation and male provisioning. The Black Cockatoos of the genera *Probosciger* and *Calyptorhynchus* exhibit the aforementioned pattern of female-only incubation and male provisioning, whereas the cockatoo genera of *Eolophus, Cacatua, Callocephalon,* and *Nymphicus* exhibit biparental incubation without males provisioning females (Rowley 1990). Among these latter species, mates must coordinate incubation shifts to ensure that their eggs receive adequate coverage and protection. Cockatiel mates that demonstrate greater coordination of incubation subsequently experience greater hatching success of fertile eggs, and those mates that exhibit greater affiliation and behavioral synchrony and less aggression subsequently display greater incubation coordination and thus hatching success (Spoon et al., in press). Kakapos also exhibit a somewhat different incubation pattern in that although the female alone broods, males do not provision incubating females or chicks (Merton et al. 1984; Powlesland et al. 1992). Additional notable exceptions include Golden Conures, in which multiple females may lay eggs in one nest and several males and females may participate in nest attendance (Oren & Novaes 1986), and Monk Parakeets, in which some form of incipient helping at the nest by individuals other than the pair members may occur (Eberhard 1998).

After hatching, parrot chicks experience a relatively lengthy period of dependence upon their parents. Compared to raptors, owls, and pigeons of equivalent body weight, parrots exhibit a relatively extended nestling period (Saunders et al. 1984). With the only known exception of the Kakapo, in which the female alone cares for her chicks, male and female psittacine parents jointly care for their young. In general, in species with female-only incubation and male provisioning, the male initially continues to provision the female who in turn feeds the newly hatched chicks; as the nestlings age, the female spends progressively more time away from the nest, returning to feed the young with the male who may also begin to directly feed the chicks (several lovebird

species, Dilger 1960; White-tailed Black Cockatoos, Saunders 1982; Thick-billed Parrots, Lanning & Shiflett 1983; Budgerigars, Stamps et al. 1985; Green-rumped Parrotlets, Waltman & Beissinger 1992; Monk Parakeets, Eberhard 1998; Glossy Black Cockatoos, Garnett et al. 1999; Lilac-crowned Amazons, Renton & Salinas-Melgoza 1999; Black-billed Amazons, Koenig 2001). Keas appear to take this pattern to the extreme in that initially the male feeds the female, who in turn feeds the young chicks, but as the chicks age the male begins to feed them directly, and by fledging the male alone feeds them and continues to do so alone for several weeks after fledging (reviewed in Diamond & Bond 1999). Although the Vasa Parrot displays a similar chick-rearing pattern in that females feed the nestlings with regurgitated food received from males, this species once again provides an interesting twist on this general pattern—only female Vasa Parrots sing, and they appear to do so primarily during chick-rearing to attract provisioning males. Females that sing more frequently or more complex songs receive more provisions from males and produce larger clutches and broods (Ekstrom 2002). In contrast to the widespread pattern of female-only incubation and male provisioning, species such as Galahs (Rowley 1990) and Cockatiels (Spoon 2002) exhibit a parental care system in which both parents incubate and feed the chicks directly.

Another important aspect of parrot reproduction is hatching asynchrony (Waltman & Beissinger 1992). Because many parrots begin incubation with the first egg but often continue to lay eggs for several days, a clutch may experience strong hatching asynchrony, resulting in chicks of vastly discrepant sizes and competitive abilities. Because of this, last-hatched chicks may die of starvation. In Green-rumped Parrotlets, all chicks in small broods experienced uniformly high survival, whereas the last and penultimately hatched chicks in large clutches experienced reduced survival, apparently due to starvation (Waltman & Beissinger 1992). A similar pattern occurs in Burrowing Parrots (Masello & Quillfeldt 2002). White-tailed Black Cockatoos offer an even more dramatic example with two eggs laid approximately eight days apart. If the first chick survives until the second egg hatches, the second-hatched chick typically dies of starvation within a couple of days (Saunders 1982). This pattern may represent insurance against infertile eggs or, at least in the case of the Green-rumped Parrotlet, may allow pairs to raise additional young in exceptionally good years.

Parrot parents may either overcome or facilitate the discrepant competitive abilities of chicks by taking an active role in the distribution of food to chicks. Studies on Crimson Rosellas (Krebs & Magrath 2000; Krebs 2001) and Budgerigars (Stamps et al. 1985) demonstrate that parents can preferentially allocate food to certain chicks and that males and females may show different feeding preferences based on age and hunger level of chicks. After fledging occurs, parents may continue to feed the chicks for several weeks or months and may continue to associate with them for several months (White-fronted Amazons, Skeate 1984; Corellas, Beeton 1985; Galahs, Rowley 1990; Major Mitchell's Cockatoo, Rowley & Chapman 1991; Green-rumped Parrotlets, Waltman & Beissinger 1992; Keas, Diamond & Bond 1999; Burrowing Parrots, Masello et al. 2002; Cockatiels, T. Spoon, personal observation) and in some cases until the parents enter their next reproductive cycle the following year (e.g., White-tailed Black Cockatoo, Saunders 1982).

SUMMARY

Parrots are often regarded as a rather uniform group of species, and in many respects they conform to this generalization. Most parrot species exhibit social monogamy and biparental care of young. In these species, pair relationships commonly endure for several breeding attempts and persist throughout the year. In addition, many affiliative and courtship behaviors characterize these relationships. However, two known and intriguing exceptions occur—lek-breeding Kakapos and highly polygynandrous Vasa Parrots, neither species of which exhibits the close pair bonds observed in socially monogamous species. In addition, Kakapo females alone care for their eggs and young, and Vasa females receive regurgitated food provisions from several males while caring for offspring. Two species, Monk Parakeets and Golden Conures, may also engage in some degree of cooperative or communal breeding. Yet, even in socially monogamous species, individuals may not display absolute sexual monogamy, and in some instances polygamous breeding groups occur. Among Australian psittacines, larger-bodied species produce smaller clutches of larger eggs with longer incubation and nestling periods. Parrots nest in cavities or chambers or at least in hollows under overhanging vegetation or rocks. Most parrots also exhibit a prolonged association with their parents and delayed sexual maturation. Another important characteristic of psittacine reproduction involves a pronounced hatching asynchrony in many species that often results in the death of the youngest chicks.

Although researchers have made substantial progress in the study of parrot reproductive behavior, successful conservation and management of these species both in the wild and in captivity depend upon a more thorough understanding of the social and reproductive requirements of parrots. At the most basic level, this requires information on the composition of breeding groups, the processes by which breeding relationships form, nest-site selection, and parental care patterns. A more in-depth but perhaps equally critical understanding includes an appreciation of the natural variability both within and between species. Unrecognized variability may thwart conservation efforts on multiple levels. Lack of such knowledge may cause difficulties in providing the social and physical environments that best promote breeding success. Similarly, that which goes unrecognized or unappreciated may be lost, fundamentally altering the behavioral and perhaps genetic composition of a species.

REFERENCES

Alderton, D. 1991. *The atlas of parrots of the world.* Neptune City, NJ: T. F. H. Publications.

Arnold, K.E., I.P.F. Owens, and N.J. Marshall. 2002. Fluorescent signaling in parrots. *Science* 295:92.

Arrowood, P.C. 1987. Duetting, pair bonding and agonistic display in parakeet pairs. *Behaviour* 106: 129–157.

Baltz, A.P., and A.B. Clark. 1997. Extra-pair courtship behaviour of male budgerigars and the effect of an audience. *Animal Behaviour* 53:1017–1024.

Beeton, R.J.S. 1985. The little corella: A seasonally adapted species. *Proceedings of the Ecological Society of Australia* 13:53–63.

Bennett, P.M., and I.P. Owens. 1997. Variation in extinction risk among birds: Chance or evolutionary predisposition? *Proceedings of the Royal Society of London, Series B* 264:401–408.

Birkhead, T.M., and A.P. Møller. 1992. *Sperm competition in birds: Evolutionary causes and consequences.* London: Academic Press.

Bluhm, C.K. 1985. Mate preferences and mating patterns in canvasback ducks (*Aythya valisineria*). In *Avian monogamy*, ed. P.A. Gowaty and D.W. Mock, pp. 45–56. Washington, DC: American Ornithologists' Union.

Bottoni, L., R. Massa, R.W. Lea, and P.J. Sharp. 1993. Mate choice and reproductive success in the red-legged partridge (*Alectoris rufa*). *Hormones and Behavior* 27: 308–317.

Brightsmith, D.J. 2005. Competition, predation and nest niche shifts among tropical cavity nesters: Phylogeny and natural history evolution of parrots (Psittaciformes) and trogons (Trogoniformes). *Journal of Avian Biology* 36:64–73.

Brockway, B.F. 1964. Ethological studies of the budgerigar: Reproductive behavior. *Behaviour* 23:294–324.

Brockway, B.F. 1965. Stimulation of ovarian development and egg laying by male courtship vocalization in budgerigars (*Melopsittacus undulatus*). *Animal Behaviour* 13:575–578.

Brockway, B.F. 1968. Influences of sex hormones on the loud and soft warbles of male budgerigars. *Animal Behaviour* 16:5–12.

Clout, M.N., G.P. Elliott, and B.C. Robertson. 2002. Effects of supplementary feeding on the offspring sex ratio of kakapo: A dilemma for the conservation of a polygynous parrot. *Biological Conservation* 107:13–18.

Collar, N.J. 1997. "Family Psittacidae (parrots)." In *Handbook of the birds of the world. Volume 4: Sandgrouse to cuckoos*, ed. J. del Hoyo, A. Elliot, and J. Sargatal, pp. 280–477. Barcelona: Lynx Edicions.

Collar, N.J., and A.T. Juniper. 1992. "Dimensions and causes of the parrot conservation crisis: Solutions from conservation biology." In *New world parrots in crisis*, ed. S.R. Beissinger and N.F.R. Snyder, pp. 1–24. Washington, DC: Smithsonian Institution Press.

Cruz, A., and S. Gruber. 1980. "The distribution, ecology, and breeding biology of Jamaican amazon parrots." In *Conservation of new world parrots: Proceedings of the ICBP Parrot Working Group Meeting*, ed. R.F. Pasquier, pp. 403–417. Washington, DC: Smithsonian Institution Press.

Derrickson, S.R., and N.F.R. Snyder. 1992. "Potentials and limits of captive breeding in parrot conservation." In *New world parrots in crisis,* ed. S. R. Beissinger and N. F. R. Snyder, pp. 133–163. Washington, DC: Smithsonian Institution Press.

Diamond, J., and A.B. Bond. 1999. *Kea, bird of paradox: The Evolution and Behavior of a New Zealand Parrot.* Berkeley: University of California Press.

Dilger, W.C. 1960. The comparative ethology of the African parrot genus *Agapornis*. *Zeitschrift fur Tierpsychologie* 17:649–685.

Dunn, P.O., and J.T. Lifjeld. 1994. Can extra-pair paternity be used to predict extra-pair paternity in birds? *Animal Behaviour* 47:983–985.

Eberhard, J.R. 1998. Breeding biology of the monk parakeet. *Wilson Bulletin* 110:463–473.

Ekstrom, J. 2002. Singing for your dinner but not for your mates: Female song and polygynandry in the greater vasa parrot. Abstract from V. Kirindy Symposium, 23 August at University of Sheffield, UK.

Enkerlin-Hoeflich, E.C. 1995. Comparative ecology and reproductive biology of three species of *Amazona* parrots in northeastern Mexico. PhD diss., Texas A&M University, College Station.

Farabaugh, S.M., E.D. Brown, and R.J. Dooling. 1992. Analysis of the warble song of the budgerigar (*Melopsittacus undulatus*). *Bioacoustics* 4:111–130.

Forshaw, J.M. 1981. *Australian parrots,* 2nd ed. Melbourne, Lansdowne Editions.

Forshaw, J.M. 1989. *Parrots of the world,* 3rd ed. London: Blanford Press.

Forshaw, J.M., & W.T. Cooper. 1981. *Australian parrots*. Melbourne: Lansdowne Press.

Garnett, S.T., L.P. Pedler, and G.M. Crowley. 1999. The breeding biology of the glossy black cockatoo *Calyptorhynchus lathami* on Kangaroo Island, South Australia. *Emu* 99:262–279.

Garnetzke-Stollman, K., and D. Franck. 1991. Socialisation tactics of the spectacled parrotlet (*Forpus conspicilllatus*). *Behaviour* 119:1–29.

Hardy, J.W. 1963. Epigamic and reproductive behavior of the orange-fronted parakeet. *Condor* 65:169–199.

Higgins, P.J., ed. 1999. *Handbook of Australian, New Zealand, and Antarctic birds. Volume 4: Parrots to dollarbirds.* Victoria: Oxford University Press.

Hile, A.G. 2002. Effects of male vocal learning on female behavior in the budgerigar. *Brain, Behavior and Evolution Abstracts* 60:62–63.

Hile, A.G., T.K. Plummer, and G.F. Striedter. 2000. Male vocal imitation produces call convergence during pair bonding in budgerigars, *Melopsittacus undulatus*. *Animal Behaviour* 59:1209–1218.

Jackson, J.R. 1963. Studies at a kaka's nest. *Notornis* 10:168–175.

Kavanau, J.L. 1987. *Lovebirds, cockatiels, budgerigars: Behavior and evolution.* Los Angeles: Science Software Systems, Inc.

Klint, T., and M. Enquist. 1981. Pair formation and reproductive output in domestic pigeons. *Behavioural Processes* 6:57–62.

Koenig, S.E. 2001. The breeding biology of black-billed parrot *Amazona agilis* and yellow-billed parrot *Amazona collaria* in Cockpit Country, Jamaica. *Bird Conservation International* 11:205–225.

Krebs, E.A. 1998. Breeding biology of crimson rosellas *Platycercus elegans* in Black Mountain, Australian Capital Territory. *Australian Journal of Zoology* 46:119–136.

Krebs, E.A. 2001. Begging and food distribution in crimson rosella (*Platycercus elegans*) broods: Why don't hungry chicks beg more? *Behavioral Ecology and Sociobiology* 50:20–30.

Krebs, E.A., and R.D. Magrath. 2000. Food allocation in crimson rosella broods: Parents differ in their responses to chick hunger. *Animal Behaviour* 59:739–751.

Lanning, D.V., and J.T. Shiflett. 1983. Nesting ecology of thick-billed parrots. *Condor* 85:66–73.

Lawson, P.W., and D.V. Lanning. 1980. "Nesting and status of the maroon-fronted parrot (*Rhynchopsitta terrisi*)." In *Conservation of new world parrots: Proceedings of the ICBP Parrot Working Group Meeting*, ed. R.F. Pasquier, pp. 385–392. Washington, DC: Smithsonian Institution Press.

Levinson, S.T. 1980. "The social behavior of the white-fronted amazon (*Amazona albifrons*)." In *Conservation of new world parrots: Proceedings of the ICBP Parrot Working Group Meeting*, ed. R.F. Pasquier, pp. 403–417. Washington, DC: Smithsonian Institution Press.

Lupo, C., L. Beani, L., R. Cervo, R., L. Lodi, L., and F. Dessi-Fulgheri. 1990. Steroid hormones and reproductive history of the grey partridge (*Perdix perdix*). *Bollettino di Zoologia* 57:247–252.

Manning, A.D., D.B. Lindenmayer, and S.C. Barry. 2004. The conservation implications of bird reproduction in the agricultural "matrix": A case study of the vulnerable superb parrot of south-eastern Australia. *Biological Conservation* 120:367–378.

Masello, J.F., G.A. Pagnossin, G.E. Palleiro, and P. Quillfeldt. 2001. Use of miniature security cameras to record behaviour of burrow-nesting birds. *Vogelwarte* 4:150–154.

Masello, J.F., and P. Quillfeldt. 2002. Chick growth and breeding success of the burrowing parrot. *Condor* 104:574–586.

Masello, J.F., and P. Quillfeldt. 2003. Body size, body condition, and ornamental feathers of burrowing parrots: Variation between years and sexes, assortative mating and influences on breeding success. *Emu* 103:149–161.

Masello, J.F., A. Stramkova, P. Quillfelt, J.T. Epplen, and T. Lubjuhn, T. 2002. Genetic monogamy in burrowing parrots *Cyanoliseus patagonus*. *Journal of Avian Biology* 33:99–103.

Merton, D.V., R.B. Morris, and I.A.E. Atkinson. 1984. Lek behaviour in a parrot: The kakapo *Strigops habroptilus* of New Zealand. *Ibis* 126:277–283.

Monterrubio, T., E. Enkerlin-Hoeflich, and R.B. Hamilton. 2002. Productivity and nesting success of thick-billed parrots. *Condor* 104:788–794.

Murphy, S., S. Legge, and R. Heinsohn. 2003. The breeding biology of palm cockatoos (*Probosciger aterrimus*): A case of a slow life history. *Journal of Zoology* 261:327–339.

Navarro, J.L., M.B. Martella, and E.H. Bucher. 1992. Breeding season and productivity of monk parakeets in Cordoba, Argentina. *Wilson Bulletin* 104:413–424.

Nespor, A.A., M.J. Lukaszewicz, R.J. Dooling, and G.F. Ball. 1996. Testosterone induction of male-like vocalizations in female budgerigars (*Melopsittacus undulatus*). *Hormones and Behavior* 30:162–169.

Oren, D.C., and F. Novaes. 1986. Observations on the golden parakeet *Aratinga guarouba* in northern Brazil. *Biological Conservation* 36:329–337.

Paranhos, S.J., and L.O. Marcondes-Machado. 2000. Breeding behavior of *Brotogeris versicolorus chiriri* (Aves, Psittacidae) in Sao Paulo, Brazil. *Iheringia Serie Zoologia* 88:61–66.

Pearn, S.M., A.T.D. Bennett, and I.C. Cuthill. 2001. Ultraviolet vision, fluorescence and mate choice in a parrot, the budgerigar *Melopsittacus undulatus*. *Proceedings of the Royal Society Biological Sciences Series B* 268:2273–2279.

Power, D.M. 1966. Antiphonal duetting and evidence for auditory reaction time in the orange-chinned parakeet. *Auk* 83:314–319.

Powlesland, R.G., B.D. Lloyd, H.A. Best, and D.V. Merton. 1992. Breeding biology of the kakapo *Strigops habroptilus* on Stewart Island, New Zealand. *Ibis* 134:361–373.

Renton, K. 2004. Agonistic interactions of nesting and nonbreeding macaws. *Condor* 106: 354–362.

Renton, K., and A. Salinas-Melgoza. 1999. Nesting behavior of the lilac-crowned parrot. *Wilson Bulletin* 111:488–493.

Rowley, I. 1990. *Behavioural ecology of the galah, Eolophus roseicapillus*. New South Wales, Australia: Surrey Beatty & Sons, Chipping Norton.

Rowley, I., and G. Chapman. 1991. The breeding biology, food, social organization, demography and conservation of the Major Mitchell or pink cockatoo, *Cacatua leadbeateri*, on the margin of the Western Australia wheatbelt. *Australian Journal of Zoology* 39:211–261.

Ryan, K.K., and J. Altmann. 2001. Selection for male choice based primarily on mate compatibility in the oldfield mouse, *Peromyscus polionotus rhoadsi*. *Behavioral Ecology and Sociobiology* 50:436–440.

Saunders, D.A. 1974. The function of displays in the breeding of the white-tailed black cockatoo. *Emu* 74:43–46.

Saunders, D.A. 1982. The breeding behavior of the short-billed form of the white-tailed black cockatoo (*Calyptorhynchus funereus*). *Ibis* 124:422–455.

Saunders, D.A., I. Rowley, and G.T. Smith. 1985. "The effects of clearing for agriculture on the distribution of cockatoos in the southwest of Western Australia." In *Birds of the eucalypt forests and woodlands: Ecology, conservations, management,* ed. A. Keast, H. F. Recher, H. Ford, and D. Saunders, pp. 309–321. Sidney Australia: Royal Australasian Ornithologists Union and Surrey Beatty and Sons.

Saunders, D.A., G.T. Smith, and Campbell, N. A. 1984. The relationship between body weight, egg weight, incubation period, nestling period and nest site in the Psittaciformes, Falconiformes, Strigiformes and Columbiformes. *Australian Journal of Zoology* 32:57–65.

Saunders, D.A., G.T. Smith, and I. Rowley. 1982. The availability and dimensions of tree hollows that provide nest sites for cockatoo (Psittaciformes) in Western Australia. *Australian Wildlife Research* 9:541–546.

Seibert, L.M., and S.L. Crowell-Davis. 2001. Gender effects on aggression, dominance rank, and affiliative behaviors in a flock of captive adult cockatiels (*Nymphicus hollandicus*). *Applied Animal Behaviour Science* 71:155–170.

Serpell, J.A. 1981. Duets, greetings, and triumph ceremonies: Analogous displays in the parrot genus *Trichoglossus*. *Zeitschrift fur Tierpsychologie* 55:268–283.

Skeate, S.T. 1984. Courtship and reproductive behavior of captive white-fronted amazon parrots *Amazona albifrons*. *Bird Behaviour* 5:103–109.

Smith, G.T., and D.A. Saunders. 1986. Clutch size and productivity in three sympatric species of cockatoo (Psittaciformes) in the south-west of Western Australia. *Australian Wildlife Research* 13:275–285.

Snyder, N.F.R., J.W. Wiley, and C.B. Kepler. 1987. *The parrots of Luquillo: Natural history and conservation of the Puerto Rican parrot.* Los Angeles: Western Foundation of Vertebrate Zoology.

Spoon, T.R. 2002. Reproductive success, parenting, and fidelity in a socially monogamous parrot (cockatiels, *Nymphicus hollandicus*): The influence of social relationships between mates. PhD diss., University of California, Davis.

Spoon, T.R., J.R. Millam, and D.H. Owings. 2004. Variation in the stability of cockatiel (*Nymphicus hollandicus*) pair relationships: The roles of males,

females, and mate compatibility. *Behaviour* 141: 1211–1234.

Spoon, T.R., J.R. Millam, and D.H. Owings. In press. The importance of mate behavioural compatibility in parenting and reproductive success by cockatiels (*Nymphicus hollandicus*). *Animal Behaviour.*

Stamm, R.A. 1962. Aspekte des Paarverhaltens von *Agapornis personata* (Aves, Psittacidae, Loriini). *Behaviour* 19:1–56.

Stamps, J., A. Clark, P. Arrowood, and B. Kus. 1985. Parent offspring conflict in budgerigars. *Behaviour* 94:1–40.

Striedter, G.F., L. Freibott, A.G. Hile, and N.T. Burley. 2003. For whom the male calls: An effect of audience on contact call rate and repertoire in budgerigars, *Melopsittacus undulatus*. *Animal Behaviour* 65:875–882.

Sutherland, W.J. 2002. Science, sex and the kakapo. *Nature* 419:265–266.

Taylor, S., and M.R. Perrin. 2004. Intraspecific associations of individual brown-headed parrots (*Poicephalus cryptoxanthus*). *African Zoology* 39:263–271.

Trillmich, F. 1976. Spatial proximity and mate specific behaviour in a flock of budgerigars (*Melopsittacus undulatus*, Aves, Psittacidae). *Zeitschrift fur Tierpsychologie* 41:307–331.

Waltman, J.R., and S.R. Beissinger. 1992. Breeding behavior of the green-rumped parrotlet. *Wilson Bulletin* 104:65–84.

Wanker, R., J. Apein, B. Jennerjahn, and B. Waibel. 1998. Discrimination of different social companions in spectacled parrotlets (*Forpus conspicillatus*): Evidence for individual vocal recognition. *Behavioral Ecology and Sociobiology* 43:197–202.

Wanker, R., B.L. Cruz, and D. Franck. 1996. Socialization of spectacled parrotlets *Forpus conspicillatus*: The role of parents, crèches and sibling groups in nature. *Journal of Ornithology* 137:447–461.

Wilkinson, R., and T.R. Birkhead. 1995. Copulation behaviour in the Vasa parrots *Coracopsis vasa* and *C. nigra*. *Ibis* 137:117–119.

Wright, T.F., and M. Dorin. 2001. Pair duets in the yellow-naped amazon (Psittaciformes: *Amazona auropalliata*): Responses to playbacks of different dialects. *Ethology* 107:111–124.

Yamamato, J.T., K.M. Shields, J.R. Millam, T.E. Roudybush, and C.R. Grau. 1989. Reproductive activity of force-paired cockatiels (*Nymphicus hollandicus*). *Auk* 106:86–93.

Zann, R. 1965. Behavioural studies of the quarrion (*Nymphicus hollandicus*). B.S. thesis, University of New England, Armidale, New South Wales.

9
Nest Box Preferences

Scott George Martin and April Romagnano

SUMMARY

Traditionally, cavity-type nest boxes are preferred over all other options for captive breeding of most psittacine species. These species indeed have greater reproductive success when they are given cavity-type boxes. The basis for this information is largely field studies. The idea of the cavity-type nest boxes is an extrapolation from the wild, where the majority of psittacine birds nest in living trees. However, one scientific study, conducted by the first author, exists in the literature and corroborates this choice. This study also gives alternatives to improve reproductive success for the naive (first-time layers), the recently non-breeding, and the floor-laying psittacine birds, instead of re-pairing or even culling these potentially reproductively successful birds. However, other studies have shown that the efficacy of nest boxes may depend upon early experience with them since Cockatiel chicks parent-reared without nest boxes, or hand-reared by humans, do not readily use cavity-type nest boxes as adults. This problem will certainly be exacerbated with increasing numbers of hand-reared psittacine birds going into captive breeding situations.

REVIEW OF THE NEST BOX SELECTION STUDY

The demand for captively bred parrots for the pet bird market is ever increasing due to the trade bans imposed in response to the threatened or endangered status of the majority of psittacine species, and due to the increasing popularity of birds as pets.[3] Birds are now the third most common pet in the United States and their popularity is growing. Further, since nearly all psittacine birds are cavity nesters in the wild, it is especially important to understand problems relating to nest box use in captivity to increase reproductive efficiency.[3].

For many temperate-zone birds, variation in the photoperiod is known to provide the most important initial cue for control of the reproductive cycle.[3, 4, 5] However, photoperiod is often supplemented by other proximate factors to initiate reproduction.[3] This is especially true for cavity-nesting parrots, for which provision of a nest box is perhaps the most important environmental stimulus available to induce reproductive development. Further, it has been shown that maximum levels of serum-luteinizing hormone in female Cockatiels is only achieved when a combination of photostimulation, nest box access, and full mate access is available.[3–5] Other studies have shown that the efficacy of nest boxes may depend upon early experience with them since Cockatiel chicks reared without nest boxes did not readily use them as adults.[4] Further, Cockatiel chicks reared in nest boxes by parents are far more likely to use nest boxes as adults, when compared to chicks hand-reared by humans and lacking early exposure to nest boxes.[3, 4] With the increase in domestically hand-reared birds that subsequently go on to be breeders, initiating successful reproduction and use of the cavity-type nest boxes are likely to become progressively problematic.

Characteristics of nest boxes such as size, shape, construction material, location, and interior light intensity all influence nest box selection in different species of psittacine birds (Figure 9.1 and Table 9-1).[1–3, 6, 7] In communal groups, Cockatiels prefer higher nest boxes, and those with smaller nest entrances, over lower nest boxes and those with larger entrances.[3] Preferential nest-site selection involving a variety of nest-site

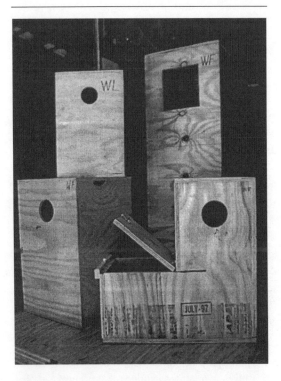

Figure 9.1. Some basic nest box types. Upper left is a vertical box (VB), as is the one below; these VBs come in various sizes depending on the species. The upper right-hand box is a horizontal macaw (HM) and is always 16″ x 16″ x 48″. The lower right-hand box is known as an L-shaped or boot box. WF stands for wire front and WL stands for wire ladder.

characteristics has been observed in several species.[1–3, 6, 7] However, occasionally individual psittacine birds may choose nesting sites that resemble neither natural nor artificially provided ones. Floor laying is an example of such an aberrant nest-site selection behavior. This behavior decreases hatchability through either egg surface or interior contamination secondary to egg soiling or minor cracks or breakage. In captive parrots floor laying is most common in the smaller species. This behavior is costly and considered maladaptive.

The etiology of floor laying is unknown, but this behavior can affect up to 25% of Cockatiel pairs in captive breeding colonies, despite the presence of conventional cavity-type nest boxes and proper long day photoperiod stimulation.[3] It is possible that such birds may have floor laid even if the two previously mentioned stimuli, cavity-type nest boxes and photostimulation, were absent. Since the etiology of this aberrant laying behavior has not been elucidated, and since it can be devastating from both a financial and a conservational standpoint, the first author conducted a study to address the nature of nest box selection in captivity. This study was composed of two experiments in which nest boxes of two different nest entrance types were offered as choices to Cockatiels with or without a history of floor laying, as well as to birds that had not laid in a previous breeding trial, and finally to reproductively naive birds. The nest box entrance types chosen

Table 9-1   Nest box types for different species

Species	Nest box type
Budgerigars, Cockatiels, Quaker Parrots, Lovebirds, Parrotlets, Grey- and Green-cheeked Parakeets, and numerous other smaller psittacine birds, Eclectus, Cockatoos of various sizes (except for Palm Cockatoos, who prefer a vertical open-top box 2′ x 2′ x 6′ [VO]), smaller Macaws, Conures, Amazons, Pionus, Caiques, hawk heads, thick-billed parrots and the lesser vasas	Will happily breed in VB boxes of various sizes
Large and medium-sized macaws and Greater Vasas	Will happily breed in HM boxes of various sizes
African Greys	Will happily breed in L-shaped or boot boxes that give a lot of privacy to the female and her young

were a small hole for the classic cavity-type nest boxes and a shelf-type entrance as the alternative.

NEST BOX SELECTION

In the nest box selection study, the nest box entrance preferences of Cockatiels were examined and recorded.[3] Some of the birds were historically floor layers, some were cavity-type layers, some had not recently laid, and the rest were reproductively naive (first-time layers).

The nest box entrances of the cavity-type nest boxes were circular and relatively small, while the entrances of shelf-type boxes were rectangular and relatively large (Figure 9.2).

The study found that birds with histories of laying in cavity-type boxes tended to choose cavity-type boxes again and repeated this preference, while those birds that were previously floor layers or had not recently laid tended to choose shelf-type boxes for their first clutches but later switched to cavity-type boxes for subsequent clutches. Hence, with reproductive experience afforded by the shelf-type nest box, these birds later, when they were more experienced layers, preferred the conventional cavity-type nest box. Reproductively naive Cockatiels were divided in their nest box preferences. Approximately one-third of the reproductively naive Cockatiels chose shelf-type boxes for their first clutches but increasingly used cavity-type boxes for subsequent clutches.

Further, it was noted that Cockatiels that laid in cavity-type boxes never switched to shelf-type boxes. Fertility, hatchability, and fledging success, defined as survival to three weeks of age, were all greater in cavity-type boxes, resulting in greater chick production.

The question that was asked, and that was clearly answered by this study, was whether there is a nest box selection preference among Cockatiels.[3] Cavity-type nest box selection was preferred by Cockatiels that had historically bred and used cavity nests. Further, naive, non-laying, and floor-laying Cockatiels also all eventually moved toward cavity-type nest boxes as their preferred nesting sites. The presence of the shelf-type nest box, however, initiated successful laying in these problem birds.

It has previously been noted that given the right materials, most all psittacine birds seek out or build cavity-type nests. This clear and universal

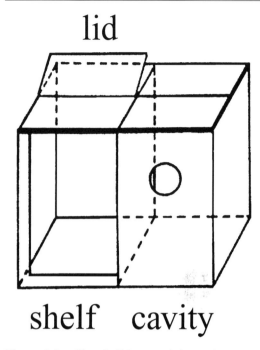

Figure 9.2. The shelf-type and the cavity-type nest box setup, used in the Cockatiel nest box selection study. They were installed side by side as depicted.

pattern leads one to believe that cavity-type nesting must be the closest to natural parrot nesting in wild populations.

WILD NESTS

According to Thompson, parrots in the wild nest in cavities that are primarily found in living trees, or they nest in cavities within dead trees.[6] It is clear that parrots prefer to lay their eggs in spaces that are cavity- or hole-like, so as to afford the eggs more protection from both predators and the environment.[6] New world birds use abandoned woodpecker nests, which are great for many of the smaller parrots. Larger parrots have a harder time finding appropriate-sized cavity nests that are abandoned.[6] Nesting cavities must accommodate the nesting female, her mate, and their potential young. Most psittacine young will grow to the size of their parents by weaning/fledging.[6]

Thompson also notes that a subgroup composed of various parrot and parrot-like species chooses nesting sites in cavities other than trees.[6] Some of these sites include tunnels in cliff sides, active and inactive termite mounds, and chambers or hollows found within the rocks on the ground. However, any parrot species that nests on the ground is more vulnerable and thus very endangered. Examples of ground-nesting psittacine birds include the Bahama Parrot and the Kakapo.[6]

CONCLUSION

The authors believe that given the results of the first author's nest box selection study and exploring the general nesting habits of different species of parrots in the wild, one can, and should, attempt to give each psittacine species a nest box choice, if the classic captive cavity-type nest boxes are unacceptable, that is, if the birds do not breed. Of course, this is assuming that the psittacine pair in question is a true pair, consisting of both a female and a male of the same species, and that they are sufficiently healthy for breeding. Hence, one should always attempt to match the natural nesting needs of captive psittacine birds first, and if this does not work, employ the shelf-type nest box choice to reintroduce or introduce the cavity-type nest box nesters, the naive, the non-layers, and the floor-laying birds to a suitable nest before thinking of re-pairing or culling birds. It is likely that most psittacine birds would benefit from a shelf-type nesting opportunity and then if also given the choice, as in the study, would likely eventually move toward cavity-type nest boxes as their preferred nesting site.

Since the etiology of rejecting the cavity-type nest box is unknown in captive, otherwise healthy true psittacine pairs, one would have to assume that experience plays a significant and growing role. It is well known that the fostering of natural behaviors, such as parental rearing in a cavity nest box if just for a brief period of time, is an approach that has been demonstrated to improve reproductive success and the general well-being of breeding psittacine birds.[7] Styles states that birds properly socialized to their own species are indeed superior in their reproductive abilities, while improperly socialized birds are much less likely to become successful breeders.[7]

The findings discussed in this chapter agree with other Cockatiel studies where the efficacy of cavity-type nest boxes appeared to depend upon early experience with them, in that parent-raised Cockatiel chicks reared without nest boxes and Cockatiel chicks hand-reared by humans and thus also lacking early exposure to nest boxes do not readily use them as adults. Hence, with the increase in domestically hand-reared birds that will subsequently go on to become domestic breeders, the likelihood of problem layers can be expected to increase.

REFERENCES

1. Clubb, S.L. 1997. "Avicultural medicine and flock health management." In *Avicultural medicine and surgery,* ed. R.B. Altman, S.L. Clubb, G.M. Dorrestein, and K. Quesenberry, pp. 101–116. Philadelphia: WB Saunders Co.
2. Johnson, T., and K. Clubb. 1992. "Aviary design and construction." In *Psittacine aviculture, perspectives, techniques and research,* ed. R.M. Schubot, K.J. Clubb, and S.L. Clubb S.L., pp. 4.1–4.12. Loxahatchee, FL: Avicultural Breeding and Research Center..
3. Martin, S.G., and J.R. Millam. 1995. Nest box selection by floor laying and reproductively naive captive cockatiels (*Nymphicus hollandicus*). *Appl Anim Behav Sci* 43:95–109.
4. Meyers, S.A., J.A. Millam, T.E. Roudybush, and C.R. Grau. 1988. Reproductive success of hand-reared vs parent reared cockatiels (*Nymphicus hollandicus*). *Auk* 105:536–542.
5. Millam, J.R., B. Zhang, and M.E. el Halawani. 1996. Egg production of cockatiels (*Nymphicus hollandicus*) is influenced by number of eggs in nest after incubation begins. *General and Comparative Endocrinology* 101 (2):205–210.
6. Thompson, D.R. 1998. "The importance of nest-boxes." International Aviculturists Society Convention.
7. Styles D. 2001. "Captive psittacine behavioral reproductive husbandry and management: Socialization, aggression control, and pairing techniques." Proceedings of the Association of Avian Veterinarians (Specialty Advanced Program), pp. 3–14.

10
Hand-Rearing: Behavioral Impacts and Implications for Captive Parrot Welfare

Rebecca Fox

INTRODUCTION

Since the Wild Bird Conservation Act of 1992 banned the importation of most wild-captured parrots into the United States, hand-rearing of domestically bred parrot chicks has become the dominant method of producing parrots for the pet trade. That hand-reared parrots are popular as pets should not be surprising: young hand-reared parrots are tame, apparently enjoy contact with humans, and seem much better adapted to life as a pet than do most parent-reared parrots (Millam 2000). Hand-reared parrots may be more likely to talk than parent-reared birds (see the "Social Behavior" section of this chapter). However, hand-rearing is time-intensive and technically demanding, and both the scientific and lay literature suggest that hand-reared birds may exhibit a number of behavioral abnormalities.

Hand-rearing requires that parrot chicks be separated from their parents for long periods of time (several weeks to several months, depending on the species). It has long been appreciated that even short-term separations are stressful (cf. Vazquez 1997 for examples in rats), and that disruptions in parental care can disrupt normal behavioral and physiological development (cf. Levine 2001; Capitanio 1986). In rat pups, maternal behavior during the first two to three weeks of life is critical to both the regulation of the pups' physiological state and to normal brain development (Meaney 2001, Levine 2001, Vazquez 1997). Even brief periods of maternal separation (greater than three hours) during the first two to three weeks of life are sufficient to produce long-lasting changes in responsiveness to stress and reactivity to novelty in rats and other mammals including mice and guinea pigs (Meaney 2001; Levine 2001; Albers et al. 2000; Vazquez 1997). These changes are primarily mediated by changes in the hypothalamic-pituitary-adrenal (HPA) axis induced by maternal separation (Francis et al. 2002; Meaney 2001; Levine 2001; Albers et al. 2000; Vazquez 1997; Biagini et al. 1998). Maternally-separated animals also experience delays in tissue growth and altered circadian rhythms, effects that are probably also mediated by increased HPA axis responsivity to stressors (high levels of glucocorticoids, which are produced when the HPA axis is activated by stress, have catabolic effects) (Biagini et al. 1998). Furthermore, maternal separation affects not only the separated animals themselves but their offspring as well. Meaney (2001) demonstrated that maternal behavior influences how rat pups will behave toward their own offspring.

Although maternal separation effects have not been directly demonstrated in parrots, some evidence suggests that these effects do occur. A study of growth rate differences in hand-reared and parent-reared chicks at Loro Parque suggests that parrots may respond to maternal separation with slower growth rates. In at least two psittacine species (*Ara rubrogenys, Pyhurra p. perlata*), hand-reared chicks show a growth-rate deficit similar to that of maternally-separated rat pups (Navarro & Castanon 2001). However, this deficit may be alleviated by leaving the chicks with the parents during the first week of life and beginning hand-rearing thereafter, suggesting some aspect of parental care during the first two weeks of life may be responsible for maintaining normal growth rates in parrots (Navarro & Castanon 2001).

Hand-reared parrots typically experience far longer periods of maternal separation than those that cause striking behavioral changes in mammals such as rats (separations of weeks to months for hand-reared parrots versus separations of hours in maternally-separated mammals in many experimental paradigms). Nursery-reared monkeys, which experience a comparable level of maternal separation to hand-reared parrots, frequently develop abnormal behaviors including self-mutilation (possibly analogous to feather picking in companion birds), increased responsivity to stress, and altered social behavior (Capitanio 1985).

Furthermore, hand-rearing deprives parrots of parental contact that may be required to establish normal social and sexual preferences. A number of studies (cf. Immelmann 1972, 1975 for reviews) have shown that the presence of parents is often a critical component of the development of normal species identity and sexual imprinting. Sexual imprinting refers to the process by which animals learn the characteristics of appropriate mates by learning the characteristics of their parents or siblings. Among parrots, Galahs (*Cacatua roseicapilla)* naturally cross-fostered to the sympatric Leadbeater's Cockatoo (*C. leadbeateri*) apparently imprint on their foster parents and associate solely with *C. leadbeateri* individuals during adulthood (Rowley & Chapman 1986). Cross-fostered Galahs also choose to mate with *C. leadbeateri*, suggesting that sexual imprinting does occur in these species and may be disrupted by changing the neonatal environment (Rowley & Chapman 1986). Anecdotal evidence suggests that sexual imprinting may occur in a number of parrot species, including Budgerigars (*Melopsittacus undulatus*) and Senegal Parrots (*Poicephalus senegalus senegalus*) (Klinghammer 1967). Thus, hand-rearing may also have negative reproductive consequences.

In this chapter, I will discuss two studies of the reproductive and behavioral consequences of hand-rearing in Cockatiels (*Nymphicus hollandi-*

cus) and Orange-winged Amazon Parrots (*Amazona amazonica*). The first study, conducted by Myers et al. (1988), examined differences in nesting behavior and reproductive success in hand-reared and parent-reared Cockatiels. The second study is part of my own research, and examined differences in social preferences, vocal behavior, and neophobia (fear of novel objects) in 3-month-old to 12-month-old hand-reared and parent-reared parrots. I will also discuss the possible welfare consequences of hand-rearing for captive parrots.

BEHAVIORAL DIFFERENCES IN HAND-REARED VERSUS PARENT-REARED PARROTS

Reproductive Behavior

Rowley and Chapman (1986) suggest that parental identity strongly influences the learning of species identity and sexual imprinting in parrots. Sexual imprinting refers to a process by which exposure to certain characteristics early in life increases an animal's preferences for those characteristics in a mate. Furthermore, habitat imprinting may be important for parrots to learn the characteristics of appropriate nest sites. Habitat imprinting refers to a process in which exposure to a particular habitat feature early in development increases preference for that feature later in life. Hand-reared parrots, which are generally reared in brooders and fed by humans, are deprived of the opportunity to learn the characteristics of appropriate nest sites and mates and can show inappropriate reproductive behavior (Myers et al. 1988). In Cockatiels (*Nymphicus hollandicus*), hand-rearing decreases reproductive success by altering both nesting behavior and normal sexual behavior (see Table 10-1), probably because maternal separation disrupts normal sexual and habitat imprinting (Myers et al. 1988).

Maternal separation (i.e., hand-rearing) disrupts habitat imprinting in both male and female Cockatiels. Some effects of hand-rearing on nesting behavior were sex-specific: hand-reared (H) males were less likely to inspect nest boxes than parent-reared (P) males, but the female's rearing condition had no effect on nest inspection (Myers et al. 1988). However, both the male's and the female's rearing condition influences where a pair chooses to lay their eggs. The mates of H-males

Table 10-1   Comparison of reproductive behavior and success in hand-reared (H) and parent-reared (P) cockatiels (modified from Myers et al. 1988)

	Nest inspection by male	Floor laying by female	Egg fertility	Overall RS*
H-male	Low	High	Lower	Lower
P-male	High	Low	Higher	Higher
H-female	No difference	High	No difference	No difference
P-female	No difference	Low	No difference	No difference

*RS: Reproductive success, defined by the number of offspring surviving to fledging.

were about three times more likely to lay eggs on the cage floor rather than in the nest box, regardless of rearing condition. Early experience in females also influences where they choose to lay their eggs—floor laying was more common in pairs containing H-females than in pairs containing P-females (Myers et al. 1988).

Hand-rearing apparently influences sexual imprinting in males more strongly than in females. H-male pairs have significantly lower egg fertility and reproductive success when compared to P-male pairs, presumably because males exhibit abnormal courtship behavior or copulation (Myers et al. 1988). However, normal sexual imprinting is apparently less critical for female receptivity, as H-females did not exhibit significantly impaired reproductive success relative to P-females (Myers et al. 1988). Because the Cockatiels used in this study were force-paired, hand-rearing may have effects on mate choice in females that were not detected (Myers et al 1988).

Hand-rearing/maternal separation causes sex-specific disruptions in normal sexual behavior in parrots. In males, nest box recognition and use are impaired, and normal copulatory behavior is probably impaired as well (Myers et al. 1988). Certainly, hand-rearing has a significant negative effect on a male's reproductive success. The behavioral disruptions in females seem to be less serious. Although hand-reared females exhibit higher levels of floor laying, the reproductive success of pairs containing H-females is not impaired relative to P-female pairs.

Social Behavior

SOCIAL PREFERENCES

Abnormal sexual behavior may be broadly related to disruptions in normal social preferences induced by hand-rearing. My recent work, which

compared the behavior of hand-reared and parent-reared Orange-winged Amazon Parrots (*Amazona amazonica*) suggests that hand-rearing alters social preferences and normal vocalizations in juvenile (3–12 months of age) Orange-winged Amazons.

Hand-reared parrots exhibit a strong preference for social contact with humans and reduced preferences for contact with conspecifics. When a hand-reared Amazon is placed in a choice cage with a human handler to one side and two parrots in their home cage to the other, the hand-reared bird will perch on the side of the cage nearest the handler significantly more frequently than predicted by chance. Conversely, non-tame parent-reared birds perch on the side of the cage nearest conspecifics significantly more often than predicted by chance. Parent-reared birds that have been tamed by occasional neonatal handling (e.g., Aengus & Millam 1999) exhibit approximately equal preference for human and conspecific companionship, suggesting that while tameness influences social preferences in parrots, hand-rearing disrupts social preferences to a much greater extent (see Figure 10.1).

VOCAL BEHAVIOR

Parent-reared and hand-reared birds also differed considerably in the extent and the speed with which they acquired human vocalizations, suggesting that hand-rearing may also disrupt normal vocal development in parrots. Three of six Orange-winged Amazons hand-reared in 2001 began mimicking human vocalizations while still in the nursery (i.e., before three months of age), and the remaining three birds began mimicking human speech in the presence of experimenters by four months of age. Of the parent-reared birds, only two of the five birds that had been tamed by

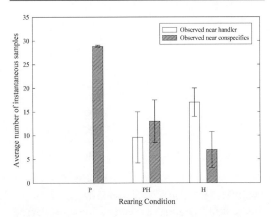

Figure 10.1. Numbers of instantaneous samples (mean ± S.E.) in which hand-reared (H), parent-reared with human handling (PH), and parent-reared (P) birds were observed perching near either a familiar handler or near a cage containing two conspecifics during a preference test. Each subject's location in the test cage was recorded every 30 seconds for 15 minutes.

Table 10-2 Human vocalizations used by 3- to 12-month-old hand-reared and parent-reared Orange-winged Amazons

Bird	Vocalizations
Valentine	"step up," "hello," "hi," "good bird," "squeak," "hi, Val," kissing noises, various whistles
Squeeker	"step up," "hello," "good bird," "good boy," "good Squeeker," "squeak," "hi, Val," "Squeeker," kissing noises, various whistles
Julian	"step up," "hello," "hi," "good boy," "good girl," various whistles, kissing noises, "brrrring!"
Andy	"step up," "hello," "hi," "good," "good boy," "good girl," "good boygirl," "good bird," "I love you," "Andy," "what doing," various whistles, kissing noises, "brrrring!"
Kelly	"step up," "hi," "good girl," "good bird," kissing noises, various whistles, "brring!"
Taylor	"step up," "hi," "good boy"
Mackenzie*	"Step up," "hi," "brrrr"
Robin*	"Step up," "hi," kissing noise

*Parent-reared bird.

neonatal handling ever mimicked human speech in the presence of humans, and they did not do so until six to nine months of age. The two parent-reared birds that did develop human vocalizations were also qualitatively the tamest of the parent-reared group. Hand-reared birds also developed far more extensive repertoires than did parent-reared birds (see Table 10-2).

The high levels of human mimicry exhibited by the hand-reared birds are probably related to several factors, of which extensive exposure to human speech and the perception of human contact as rewarding are probably the most pertinent. Early removal from the nest also seems to prevent the learning of species-typical vocalizations (hand-reared birds do not develop the loud high-pitched call typical of Orange-winged Amazons until they have been housed with normally vocalizing birds for at least a week), and human sounds may thus occupy a larger-than-normal part of hand-reared birds' repertoires.

Research by Pepperberg et al. (1998) and West and King (1990) suggests that the learning of human vocalizations by mimetic species such as parrots and starlings is heavily dependent on social interaction with humans. Hand-reared birds, which are fed as many as five times/day or more

during the first few months of life, have much more extensive contact with humans than do parent-reared birds: even those birds that have been reared under neonatal handling paradigms are only handled five times/week for approximately 20 minutes/session. Because the hand-reared birds have more extensive contact with humans, they also have more opportunities to learn human vocalizations. It also seems reasonable that those birds that find human attention especially rewarding will be more likely to use human vocalizations in the presence of people (e.g., Pepperberg 1999). The hand-reared Orange-winged Amazons in this study appeared to use human vocalizations to elicit human attention. They typically vocalized when an experimenter or handler entered the room, and they often used human vocalizations during handling sessions. These vocalizations generally elicited increased attention, or at least a vocal response, from the human handlers. The parrots' human vocalizations were typically accompanied by excited displays such as rapid pupil dilation and contraction ("pinpointing"), head and neck feather erection, and tail fanning. Parrot "speech" is likely related to extensive exposure to human speech and reinforced by operant conditioning in which human attention serves as the reward. Hand-reared birds are, in general, more likely to talk and less likely to exhibit normal vocalizations than are parent-reared birds, even those that have been tamed by neonatal handling.

Neophobia

Maternal separation and hand-rearing affect not only social preferences and learned vocalizations but may also change the developmental trajectory for certain behaviors. Neophobia refers to the avoidance of novel objects and/or foods by animals and is related to animals' reactivity to novelty (cf. Meaney 2001). Less neophobic animals will approach a novel object more readily than more neophobic animals and will exhibit higher levels of exploratory behavior in a novel environment. Neophobia probably represents an adaptive response for avoiding potentially poisonous food items and predators, and, at least in ravens, seems to develop after juveniles are weaned and their food preferences have solidified (Heinrich 1998).

In order to distinguish neophobia from a lack of interest in novel items, I tested hand-reared and parent-reared birds by presenting them with a dish of peanuts (a highly favored food) over which a novel object had been hung. Novel objects included a green plastic mug, a blue toy dump truck, a large black cooking spoon, and a toy elephant. The birds' latency to approach the dish/novel object combination was measured and used as an index of neophobia. More neophobic birds would presumably take longer to approach the dish /novel object combination than would less neophobic birds.

After a two-week habituation period in which the birds were habituated to the dish of peanuts alone, five consecutive tests in which the birds were presented with the dish and a novel object were administered approximately ten days apart when the chicks were approximately 135–180 days old. Striking differences in neophobia were apparent in parent-reared and hand-reared birds throughout most of the testing period (Figure 10.2). Parent-reared birds were already somewhat neophobic by 135 days and showed latencies of a

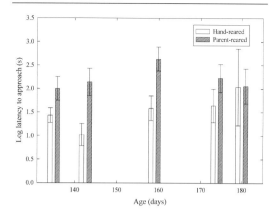

Figure 10.2. Latencies (mean ± S.E.) to approach and feed from a dish of favored food in the presence of a novel object for parent-reared and hand-reared birds in a series of five tests administered between the ages of 135 and 180 days. Data were log-transformed to homogenize variance. Repeated-measures ANOVA showed that latencies differed significantly between parent-reared and hand-reared birds ($F_{1,17} = 9.25$, $P = 0.007$).

several minutes to approach the dish + object combination. Conversely, hand-reared birds approached the dish + object combination within a few seconds. Neophobia (latency to approach the dish + novel object combination) peaked at 160 days in parent-reared birds and then began to decline, but neophobia remained low in hand-reared birds until 180 days, when hand-reared birds abruptly began reacting fearfully to novel objects. However, the behavior of hand-reared birds at one year of age suggests that hand-rearing only delays the onset of neophobic behavior in hand-reared birds but does not permanently alter the level of neophobia; 12-month-old hand-reared and parent-reared birds behave very similarly in response to novelty. When presented with a novel toy, 12-month-old hand-reared and parent-reared birds displayed comparable levels of fearful behavior when their behavior was scored on a scale of 0 (approach toy) to 5 (frantic attempts to escape) (Figure 10.3).

The differences in neophobia may be due either to delayed maturation in the hand-reared birds or to a more generalized habituation to novelty. Research in rats has shown that maternal separa-

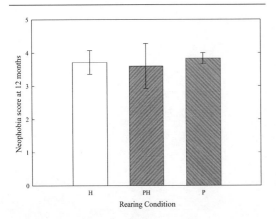

Figure 10.3. Neophobia scores (mean ± S.E.) for parent-reared (P), parent-reared with human handling (PH), and hand-reared (H) birds when presented with a novel object at 12 months of age. A score of 0 represents immediate approach to the toy, while a score of 5 represents frantic attempts to avoid the toy. Neophobia scores did not differ significantly between the three rearing conditions.

tion early in life acts to disrupt or delay the maturation of certain regions of the amygdala that relate to stress reactivity and responsivity to novelty (Vazquez 1997, Levine 2001). In birds, the medial archistriatum controls fearfulness and reactivity to novelty, and lesions of the medial archistriatum greatly reduce fearfulness in wild birds (Butler & Hodos 1996). Similar effects are seen in rhesus macaques with neonatal lesions to the central nucleus of the amygdala, who exhibit very low levels of behavioral inhibition in response to stimuli that induce fearful behavior in normal macaques (Prather et al. 2001). It is possible that maternal separation affects the maturation of the medial archistriatum in parrots, leading to greatly reduced levels of neophobia in parrots. However, hand-reared birds also generally experience higher levels of novelty (different caregivers, more extreme changes in light level, exposure to a greater variety of objects, etc.) during the nestling period than do parent-reared birds, which remain in a dark nest box until fledging. The reduced neophobia displayed by young hand-reared birds could simply reflect an adaptation to novelty.

After weaning, the parent-reared and hand-reared birds were housed under identical conditions, so the disappearance of behavioral differences between the two groups may be related to a phenomenon described by Francis et al. (2002), in which environmental conditions (in this case, enrichment) can reverse the effects of maternal separation in prepubertal rats. Alternatively, although the birds were provided with toys, the toys were changed relatively infrequently (every few months), and the level of novelty experienced by the hand-reared birds may not have been sufficient to maintain low levels of neophobia that they exhibited at the beginning of the study.

Summary

From a behavioral perspective, hand-rearing reliably produces tame, human-habituated birds that tend to talk more than do parent-reared birds. For this reason, young hand-reared birds are quite appealing as companion animals. However, hand-rearing is also a potent disrupter of normal behavioral development in Cockatiels and Orange-winged Amazons (see Table 10-3). Hand-rearing can cause abnormalities in sexual behavior and nesting, especially in male Cockatiels. These abnormalities are probably related to abnormal sexual and habitat imprinting (Myers et al. 1988). Anecdotal evidence suggests that hand-reared parrots frequently imprint sexually on humans and may even prefer to court their owners over conspecifics. Certainly, hand-rearing alters social preferences to a much greater degree than does

Table 10-3 Summary of behavioral differences between hand-reared and parent-reared Cockatiels and Orange-winged Amazon parrots

	Nest recognition	Social preference	Human vocalizations	Onset of neophobia
Hand-reared	Poor	Humans	Common	6 months of age
Parent-reared	Normal	Con-specifics	Rare	On or before 4.5 months of age

taming by neonatal handling, with hand-reared birds showing a much stronger preference for human companionship than neonatally-handled birds. Hand-reared Orange-winged Amazons also show developmental differences in neophobia, with hand-reared birds developing a fear of novel objects much later than parent-reared birds. However, when parent-reared and hand-reared birds are housed under identical conditions, differences in neophobic behavior disappear by the time the birds are 12 months of age.

IMPLICATIONS FOR PARROTS IN CAPTIVITY

Breeding Programs

Because of restrictions on the importation of wild parrots imposed by the Wild Bird Conservation Act, the success of breeding programs in the United States (both for conservation purposes and for the purpose of producing parrots for the pet trade) rests on the continued availability of reproductively competent domestically raised parrots. Because hand-reared Cockatiels show a number of abnormalities in reproductive behavior and the reproductive success of hand-reared Cockatiels paired with hand-reared Cockatiels is extremely low (Myers et al. 1988), it is likely shortsighted to emphasize the production of hand-reared birds over more reproductively normal parent-reared birds. The loss of wild-captured breeding stock to age or disease could be disastrous, especially for those species that are rare or difficult to breed in captivity, unless healthy, reproductively normal parent-reared birds are available to replace them.

However, Myers et al. (1988) also showed that the reproductive success of hand-reared birds (at least Cockatiels) can be improved by pairing them with a parent-reared, reproductively normal partner. This is particularly true for female parrots (Myers et al. 1988). Careful pairing of hand-reared birds with more experienced parent-reared mates may help to mitigate the effects of hand-rearing on reproductive behavior. Unfortunately, hand-reared birds may also be more difficult to pair than parent-reared birds, since they exhibit greatly reduced preference for conspecific companionship.

Companion Parrots

Young hand-reared parrots seem like the perfect pet: tame, talking parrots that have little fear of new things and are quite willing to interact with humans. However, hand-rearing may also be at the root of a number of behavior problems in companion parrots.

Hand-rearing alters Orange-winged Amazons' social preferences and sexual behavior and may lead to hand-reared parrots inappropriately directing sexual behavior (both courtship behavior and aggression) toward humans. Anecdotally, sexual aggression directed at humans is common in a number of parrot species, especially in male amazon parrots and male cockatoos. Similarly, parrot owners often report that their parrots regurgitate for them or attempt to masturbate against their owners' hands or bodies. Although a strong social preference for humans may be endearing in a parrot chick, sexual aggression and inappropriate sexual behavior can be problematic in older birds.

Hand-rearing may also be related to the "phobic" behavior that has been recently described in pet parrots. In the lay literature, phobic behavior is defined as a behavior pattern in which "a previously tame and affectionate parrot 'suddenly' seems afraid of almost everything and everyone" (Blanchard 2001). This sudden, apparently inexplicable, fearfulness usually appears in hand-reared birds around the age at which they would typically become independent of their parents in the wild (Blanchard 2001). "Phobic" or anxious parrots often injure themselves trying to avoid aversive stimuli, often breaking blood feathers and injuring their keels in repeated falls (Clark 2001). Obviously, the sudden appearance of such extreme and apparently unexplainable fearful behavior in a previously fearless bird can be disconcerting and would certainly appear pathological.

This pattern seems analogous to the pattern observed in the Orange-winged Amazons, in which hand-reared birds exhibited markedly low levels of neophobia for at least two months longer than did parent-reared birds. Furthermore, the onset of neophobia in the hand-reared birds was quite sudden. In the week between the fourth and fifth novel object tests, hand-reared birds' latencies to approach the novel object/dish combination showed a striking increase (Figure 10.2). Although this sudden appearance of avoidance behavior may seem startling, the fact that hand-reared and parent-reared birds react almost identically to a novel toy at 12 months of age suggests that this "sudden" fearfulness may actually represent normal, if delayed, maturation. Although "phobic" behavior may not actually be pathological, the lay literature (cf. Blanchard 2001; Clark 2001) suggests that pet owners find it extremely disturbing, and the increased chance of injury during this "phobic" period is a very real risk.

CONCLUSION

Hand-reared parrot chicks are endearing, often talkative, and fearless. However, this period of outgoing fearlessness is only temporary. By one year of age, hand-reared and parent-reared Orange-winged Amazons behave identically in response to a novel object, suggesting that the period in which hand-reared birds appear particularly well adapted to captivity may only be temporary. Furthermore, hand-reared Cockatiels show serious deficits in reproductive behavior that are probably related to abnormal sexual and/or habitat imprinting (Myers et al. 1988). Abnormal sexual imprinting and a strong social preference for humans may cause behavior problems in pet parrots, which are probably more likely to inappropriately direct sexual behavior at their owners. Hand-reared birds may exhibit other behavior problems as well, most notably so-called "phobic" behavior. Hand-rearing is also time intensive (hand-reared parrots often must be fed several times a day for several months), technically demanding, and risky (aspiration of hand-rearing formula can kill or sicken chicks very quickly).

However, research has shown that occasional (four to five times/week for 30 minutes) handling of parent-reared Orange-winged Amazon chicks between two weeks of age and fledging also produces tame chicks that are less responsive to stress than birds that have been parent-reared without handling (cf. Aengus & Millam 1999). Because neonatally handled birds that remain in the nest have much more contact with parents and siblings than they do with humans, it is also likely that they will show normal reproductive behavior at maturity (Aengus & Millam 1999). Neonatal handling also requires far less time, effort, and expense (in terms of hand-rearing supplies and equipment) than does hand-rearing and may represent a viable alternative for producing parrots for the pet trade.

REFERENCES

Aengus, W.L., and J.R. Millam. 1999. Taming parent-reared orange-winged amazon parrots by neonatal handling. *Zoo Biology* 18: 177–187.

Albers, P.C.H., P.J.A. Timmermans, and J.M.H. Vossen. 2000. Effects of frequency and length of separation bouts between mother and offspring on later explorative behaviour of young guinea-pigs (*Cavia aperea f. porcellus*). *Behaviour* 137:1487–1502.

Biagini, G., E.M. Pich, P. Carani, P. Marrama, and L.F. Agnati. 1998. Postnatal maternal separation during the stress hyporesponsive period enhances the adrenocortical response to novelty in adult rats by affecting feedback regulation in the ca1 hippocampal field. *International Journal of Developmental Neuroscience* 16:187–197.

Blanchard, S. 2001. Working with phobic parrots. *Companion Parrot Quarterly* 54:43.

Butler, A.B., and W. Hodos. 1996. *Comparative vertebrate neuroanatomy*. New York: Wiley-Liss.

Capitanio, J.P. 1986. "Behavioral pathology." In *Comparative primate biology. Volume 2A: Conservation and ecology,* ed. G. Mitchell and J. Erwin, pp. 411–454. Alan R. Liss, Inc.

Clark, P. 2001. A vicious cycle: Helping the anxious parrot. *Companion Parrot Quarterly* 54:70–79.

Francis, D.D., J. Diorio, D. Liu, and M.J. Meaney. 1999. Nongenomic transmission across generations of maternal behavior and stress responses in the rat. *Science* 286:1155–1158.

Francis, D.D., J. Diorio, P.M. Plotsky, and M.J. Meaney. 2002. Environmental enrichment reverses the effects of maternal separation on stress reactivity. *Journal of Neuroscience* 22:7840–7843.

Heinrich, B. 1998. *Mind of the raven: Adventures and investigations with wolf-birds*. New York: Cliff Street Books.

Immelmann, K. 1972. Sexual and other long-term aspects of imprinting in birds and other species. *Advances in the Study of Behavior* 4:147–174.

Immelmann, K. 1975. Ecological significance of imprinting and early learning. *Annual Review of Ecological Systems* 6:15–37.

Klinghammer, E. 1967. "Factors influencing choice of mate in altricial birds." In *Early behavior: Cooperative and developmental approaches,* ed. H.W. Stevenson, pp. 5–42. New York: Wiley.

Levine, S. 2001. Primary social relationships influence the development of the hypothalamic-pituitary-adrenal axis in the rat. *Physiology and Behavior* 73:255–260.

Meaney, M.J. 2001. Maternal care, gene expression, and the transmission of individual differences in stress reactivity across generations. *Annual Review of Neuroscience* 24: 1161–1192.

Millam, J.R. 2000. Neonatal handling, behaviour, and reproduction in orange-winged amazons and cockatiels *Amazona amazonica* and *Nymphicus hollandicus* at the Department of Animal Science, University of California. *International Zoo Yearbook* 37:220–231.

Myers, S.A., J.R. Millam, T.E. Roudybush, and C.R. Grau. 1988. Reproductive success of hand-reared vs. parent-reared cockatiels (*Nymphicus hollandicus*). *Auk* 105:536–542.

Navarro, A., and I. Castanon. 2001. Comparative study of the growth rates of hand-raised and parent-raised psittacids in Loro Parque Fundacion. *Cyanopsitta* 60:12–16.

Pepperberg, I.M. 1999. *The Alex studies*. Boston: Harvard University Press.

Pepperberg, I.M, J.R. Baughton, and P.A. Banta. 1998. Allospecific vocal learning by grey parrots (*Psittacus erithacus*): A failure of videotaped instruction under certain conditions. *Journal of Comparative Psychology* 109:182–195.

Prather, M.D., M.L. Lavenex, W. Mauldin-Jourdain, A. Mason, J.P. Capitanio, S.P. Mendoza, and D.G. Amaral. 2001. Increased social fear and decreased fear of objects in monkeys with neonatal amygdala lesions. *Neuroscience* 106:653–658.

Rowley, I., and G. Chapman. 1986. Cross-fostering, imprinting, and learning in two sympatric species of cockatoo. *Behaviour* 96:1–16.

Vazquez, D.M. 1997. Stress and the developing limbic-hypothalamic-pituitary-adrenal axis. *Psychoneuroendocrinology* 23:663–700.

West, M.J., and A.P. King. 1990. Mozart's starling. *American Scientist* 78:106–114.

11
Behavioral Development of Psittacine Companions: Neonates, Neophytes, and Fledglings

Phoebe Greene Linden with Andrew U. Luescher

Once you have flown,/ you will walk the Earth with your eyes turned skyward;/ for there you have been,/ and there you long to return.

—Leonardo DaVinci

INTRODUCTION

Psittacine development progresses along a predictable path wherein certain behaviors become apparent in the young birds as parallel physical attributes mature. Simply put, when their eyes open, they begin to see, so eye-opening time is the ideal time for human caretakers to provide environmental enhancements that encourage visual acuity. Likewise, when we see pre-fledglings flap their fully feathered wings and hover over a perch, we provide an environment suitable for safe fledging. The fledging process itself contributes in many ways to long-term success for psittacine companions because during fledging, early behaviors culminate in a fully active animal totally engaged in and interactive with its environment, including human caretakers.

The environment is thought to have a strong impact on young animals, and experiences during a relatively short period early in the animal's life may have lasting effects on how the animal will react later in life (Levine 1962; Escorihuela et al. 1995). This also holds true for parrots (Coulton et al. 1997; Nicol & Pope 1993; Sheehan 2001).

No matter the stage—from egg to aviary—the environment provided to domestically situated psittacine birds is largely controlled by humans, with the notable exceptions of weather and nature.

We offer reinforcement suitable for us, not them, when we enrich our home-based situations to encourage desirable and ignore undesirable behaviors. In the ideal environment, changes are expected, welcomed, and result in an increase in positive behavior. Ridley suggests that genes and behavior are interdependent in that genes are "active during life; [genes] switch one another on and off; they respond to the environment" (Ridley 2003).

I intend to describe the initial behaviors of psittacine hatchlings, or neonates, who kick themselves free of their eggs and quickly grow into fuzzy babies. Next, their eyes open and they begin to look at the world around them. Soon their legs are capable of carrying their body weight; they learn to climb onto the edge of a box to look around, flap their growing wings, and vocalize with their neighbors. By the time they fledge, they actively participate in their surroundings, and it's this environment that becomes the testing and proving grounds of companion behavior. Invariably, the most "thoughtfully arranged environments" (Friedman 2002) where parrots live show telltale signs of birds. Play gyms in the family room, organic pellets in the cupboard, a perch in the shower; parrots have a way of taking over our homes with the same ease that they capture our attention with their showy plumage and antics.

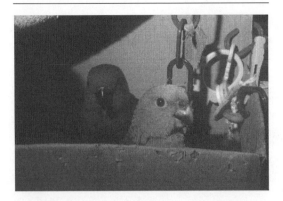

Figure 11.1. Neophyte parrots such as this young Amazon and Eclectus look out of their towel-covered box. (Photo by Layne David Dicker, courtesy of Santa Barbara Bird Farm.)

THOUGHTFUL ARRANGEMENT OF THE ENVIRONMENT

From hatchling to fledgling, young psittacines methodically use a thoughtfully arranged environment to set in motion a fascinating series of identifiable developmental progressions that respond to experience through constant reorganization and rebuilding (Ridley 2003; Figure 11.1). Under the right conditions, tiny neonates who seem helpless grow into competent fledglings. As they grow, the skills of psittacine birds are demonstrated through learned behaviors. We will examine only the most observable in this text.

Thoughtful caregivers keep the environment suitable for keen interaction with the birds as they change and develop. For example, we put away baby cuddle toys and boxes to make room for fledgling landing spots when fledging is imminent. We offer diets for a variety of age-appropriate circumstances; we'd no more encourage a 15-month-old cockatoo to take food from a syringe than we'd expect a newly hatched baby to chew through a guava branch. Friedman suggests that the developmental process should be one rich with opportunities to "select and strengthen dendrites for companion behavior and let others for free-ranging behavior fall off the brain-tree" (S.G. Friedman, personal communication, 2003). As a caregiver of young psittacine birds, I think often about which behaviors seen in young birds enhance, and which detract from, lifelong com-

panionship with humans. Once we find out what is reinforcing to our birds—depending upon their age and circumstance—and provide those items and interactions, we can deliberately select behaviors that increase a bird's success in the environment of the human home.

Although this chapter concerns itself with youngsters, it is also pertinent to adult companions. The rigorous environmental, nutritional, and interactive demands that neonates make are mimicked by the equally unapologetic demands made by highly functioning psittacine adults. Babies require warmth, humidity, food, and care in carefully calibrated amounts without which a panoply of complications can result. Psittacine caregivers are wise to avail themselves of species-specific neonatal protocols when rearing babies. As we observe our neonates, we want to encourage behaviors identified as desirable in companions and discourage those that undermine companionship. In these ways, I suggest that appropriate experiences in early developmental periods can help acclimate birds toward growth into successful companions.

This approach fosters more bird-like attributes than those historically accepted in many homes because this formula encourages birds to fly, forage for food, make predictable but not persevering noises, be reasonably social to strangers and continue to make decisions regarding their daily actions and reactions. Avian companions I have raised fly to people of their own volition, because they desire interaction. This methodology does not result in cookie-cutter companions but the reverse. When raised in environments tailored toward their growth, psittacine companions develop individual personalities, preferences, and propensities.

A Case Study of One

I describe the 240+ psittacine species currently identified by scientists as one group with specific references made to individual birds as experience and space allows. Behavioral scientist Susan Friedman, PhD, advises that each student of behavior examine his or her subjects best when the subjects are considered "a case study of one" (Friedman 2002). When we account for individuality in this manner, we include considerations of the specific set of genetics and environmental influences in order to see each animal distinct from others. This is not to say, however, that knowledge accumulated over years from many subjects is superfluous. Indeed, experience both widens and hones our abilities so that careful observers consider more influences on individual behavior, not fewer.

Designed to Be Wild; Bred to Be Captive

For many years I actively cared for psittacine neonates, some only minutes from the egg. Others benefited from early parental care. What follows are my observations of these companions who are designed to be wild and fly but who are bred to be tamed and clipped.

One large contrast between wild and domestic parrots, for example, is that wild psittacines eventually achieve total independence from their parents but captive psittacines do not gain such freedom from their caregivers. Parrots in domestic situations remain dependent upon their caregivers, who may sometimes supply and sometimes withhold rewards. Often, reinforcements offered to captive parrots are commensurate with human values, not psittacine sensibilities. Sometimes captivity and companionship mingle uneasily for parrots and people, especially for persons who are unaware of the lifelong dependence inherent in caring for such a potentially long-lived animal companion. This enforced dependence motivates us to scrutinize behavior at its elemental level—the observable—in order to improve the fate of tamed captive psittacine companions.

NEONATES

Because they hatch blind and mainly naked, psittacine neonates are designated *altricial* birds. They differ from *precocial* birds that see, walk, and forage within hours of hatching by being lastingly reliant upon care and teaching instead of quickly independent.

Their seeming helplessness, however, does not indicate that psittacine neonates are inactive—on the contrary. The hatching process is vigorous and demands that before hatching, psittacine chicks maneuver, rotate, pip the eggshell, push against the egg, and even vocalize (Abramson et al. 1995). The hatching process itself can take an extraordinarily long time, "up to 79 hours from pipping to fully hatched," reports Abramson for one Hyacinth Macaw (*Anodorhynchus hyacinthinus*)

(Abramson et al. 1995). Some pre-nestlings nap during the long hatching process. Although most hatch sooner than Hyacinths, all who emerge in optimal health have absorbed the yolky nutrients that provide the first fuel needed for growth and vigor. I have held and vocalized with hatching eggs and have watched twisting, pushing babies emerge from their egg. They often move to a place away from the cut edge of the broken shells and immediately fall asleep to recover from hatching exertions.

The first dropping excreted by neonates I note because it signals that the digestive system functions. Once the babies wake, they are ready to eat an appropriately thinned-down formulated diet.

Because they sleep so much, newly hatched psittacine birds might again seem inactive. However, even this early in development, their nascent readiness to act in response to the increasingly complex environments they will encounter as they grow becomes apparent. When they are awake, chicks even two days old will stand straight up on their haunches and repetitively vocalize when hungry. They push their sightless heads toward something to touch, lift their rumps off the towels upon which they sit, and open their beaks wide. When the flanges (sides) of their beaks are touched, the babies pump up and down to indicate their reflexive readiness to eat. Though I hand-fed from day 1 less than 25 incubator-hatched birds, all were responsive to early stimuli. Their tightly closed eyes, undeveloped muscles, and inability to thermo-regulate indicate developmentally normal physical limitations. Early sensitivity to vocalizations, food, and gentle touch massage all indicate that, as Friedman writes, "the feedback loop between behavior and the environment begins" (S.G. Friedman, personal communication, 2003).

When the proper types of comfort are provided and when the babies are healthy, some behaviors of psittacine neonates are contextually related such as snuggling/sleeping, pumping/eating, and wiggling/pooping. Snuggling precedes sleeping, pumping precedes eating, and wiggling precedes pooping. Backing up, a few quick wiggles of featherless rumps and tails, a suspenseful pause, the emergence of a well-formed broken string of fecal matter surrounded by white urates and clear urine—these are endearing and notable actions. These motions are generally accompanied by a sound that ranges from a soft sigh to a tiny grunt. Hatchlings that remain healthy and behave in the manners just described are considered well on their way toward further development.

In contrast, chicks who are dehydrated, ill, too cold, or too warm behave differently. If fed an inappropriate or inadequate diet, if housing is suboptimal, or if health is questionable, neonates will regurgitate, shiver or pant, cry, stay awake after feeding, and act either listless or hyper. Droppings may be viscous, scant, or smelly. Babies who demonstrate these behaviors and types of elimination need immediate medical evaluation.

Overall, biological parent birds are the optimal caregivers for psittacine neonates. When they respond competently to neonates' demands, adult pairs make the best psittacine early caregivers. A cockatoo hen, for instance, who wakes at midnight in order to deliver just one bite of perfectly mixed food at its most palatable temperature to her drowsy baby is the creature most suited to that job. Aviculturists are wise to consider ways to increase parenting behaviors in captive pairs rather than resorting to labor-intensive and sometimes detrimental artificial incubation and raising of hatchlings.

Adept parent birds handle hatchling neonates with ease. In contrast, aviculturists who artificially incubate have alarms bleeping them awake in the dead of night so they can carefully prepare the correct food, check its temperature, wake sleeping chicks, feed them, clean the substrate, return the chicks to the brooder, and hope sleep returns. I found hand-feeding from day 1 deleterious to my health. In addition, we generally know that parent-raised babies are fitter, fatter, and calmer than birds human-raised from day 1. Christine Sellers, DVM, considers all psittacine babies fed by humans from day 1 to be "at least somewhat compromised" (C. Sellers, personal communication, 1998) when compared to parent-fed chicks.

Because we don't want to allow yelling for food to become reinforced by the provision of food, we don't feed neonates when they yell for food. We feed upon early demand, when chicks wake and are hungry, before they cry. A baby monitor alerts us during the night and we respond efficiently (if groggily) in order to avoid teaching our birds that, if they scream loud and long, their most basic needs are met.

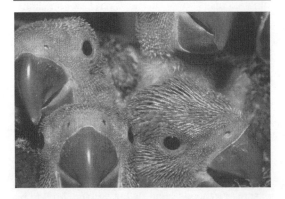

Figure 11.2.   Healthy neophytes, such as these Alexandrine chicks, have bright eyes and appear inquisitive during their busyness. See also color section. (Photo by Alice J. Patterson, courtesy of Santa Barbara Bird Farm.)

NEOPHYTES

Once babies' eyes open, I call them "neophytes" because many of their behaviors are new (Linden 1999b; Figure 11.2). As their bodies grow, their behaviors both increase and expand daily. This is an ideal time for practitioners to quite deliberately promote certain behaviors and deter others.

We are active participants in and enrichers of the growing parrot's environment. The primary (unlearned) reinforcers—finding comfort, getting food, taking rest—are in place and now the psittacine caregiver begins to control his or her contingency on the young parrot's behavior in order to encourage companionable characteristics and to diminish others. By preventing their success, we can help deter behaviors that do not promote health and happiness in captivity while we actively provide reinforcement for behaviors that do. Simultaneously, we promote captivity-related beneficial behaviors, dissuade non-companionable behaviors, and arrange the environment for success.

Just as we keep a careful eye on humidity, temperature, and substrate for the neonate, we do the same for the neophyte, with appropriate amendments. Neophytes develop properly in environments large enough for flapping, climbing, hiding, and tumbling; where chances for social interaction with other birds and with humans abound; where diets conducive to foraging are introduced; where opportunities to touch and be touched are prevalent; and where the important lifelong skills of preening and bathing are introduced and demonstrated. Enrichment at this stage is important to prevent abnormal behavior such as feather picking (Meehan & Mench 2002; Meehan, Millam, & Mench 2003). In the following paragraphs I describe the types of environments that promote these behaviors.

Healthy neophytes grow larger and more interactive by the moment. At five weeks old, for example, our African Greys (*Psittacus erithacus*) are downy-covered lumps that dreamily raise their heads for feeding. By six weeks, these same babies begin a cautious walk toward light; they touch colored fabrics, foods, and toys with their beaks; and they even begin to preen themselves and clutchmates. By seven weeks old, they pick up foods in their beaks, vocalize in response to cues, and stare steadily at the sights within their view. They also quickly scamper back to a darkened corner of the box if they are startled in any way. For this reason, we (aviculturists Abramson, Cravens, Linden, and Speed, among others) raise babies in containers that provide both privacy and places for peeking out. Sheltered areas for rest may be important to reduce skeletal problems in young growing birds (Harcourt-Brown 2004). We want to encourage birds to look out at the world when they feel safe to do so and to seek and readily find comfort when they need it. We give them environments where they can escape from feel-

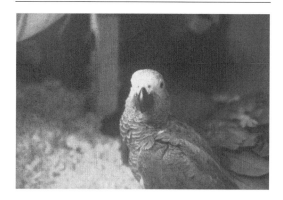

Figure 11.4. The comfort and security of the cardboard box allow opportunities for this young Grey Parrot to either peek out, hide, nap, or play. (Photo by Liz Wilson, courtesy of Santa Barbara Bird Farm.)

ings of helplessness, fear, and lasting discomfort and experience quick recoveries from upset and trauma (Figure 11.3).

Along with visual development, neophytes increase their physical development. Birds who only a week ago mainly slept, ate, and pooped now start to look at, touch, and move toward stimulation (Figure 11.4). We watch them as they watch their environment and its inhabitants—us. Their ears are open too—we want them to hear pleasant sounds because we know that psittacine adult voices can ratchet up volume, tempo, and pitch. Therefore, we keep the neophytes' habitat as free as possible of screeching and/or meaningless droning repetitive noises. I once saw a video of young parrots being fed in a large institutional environment where feedings were dispensed according to a rigid schedule. Long before "feeding time," some of the birds started screaming and the unheeded screams escalated into piercing noises that quickly woke the other babies, all of whom screamed until the ear-plugged hand feeder entered the room at the appointed time, wordlessly fed the birds, then left. This early experience allows screaming to continue unabated too long because thereby, "function is established between behavior and consequence" (S.G. Friedman, personal communication, 2003). Screaming for food—or for any need—is largely avoidable and not beneficial for birds who, as adults, routinely lose their homes because of loud endless noise

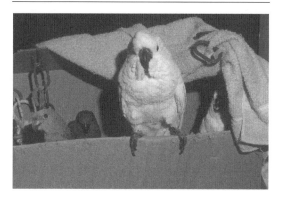

Figure 11.3. Before fledging, this young Moluccan Cockatoo tests her feet and balance when she climbs onto the edge of the box she shares with other psittacids. (Photo by Layne David Dicker, courtesy of Santa Barbara Bird Farm.)

making. Instead, we want to reward hungry birds with their food when they make those first "acceptable" noises. Development incorporates not only food and feedings, however.

Slowly, steadily, over the next few weeks, psittacine birds increase the amount of time they spend looking out of their containers and decrease the amount of time they spend hiding and sleeping. However, they still need to both sleep and hide so dual-function containers that afford both dark and peeking-out sections continue to be used. Inside the box, we add toys and bowls of colored foods for touching and visual interest because we want to promote curiosity and exploration as we lessen the numbing effects of blank environments (Meehan & Mench 2002). We also touch the babies to replicate parental contact and to acclimate the birds for future handling. Aviculturist Katy McElroy's videotape of Moluccan Cockatoo (*Cacatua moluccensis*) parent birds as they care for a hatchling is surprising because it shows lavish amounts of attention directed to one lone chick (McElroy 1998).

Neophytes' observable behaviors include looking, touching, and moving but now these behaviors are *more* looking around, *more* touching of objects with the beak, and pronounced increases in physical activities like eating, preening, and their first unstudied attempts at exercise.

Neophytes Exercise

At the beginning of the neophyte stage, psittacine wings are just beginning to produce long viable flight feathers, and neophytes regularly flap these stubby wings (Harcourt-Brown 2004). Eclectus Parrots (*Eclectus roratus*) are not the only ones to put their little heads down in the substrate, firmly plant their feet, and flap their wings repeatedly. African Greys, *Psittacula*, Cockatoos, Amazons, and Macaws do the same. Their bottom-heavy physiques serve as ready ballast during these flapping exercises.

In preparation for flight, psittacine birds start to hop, jump, and strut. Amazons are especially good at strutting. They push their chests out, hold heads high and wings akimbo—then pounce on toys or roll on their backs for tummy tickles. All pre-fledged psittacine birds should be given ample opportunity to exercise their legs and feet for the sheer joy of it, and as good preparation for landings after flight.

Pre-fledged birds also need to practice climbing. Up the sides of their containers they climb and perch on the edge. Soon, they are climbing and flapping, then flapping while climbing. At first, they grip tightly onto the perch. Later, they can be seen flapping vigorously while hovering a bare inch from the perch, as they test the formative abilities of their untried wings.

Neophytes Interact

Neophytes act independently. They also mingle with each other. Increasingly, they actively participate in their environments and interact with their caregivers. Environmental enrichment early in life will increase the motivation for exploration and reduce neophobia (Nicol & Pope 1993; Holsen 1986). Early environmental enrichment also fosters species-typical behavior and reduces abnormal and detrimental behavior (Clayton & Krebs 1994; van Hoek & King 1997; Coulton et al. 1997). Enrichment also positively influences brain development (e.g., Turner et al. 2002; Rosenzweig & Bennett 1996; Rosenzweig 1984) and learning ability (Winocur & Greenwood 1999; Cooper & Zubek 1958; Renner & Rosenzweig 1987). Housing young birds in pairs has been shown to be beneficial compared to single-bird housing. Pair-housed birds were more interactive with the environment, less fearful, and engaged more in adaptive behavior and performed less detrimental or abnormal behavior (Meehan, Garner, & Mench 2003). Gentle early handling imposes a mild stress on the young bird but is beneficial because it reduces detrimental reaction to non-avoidable chronic stress while intensifying potentially life-saving reactions to acute stress (Levine 1960/1973). The more early stimulation is provided to the young animal, the greater the decrease in emotional reactivity (Denenberg 1969).

Some of the behaviors we see in neophytes include these:

Independently, they look at, approach, and finally touch objects housed in their boxes. Later, in preparation for fledging, they run, hop, and practice flapping.

They snuggle, eat, and sleep with each other. Sometimes they pump on each other's wing tips or other body parts in simulated feeding motions. If one wakes, is hungry, and begins moving, the others quickly wake and homogenous squirming ensues, soon accompanied by food begging sounds.

They vocalize in response to their caregivers and often assume the feeding posture: flat bottom on the substrate, neck extended, beak open wide. They also will sit still and even nap while being held and softly touched.

Neophytes Eat

Neophytes remain on formulated diets with appropriate amounts administered according to the best species-specific schedules. The *method* of delivery of foods matters little as long as the *caliber* of the feeding experience is positive, unrushed, and as infused with interaction as it is with nutrition. Syringe, paper cup, spoon, or by hand—the implements that deliver food are not nearly as important as is the undivided attention of the deliverer. We want to instill the ideas that eating with a group is fun, that eating a variety of foods is even more fun, and that eating it, shredding it, pulverizing it, and wasting it are the best fun ever.

Here's how a feeding of neophytes typically occurs at my house:

A box inhabitant stirs and so I scrub my hands, then start to warm the food. As neophytes wake, one flaps and falls over, another just flaps. Most stretch upon waking and some practice making a step or two, but not always with forward motion. The oldest birds advance toward the opening first and it is usually a pin-feathered head that greets me.

I peel back the towel in response to their postures and body language. I then establish vocal and physical contact with the neophytes. For example, if one still sleeps, I take care to be quiet until the baby wakes; then vocalizations remain soft and actions deliberate, predictable, and modified to soothe, not alarm. As the feeding begins, one baby invariably stands front and center. This is most likely the oldest or most-developed chick. In a mixed clutch box, for example, an older macaw might be less developed than the younger Grey. The Grey, in this instance, would be first to the feeding.

Round-robin type feeding (where each bird gets a predetermined number of morsels or strict measure of cc's in a set rotation) is anathema to me. I feed based on individual assessment of each baby in my care. If one ate a small break-

fast, I depend upon that chick to be extra receptive to the mid-morning meal. As already noted with feeding utensils, hand feeders develop, refine, and practice the hand-feeding technique that works best for them and the babies they nurture. Some colleagues feed exactly measured amounts, others use a syringe or spoon, and still others feed in regimented order, but those aspects of hand-feeding are of limited consequence except if they expedite careful record-keeping. The individual identity of each baby under human care is of primary importance, as is that individual's progress, health, and comfort and the hand feeder's ability to track and encourage these important measures of wellness.

Neophytes Touch

I feed by hand because that's what I like to do. I hold real pieces of softened formulated diet between my fingers, which touch the babies approximately where and how parent birds use their beaks to touch babies' beaks while feeding. It would seem like each feeding would become more automatic than the next, but the reverse is true for me. With each feeding, neophytes change, albeit slightly. Over a week, cumulative small adjustments make a huge difference in the feeding technique. One day the baby macaw swallows the food whole, the next day she mouths each piece. Some pump on fingers or utensils, some seem to grab food from the air if it's tossed in their general vicinity. My job includes watching for these subtle shifts as babies use their beaks and tongues to eat, preen, and touch more objects.

An important skill begins at this stage when we teach psittacine neophytes how to interact with and touch human hands. I enjoy reinforcing them when they touch me in appropriately gentle ways, just as they provide me with valued reinforcement by being happy to see me, eager for the food, and solicitous of my touch. I learn about each of them through tactile connection, and they learn that when they repeatedly reach for a human hand, rewards they value result.

Neophytes Preen

The variety of preening-like skills displayed in this early stage of development is surprising. The current epidemic of feather-picking in companion parrots (Jenkins 2000) is a bleak situation that has so far resisted solution. Because all possibilities for improvement are welcome, hand feeders are well advised to encourage early beak/tongue co-ordination. For example, the ability to pull a many-segmented item through the beak is a good one that neophytes can practice with carrot tops, Italian parsley, and other leafy green food items. These skills practiced with greens benefit young birds who lack parental or sibling preening and must solo preen.

Preening and eating skills begin to overlap. Neophytes offered fresh wet greens touch, lick, preen, and shred them. At first, they don't ingest palpable quantities of these offerings but inges-tion is not the goal here, practice is: we want them to generalize preening of greens into preening of feathers. We note how they use their tiny tongues and already surprisingly dexterous beaks to ex-plore the fissures and intricacies of carrots tops, dandelion greens, or chard. Substantive pieces of fresh vegetables, especially greens, provide visual as well as tactile stimulation to the increasingly active neophytes. Six-week-old Greys (*P. eritha-cus*) avidly lick wet green leaves while Eclectus (*E. roratus*) drink the droplets as they fall. Cock-atoo neophytes (*Cacatua*) will preen carrot tops and baby macaws (*Ara*) will boldly shred ro-maine. Little tongues and beaks move quickly in repetitive measured motions. Fine motor skills are solicited, practiced, and enhanced when we pro-vide appropriate enrichments such as greens and toys (Figure 11.5).

A plethora of enrichment may ameliorate some feather-destructive behaviors, especially those tied to lack of preening practice, motivation, or materi-als (Meehan, Millam, & Mench 2003). We encour-age neophytes to preen inanimate objects when we can first influence those early attempts to preen. We provide them with enrichments so they can practice these activities with diligence. Further study may indicate whether or not the mastery of early tongue-beak-preen skills correlates with later lack of feather-destructive behaviors.

Early preening actions allow neophytes to prac-tice physical skills. Twist and balance of supple spines is challenged as the neophytes bend over, lean down, and nibble at the sheaths of their early feathers. Surprisingly nimble, neophytes ruffle their budding feathers with deliberation, although sometimes they tumble over when they do so. When offered enrichments such as greens, they

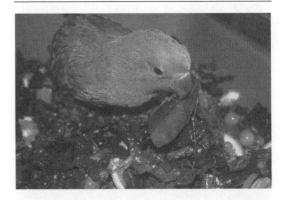

Figure 11.5. The young Eclectus male discov-ers that fledging means not only flying through the air but also landing in interesting spots. Once in the food tub, he selects a freshly cut guava leaf as his morsel of the moment. (Photo by Liz Wilson, courtesy of Santa Barbara Bird Farm.)

stretch their necks long in order to grab a hanging leaf as they jostle together for access to the cho-sen particle. Often, they perform the same mo-tions on the feathers as they do on the greens: lit-tle repetitive nibbles.

At this stage, we want to encourage potential young companions to eat healthy foods, to touch and accept touching from human hands, and to preen themselves and each other. Therefore, we add reinforcement appropriate to their increasing proficiencies. In so doing, we encourage observ-able behaviors with an eye toward long-term suc-cess. Because the neophyte stage passes quickly, we find ourselves changing reinforcers often, even daily. We encourage exercise, interaction, good eating skills, nice touching behaviors, and solid preening actions when we arrange the envi-ronment so that the neophytes are positively rein-forced by participating in these activities.

Once psittacine birds reach the stage where they are ready, many of the behaviors already ob-served begin to shift unmistakably toward the ul-timate psittacine activity—flying. Precursors to fledging including exercise, interaction, and diet, and all culminate in a series of events that lead to self-propelled airborne flight complete with take-offs, landings, mid-air turns, and recall. I have ex-perienced great joy while fledging psittacine birds.

FLEDGLINGS

Fledging principles are best guided by neither hard right-wing nor hard left-wing practices. Hard right-wing thinking assumes that birds who do not fledge don't miss the experience. Hard left-wing thinking—that all birds must fly all the time, preferably "freely" outside—is equally unsupportable for all but a minority of psittacine caregivers. Like the obsolete one wing only clip, either hard direction results in a crash. We can achieve a balanced approach to fledging, one where the birds get a chance to experience their personal kinesiology and are adequately prepared for life and are then later suitably confined by well-measured standards of domesticity.

A balanced fledging program includes assessment of the physical characteristics of all who will participate in the young psittacine's domestic flight. Caregivers, children, dogs, cats, and visitors all participate in the equation.

A program that balances the bird's capabilities in a thoughtfully arranged environment can be achieved, but it takes total "flock" cooperation as well as knowledge about the domestication process. Domestication is in its earliest stages with parrots, most of whom are only one generation out of the jungle. Price writes, "Domestication is a process of adaptation to the captive environment that includes both genetic changes occurring over generations and environmentally induced developmental events (such as taming) that occur within the lifetime of an individual" (Price 1984). Further, the "capacity to perform the behaviors seen in the repertoire of wild counterparts remains, although the threshold for performance may be altered" (Price 1999). It is this behavioral threshold that caregivers must consider for giving parrots the richest experience possible as our companions.

Before I describe my limited domestically based fledging experiences, I must give credit to two major flight-related influences, one human, one psittacine. The former is Eb Cravens, an aviculturist in Hawaii whose articles published in the late 1980s recounted experiences with birds in flight both indoors and outdoors (*AFA Watchbird,* "Birdkeeping Naturally," 1988–1990). Cravens's writings continue to influence many. The psittacine influence on my fledging program, described next, comes from a flock of feral amazons.

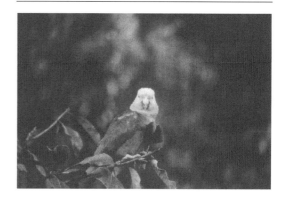

Figure 11.6. The naturalized Double Yellow-headed Amazon, a proven male, keeps lookout for his fledglings amid the trees at the Santa Barbara Bird Farm, where the wild flock's daily activities are noted. See also color section. (Photo by Harry A. Linden, courtesy of Santa Barbara Bird Farm.)

OBSERVATIONS OF WILD FLEDGLINGS

A Brief History of a Feral Flock of Amazon Parrots

A flock of amazon parrots, currently nine in number, visits our property and inspires countless hours of observation. Our aviary inhabitants greet their free-flying counterparts with recognizable yells while my spouse, Harry, and I quickly fill feed bowls to further reinforce their visits. Harry's interest in this flock goes back nearly 25 years to when he first watched a Double Yellow-Headed Amazon (*Amazona ochrocephala*; Figure 11.6) and three Lilac-crowned Amazons (*Amazona finschi*) forage in a tree located close to the freeway, seven miles from our house. This obsolete viewing area is now covered in concrete, the tree long replaced by urban blankness, and the flock has moved its foraging areas further up the mountains. Fortuitously, they include our property in the hills in their chosen territory. They make brief stops at the feeding stations we supply for them but it's clear to us that their territory is vast because sightings extend for at least 35 miles in every land-based direction from our property or from their nesting sites, which we believe are close by. We have yet to find their nesting sites, although we look with diligence. We have watched wild pairs visit two different sites. As the frequency of their visits increase, so does our anticipation. We have watched them gnaw at and enlarge openings, sit inside good nesting areas, and even mate close by. However, even after weeks of fixing up, they have left these observable sites for places still undiscovered by us. Clearly, these observations—made in our backyard and the surrounding rural areas—do not constitute a scientific study. The flock's almost daily visits give us limited information on their many activities but we avidly watch them anyway.

Initially, this flock was formed of probable escapees from local aviaries or homes. The Double Yellow-headed Amazon (*Amazona ochrocephala tresmariae*), who we later discovered was a male, and his chosen Lilac-crowned Amazon (*Amazona finschi*; Figure 11.7) hen were the first to reproduce. Although they both disappeared during the winter of 2001, they produced many offspring, three of whom still visit. There are two other Lilac-crowneds initially referred to as "the sentry" and "the babysitter." We assumed they were the same sex because we never saw interaction between them but they eventually proved themselves a viable pair. They've fledged five babies, one of whom still frequents our property. Over the years, the *A. O. tresmariae* and *A. finschi* pair produced eight hybrid chicks that we watched fledge, three of whom still visit. Undoubtedly, both pairs have produced babies who never made it to the fledging grounds we observe in our backyard and surrounding mountains and valleys, and so these are not included in this count nor meant as a commentary on fertility. These numbers do, however, reflect survivability after successful hatching and fledging for this group of birds.

How We Determine Unseen Nesting Schedules

Gravity bound, we humans are locked into limited observations from which we make suppositions that sometimes prove out, sometimes do not. Since these birds have never—so far—nested where we can see them, we have to calculate their seasonal schedules.

For example, we assume that these wild birds go to nest when the hens begin to miss the twice-daily feedings. When the hens stop coming, we mark this date on a calendar kept for this purpose. At the same time that the hens cease their visits, we consistently make two interesting ob-

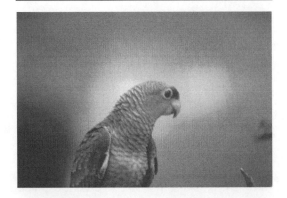

Figure 11.7.   This Lilac-crowned Amazon fledgling received flying lessons from her parents and older siblings. (Photo by Harry A. Linden, courtesy of Santa Barbara Bird Farm.)

servations. First, the male birds come more frequently than the normal dawn and sunset times. Second, at the same time the hens stop coming, the males' beaks become encrusted with food, presumably from feeding the roosting hens, undoubtedly a messy process, at least for these pairs of birds.

Now, the males make their way in solitude and go from place to place among the feeding stations as they peer into each food cup. If we do not provide extra food quickly enough (our schedules must change to accommodate theirs), they call or pace while looking closely at the door from which their food servers emerge. One feeding male comes right to our windows and peers inside, yells loudly, then waits, several times a day. Other times the males sit camouflaged by a tree in absolute silence, depending on the hawk status and their hunger.

Approximately four weeks after the hens stop coming, males increase their visits and the intensity of their solicitations aimed at us. We note that the males have even messier beaks. At this time, the feeding males have very little interaction with other flock members; they eat quickly and fly away, often only to return an hour or so later, seemingly impatient and important. As I stand in my carefully disinfected kitchen, I watch the males with their food-coated beaks gobbling food to feed to undoubtedly equally untidy hens. We mark this date on our calendar with the note "probable hatch."

About eight weeks after the probable hatch, the mother birds show back up at our feeders. The hens' beaks are also noticeably soiled, but the mother birds are decidedly less active than the males. If other parrots are present, the feeding hens hang around the food stations and preen themselves while the males fly away, then back, then away again.

Day of Celebration: A Wild Fledgling Appears

With amazons, we expect fledging at approximately 10.5 weeks after our probable hatch date. Ten days to three weeks after that day, if fortune is with us, we see a wild fledgling, new to the property. Actually, we hear about new arrivals well before we see them because all of our aviary and pet birds comment—loudly, as if heralding a great event—on the first sighting of a new parrot. These enthusiastic greetings continue for several days and are soon enough answered by the fledglings' own contributions to flock communication, food begging, and calling.

These wild-hatched fledglings make few food begging noises, but they do make some, especially early in the fledging process. Mostly they are closely attended and thus excessive noises are unnecessary. In particular, the father birds are consistently attentive. Rarely do we hear prolonged food begging noises that, with amazons, consist of distinctly resonant honking noises, identifiable nearly a mile from the source.

We watch fledglings in the fruit trees as they watch their parents and older siblings. The more experienced birds march through the foliage, select an orange, for instance, take a single bite of it, drop it, and continue on their way. The large dark eyes of the fledglings are riveted on these feeding activities and we watch them similarly mesmerized. Field glasses allow us to see the details of their faces, marked by dark eyes, unmistakably untidy beaks, and individualized features.

After several observational sessions, we see the fledglings bounce along flexible tree branches and make their initial attempts at independent feeding. During the next weeks, parent birds continue to feed the wild fledglings, but with decreasing frequency. The fledglings increase their independent foraging and eating activities (Figure 11.8).

The begging and honking noises also diminish and are replaced by tremendous amounts of airborne activities. Often, we worry that the fledg-

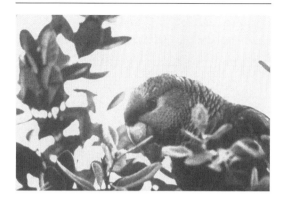

Figure 11.8. Another hybrid chick from a proven disparate and now long-missing pair. (Photo by Harry A. Linden, courtesy of Santa Barbara Bird Farm.)

lings aren't eating enough, because they fly and fly and spend measurably less time actually at the feeding stations than do older flock members. They alleviate our fears when their flight proficiency increases day by day. Therefore, foraging, eating, and flying sessions increase in frequency and duration.

After the morning feeding, fledglings will wait on a branch and are eventually met by one flock member who takes them through the sky, across the valley, and back to landing perches. These daily flying lessons occur for about two weeks. During this time some of the successful fledglings follow their flight instructor, coordinate themselves, and keep up with physical demands of flight. Unfortunately, others do not.

The Wild Fledgling Who Didn't Come When Called

In 1998, we observed two hybrid fledglings and noted them as healthy looking. One stayed close by the parent birds but the other was late to arrive and missed several gatherings altogether. One day I heard both parent birds as they sat on a high exposed tree branch and called long and loudly. After ten minutes, the fledgling arrived and they all eventually ate. Two days later, the parent birds resumed their loud calling and the tardy fledgling eventually arrived. The next day, the parent birds called but the fledgling didn't come. The next day, the parent birds did not call and the fledgling was never again seen.

Whenever there is excess vocalization, trouble

is often brewing. I am usually heartened by how little noise the wild fledglings make. Mainly, their needs are met, quietly. When they play in trees, however, they play loudly, usually with each other or with older siblings. Games such as "get your tummy," "hang from one toe while yelling," and "swing on a branch" seem to be flock favorites. One such fledgling, however, didn't play such games and frankly confounded us when he or she did not stop making food begging noises.

The Wild Fledgling Who Cried

Well after the other fledglings had stopped making food-solicitation noises, a particular fledging bird repetitively honked morning and evening. Whole hours went by punctuated by the noise yet we never saw this fledgling come to the feeding stations. Field glasses afforded me views of this young amazon (*A. finschi*) who usually had an older sibling in a nearby branch and who begged and begged for food. According to our calculations, this bird was nearly nine months old before he or she was seen no more and the noises ceased.

HOME-BASED EXPERIENCES WITH FLEDGING

Many years ago when I first raised psittacine birds, it was not unusual to clip their wings on the day of their first flight. After all, it is highly inconvenient, usually messy, and sometimes dangerous to have young birds taking off and landing with abandon. However, because many of our pet companions are in full flight, it seems unfair to clip the babies who repeatedly indicated their readiness to fly (Figure 11.9). While the older pets capable of flight stay on their perches and preen, chew toys, or just hang out, fledglings quiver, flap, look for landing spots, and seem raring to go. After several seasons of clipping birds, it became apparent that early wing clipping is anathema to their genetic impulses. The challenges became clear: to promote flight so that the benefits associated with fledging are experienced (Linden 1998) while simultaneously increasing the characteristics that contribute to successful captivity. Concurrently, we want to overlap behaviors that encourage daily explorations of vast habitats and far-ranging food foraging excursions with skills that include shorter-distance controlled flight and foraging in a cage, aviary, or other designated habitat. Because these not-yet-

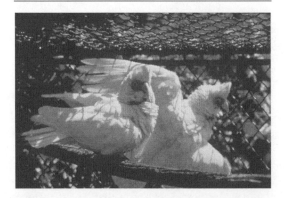

Figure 11.9. Fledgling aviaries should be large enough for the parrots to fully extend their wings in many directions and then fly and land, not merely hop and leap. The aviary enjoyed by these Slender-billed Cockatoos is 15' x 15' and sits amid loquat, orange, and nectarine trees. (Photo by Layne David Dicker, courtesy of Santa Barbara Bird Farm.)

domesticated animals surely share their wild counterparts' "behavioral capacities and response thresholds" (Meehan, Millam, & Mench 2003), they can be expected to be highly motivated to perform behavior associated with food procurement in the wild even though captive feeding methods may meet their nutritional needs. For parrots, foraging is its own reward.

Gradual clipping remains a viable alternative for many companion birds and leaves them somewhere between fully flighted and fully clipped. Birds should be left in full flight for as long as possible but after a time, in order to achieve balance between wild and domestic success, many need to be trimmed at least somewhat. In a gradual clip, only the first four to six feathers are trimmed so that some flight is possible and encouraged. In this clip, clients are advised that their birds *can fly* and indeed birds so trimmed often fly in a straight line from a play gym to a waiting hand, for instance. A well-tended home policed by vigilant responsible clients must be coupled with well-behaved birds in order to allow for successful partial or full flight (Linden 1998).

The Fledgling Aviary

The boon to any home-based fledging program is a well-equipped and commodious (Cravens 1990)

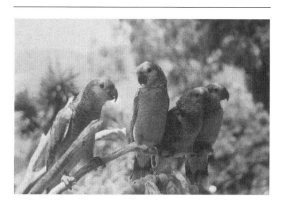

Figure 11.10. The author's one-year-old Blue-fronted Amazon, Bucket, meets his prospective mate, Bonnet, for the first time as she sits on a perch with her clutch mates. Fifteen years later, they are still together. See also color section. (Photo by Margaret Ames, courtesy of Santa Barbara Bird Farm.)

fledgling aviary (Figure 11.10). We include inducements to exercise such as rope and natural perches, multitudes of bowls, colorful toys, foraging opportunities, and showers in the aviary. Of course, the human attendant is usually the most favored enrichment. We resist the temptation to stuff the aviary so full of toys that the birds do not have room to spread their wings and fly. Here, they continue to practice the lessons they first learned in the house: fling food around, find a sibling to tickle, fly to a waiting hand, follow me to another side of the flight cage, land in lots of places. When they miss a landing spot, the birds learn to right themselves up, shake off the fall and resume action newly informed. Their learning curve is amazingly fast as long as the environment supplies thoughtfully arranged enticements and continual reinforcement.

How Fledglings Exercise: Physical Benefits of Fledging

Most obviously, we see that psittacine birds who successfully complete a fledging process attain a robust physique. Birds who fly develop pectoral muscles that are firm when palpated. They stand tall, walk and hop across moving branches, forage for foods, and eat just the right amounts. During fledging, athletic abilities are strengthened—healthy respiration, strong musculature, smooth

coordination (Linden 1998) and life-enhancing eating habits result.

Strength, endurance, climbing skills, and landing abilities blossom during fledging and positively influence confidence. Without confidence, wild psittacids would become overdependent burdens on flock mates; those lacking confidence would surely not survive. Coordination comes from using personal kinesiology; coordination leads to confidence, a distinct psychological hallmark of well-actuated beings (Linden 1999a). Domestic parrots also benefit from confidence when they amuse themselves with independent play, napping, preening, and foraging. Abilities to self-occupy are highly desirable in adult psittacine companions and are the result of these formative experiences.

How Fledglings Interact: Social Benefits of Fledging

Early experiences with flight introduce young birds to the necessity of social skills because healthy fledging includes flock activities where many participate. Aunts, uncles, cousins, grandparents, older siblings—surely all influence the young fledglings. In addition to the social experiences inherent with hand-rearing, birds learn critical social lessons when fledging. The importance of following instructions and careful observation of others and the environment are reinforced. Surely well-traveled psittacine fledglings run into many new acquaintances where they experience deferment and well-modulated assertion. They learn to leave unsavory situations, propelled by their physical strength. During this time, fledglings learn to come, follow, and obey flock signals. They also balance dependence—being with the flock—with independence when they make their own decisions, try a new path, or stop at the berry patch for an unscheduled snack. During fledging, a healthy mix of dependence and independence is tried and amended according to experience.

How Fledglings Learn: Mental Benefits of Fledging

If we want to replicate a full fledging process in the domestic psittacine—one that includes important lessons learned by wild psittacines—the challenges are many. Wild birds definitely have a much richer fledging experience than birds confined in homes, but these rich experiences are not without dangers, as illustrated by the death rate of naturalized parrots. Still, in the ideal world, once they land on the branch of a tree, wild psittacine fledglings look around their immediate habitat—they take in the lay of the land, so to speak. They watch the sky and ground for predators, calculate the distance to the feeding stations, gauge angles of descent and ascent, and watch a bug crawl along the vein of a leaf. Once airborne, these observations and calculations continue as they fly in fluid formation with the flock and learn the times, places, and circumstances under which to land, keep going, or flee with alacrity. Certain calls percolate during flight—these are not eating noises, nor are they standard calling noises. The calls made during flight use another vocabulary and volume altogether.

In contrast, domestically situated parrots often cope with fully clipped wings (enforced disablement) and are confined in a cage for consecutive hours where they endure hours of quiet sedentary solitude. We combat these domestically inflicted negatives—as best as possible—through home-based fledging and full-time human attendants.

How Fledglings Eat: The Benefits of Foraging

Right before they fly, fledglings' appetites decrease in concert with an increase in the time they spend exercising and exploring. At this time, fledglings' eating skills center around foraging excursions.

I used to chase after fledglings and beg them to stop flying in order to eat. Now I encourage them to come find the food I've placed in a variety of locations (Figure 11.11). In this way, we induce hours of busy time while we check unnatural sedentary behaviors.

Psittacine fledglings remain unweaned for varying amounts of time. From the time they fly to the time they wean is specific to the various species. Moreover, it's frequently reported that babies wean on individual schedules as well. "Weaning is the process by which birds learn to eat on their own without the assistance of their parents. Once a bird reaches its peak weight, it begins to eat on its own, perch, fly, and finally wean" (Abramson et al. 1995). Therefore, fledging and weaning are both processes that birds undergo somewhat concurrently.

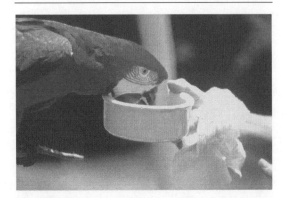

Figure 11.11. Rosie, a one-year-old Green-winged Macaw, occasionally needs encouragement to eat foods selected by her caregiver. A handheld bowl and lots of verbal interaction assist her in making good food choices. See also color section. (Photo by Layne David Dicker, courtesy of Santa Barbara Bird Farm.)

How Fledglings Touch: The Benefits of Busyness

Fledglings use their tongues to explore foot toys, fissures, and food. Their beak strength also increases and they repeatedly try to bite, gnaw, and chew on whatever is handy. Usually, human hands are most handy. This is the ideal time to discourage the propensity young birds have for chewing what's attached to nerve endings and to encourage chewing, instead, appropriate inanimate objects. We supply the environment with many items appropriate for chewing: soft wood, fresh tree branches, untreated wicker baskets, species-appropriate toys. We stock our pockets with surprises sure to please inquisitive beaks.

Whenever young birds are intent upon playing with a toy, we let their attention remain riveted on that object (Figure 11.12). We do not interrupt a busy bird. Instead, we wait for the play session to be over, then we praise the results of the bird's activity. Hopefully, this is a pile of pulverized organic materials.

Many fledglings enjoy cuddling sessions and these are certainly part of many long-term human/psittacine relationships. However, it's easy for trimmed birds, especially cockatoos and macaws, to want, to like, then to vocally demand, an amount of physical contact incompatible with human time allowances. Psittacines who scream

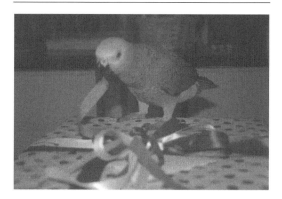

Figure 11.12. This young African Grey Parrot tries her beak at unwrapping a birthday gift. (Photo by Phoebe Greene Linden, courtesy of Santa Barbara Bird Farm.)

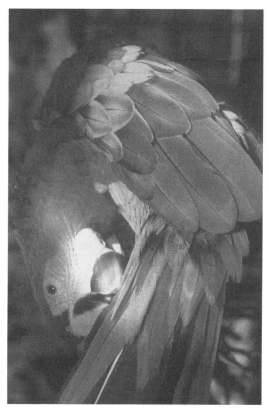

Figure 11.13. The art of preening occupies many moments in parrots' daily lives. Human caretakers can promote preening with praise and by giving parrots the baths and space necessary for expansive preening sessions. See also color section. (Photo by Kelly Flynn, courtesy of Santa Barbara Bird Farm.)

for attention do so because they have been reinforced for it in the past, and this noise usually happens on a schedule that conflicts with human-based reality. Therefore, it's best to keep touching, cuddling, and holding sessions on a fluid schedule. However, most well-trained humans do recognize and at least intermittently (and happily) reinforce companion birds who appropriately request neck rubs. Neck, head, and face scratching are favored areas for physical interaction and most socially comfortable birds will accept assistance in preening these areas. Additionally, we want to regularly touch birds' toes, feet, and legs in order to acclimate them to nail trims and blood draws. We want to familiarize psittacine birds with handling by touching them and by allowing them to touch us.

How Fledglings Preen: The Benefits of Good Hygiene

Fledglings need lots of space in order to properly preen. Preening in a cage is akin to a person doing jumping jacks in a broom closet. When given showers and plenty of space, fledglings learn to preen their own tails, wings, and backs (Figures 11.13 and 11.14). The results are breathtaking for caregivers and may provide psittacine companions with lifelong preening skills as an additional line of defense against boredom.

Height Inconvenience: A Lesson of Fledging

Now that our psittacine fledglings exercise, interact, learn, eat, touch, and preen appropriately, it's

time for them to practice some manners that help them integrate into a human flock. I teach two lessons that are important to me: (1) How to step down from tall heights, and (2) how to land on places that are not my head. As an adjunct to Dr. Friedman's discussion about height dominance in chapter 14, I'd like to add the results of my own observations on this topic.

Previously, I went along with the construct "height dominance" because I observed that the wild parent birds would not feed fledglings who stood above them. Obviously, it's inconvenient for parent birds to regurgitate uphill. They ignore the solicitation of babies who are overhead and instead feed those on the downward slope closest to

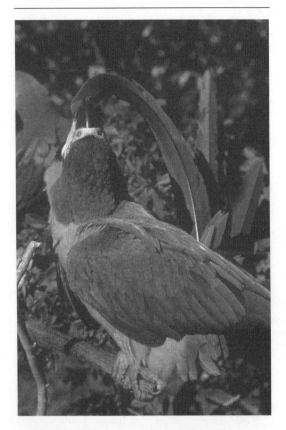

Figure 11.14. Young Blue-and-gold Macaw twists and reaches as she preens her tail feather while outdoors. See also color section. (Photo by Kelly Flynn, courtesy of Santa Barbara Bird Farm.)

their beaks. The parents favor this position for its ease and the fledglings favor it for results: they learn to sit slightly below or right next to parents and get fed; sit above and go hungry. Begging babies who sit overhead are not trying to dominate their parents, they just demonstrate their position on the learning curve. Undoubtedly, arboreal animals such as parrots enjoy sitting in trees and sometimes the view is best from the highest branches. That doesn't mean, however, that hanging out in the middle branches is submissive any more than foraging in the middle dense foliage is useless.

For me, the inconvenience of reaching overhead to grasp parrots that fly to the tops of curtain rods or ceiling beams is a deterrent. In the past, I was concerned that parrots—even young fledglings—

would try to dominate me if they got above my head, so I anxiously removed them from all these preferred (to them) places. In 2003, however, I tested a new theory explained by Dr. Luescher who thought that birds were reluctant to step on fingers that came from below because this hand position was unfamiliar to them (A.U. Luescher, personal communication, 2003). This made great sense to me—a hand that is offered palm up or with the flat ridge presented at chest level certainly looks very different from waggling fingers proffered from below.

I decided to train my fledglings and my mature companions to see if they would accept bunched fingertips that come from below as a suitable step surface. Once I stopped grabbing for their toes, it took, on average, three tries before all would step onto this new finger configuration. I realized that previously they weren't trying to dominate me, they were just unsure of such a strange stepping place and needed training in order to accept it. I learned that having birds perched overhead doesn't make them dominant any more than it makes me submissive, but it does remain inconvenient.

Still, in order to supply them with a fledging experience commensurate with their needs, not mine, I modified places that were previously "off limits" into new landing spaces. The top of the refrigerator, tops of cages, and even the top of my grandmother's antique secretary (covered with washable padding) became takeoff and landing spots for the 2003 fledglings: four Greys, two Macaws, two Cockatoos, two Amazons, and one Derbyan (*Psittacula derbiana*) Gidget. Without exception, these birds learned to step up as readily from these overhead places as they did from chest-level places when they received rewards they valued for doing so. Although they now readily step from overhead places, it's still inconvenient for me to stand on tiptoe with my arm stretched as far as it will go in order to get the birds to come to me. Instead, I decided to teach them to fly *down* from their lofty perches (Cravens 2001).

It proved simple to train the fledglings to fly down. Keeping them from landing on top of my head was more difficult. Apparently, the combination of slippery hair and a dome-shaped landing surface necessitates the use of eight sharp nails to secure good touchdown. Rather quickly I knew that I would need to enrich the non-head environment in order to save my scalp. Alternate landing spots were created: baskets weighted in the bottoms were placed all over and the birds were densely reinforced for landing on them. Similarly, I became adept at shooting my hand up in the air right behind my head to intercept the parrot landing gear. Birds who landed on my hand or on basket handles were reinforced with tickles and praise; those who landed on my head were silently set down elsewhere. In four days, the head landing incidents disappeared while the overall landings increased.

Psittacine Companions Who Never Fledged and Who Do Not Fly

Sadly, the majority of psittacids raised for the companion market will not experience a true fledging process and may never actually fly because their environments are not provisioned for such development. Space, time, and commitment limitations abound, and some aviculturists, evidence to the contrary, contend that fledging is unnecessary or extravagant. The question remains: Can a suitably developed psittacine companion who never flies remain a viable lifelong pet? The answer to that question depends, of course, on what environments shape the experiences during the time of development normally occupied by flight and after.

If caregivers can turn on the impulses for exercise, interaction, eating, foraging, touching, and preening that normally activate during flight, then yes, the result can be a well-developed companion. Persons who decide to not fledge birds obligate themselves to construct experiences commensurate with fledging wherein parrots exercise, interact, learn, and forage in equivalent ways. When deprived of flight, many birds use repetitious behaviors like yelling and overpreening as substitute actions and therefore require competent redirection. Clipped companion birds can be reinforced for athletic exercises other than flight such as climbing, swinging, and flapping. However, flapping stubby clipped wings is not nearly as satisfying as flapping full luxuriant wings, and so clipped birds must be appropriately and extravagantly enticed and reinforced to keep up the exercise needed for cardiovascular, respiratory, and muscular health.

Even clipped birds can learn to interact socially so long as they are taught that they need not bite in order to drive away unwanted attentions. Flighted birds flee from unsolicited interest and so find biting largely unnecessary, but clipped birds, lacking escape, often bite to drive away perceived intruders and other annoyances. The social interactions of clipped birds often land on the side of "overdependent" because, lacking their own resources for exploration, they depend upon human caregivers for entertainment, transportation, and to save them from less-favored persons. Therefore, conscientious caregivers of clipped companion parrots provide rope walkways and a variety of play gyms and daily activities to ensure well-adjusted lifelong companions who can both avoid and seek out social interaction, depending on what is reinforcing for the birds, not for the humans.

Of course clipped psittacids can develop healthy eating habits, but their environments also need to be thoughtfully arranged to stimulate foraging, shredding, and mulching behaviors. Companions who get only one neatly prepared bowl of food must be given other enrichments that encourage movement and action.

Many clipped companion parrots tolerate touching and learn to touch their primary caregivers with gentle ease, but lacking diversity in experience, they can become more limited as years go by. Because they are stuck on perches, clipped birds are often the unwitting recipients of unwanted touching by strangers and may learn to eschew touching as a result. Similarly, flighted birds also avoid unneeded, unwanted, and unappreciated touches, the value of which seems to be distinctly human, not avian. With few exceptions, humans like to touch birds more than most birds like to be touched by humans. Many psittacids—clipped or unclipped—learn to tolerate touching, but few enjoy it into adulthood. Nevertheless, both clipped and flighted birds can and do touch humans in very positive ways by stepping up on the offered hand, by taking treats nicely, and by sitting on laps, chests, or shoulders during relaxation times (Figure 11.15).

Clipped birds can develop very good preening skills, especially when they are supplied with large outdoor play gyms that they occupy under close supervision. Nevertheless, the immediate scrutiny needed to guard defenseless clipped birds from danger often diminishes the freedom

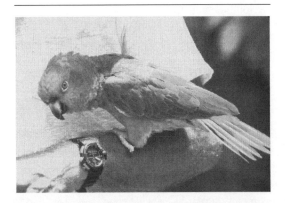

Figure 11.15. Pauly, a mature Yellow-naped Amazon male, sits protectively on his human caregiver's arm. The healthy glow of good nutrition and hygiene are evident in his colors and feather condition. (Photo by Layne David Dicker, courtesy of Santa Barbara Bird Farm.)

of large outdoor perches. Such supervision need not diminish good preening skills. Just like we leave alone birds intent upon toy destruction in order to pursue their goal, we also leave birds who are preening to their own devices.

It's difficult for clipped birds to develop a sense of independence when they must be constantly monitored. However, flighted birds require commensurate supervision since it's not feasible to have fully flighted animals zooming heedlessly around one's home. Therefore, we must conclude that all birds in captivity need good supervision in thoughtfully arranged environments.

SUMMARY

Psittacine neonates, neophytes, and fledglings all benefit from thoughtfully arranged environments that reinforce desirable companion characteristics and skills. As development progresses, we see psittacines respond to their environment through constant reorganization of observable behaviors. Domestically situated psittacines, whether flighted or clipped, remain dependent upon their caregivers to supply their environment with enrichment and rewards that are valuable to them.

During fledging, I see many of the characteristics I value in companion birds come to fruition. Exercise, interaction, foraging for foods, touching, and good preening skills obliterate (or at least greatly reduce) screaming, picking, biting, and

other cage-bound type behaviors. Surely the greatest challenges are still ahead of psittacine caregivers as we reinforce our psittacid companions for adapting to our environment while simultaneously enriching that environment in order to accommodate greater portions of their wildness.

REFERENCES

Abramson, J., B.L. Speer, and J.B. Thomsen. 1995. *The large macaws,* pp. 177, 204. Fort Bragg, CA: Raintree Publications.

Clayton, N.S., and J.R. Krebs. 1994. Hippocampal growth and attrition in birds affected by experience. *Proceedings of the National Academy of Science USA* 19:7410–7414.

Cooper, R.M., and J.P. Zubek. 1958. Effects of enriched and restricted early environments on the learning ability of bright and dull rats. *Canadian Journal of Psychology* 12:159–164.

Coulton, L.E., N.K. Waran, and R.J. Young. 1997. Effect of foraging enrichment on the behavior of parrots. *Animal Welfare* 6:357–363.

Cravens, E. 1988–present. Various columns and articles as published in *AFA Watchbird, Parrots, Original Flying Machine,* and others.

Cravens, E. 2002. The backyard aviculturist. *Original Flying Machine* 2:58–59.

Cravens, E. 2002. The links between mental alertness and flight. *Parrots* 55:12–13.

Denenberg, V.H. 1969. Open field behavior in the rat: What does it mean? *Annals of the New York Academy of Sciences* 159:852–859.

Escorihuela, R.M., A. Fernandez-Teruel, A. Tobena, N.M. Vivas, F. Marmol, A. Badia, A., and M. Dierssen. 1995. Early environmental stimulation produces long-lasting changes on ß-adrenoceptor transduction systems. *Neurobiology of Learning and Memory* 64:49–57.

Friedman, S.G. 2002. "Living and learning with parrots." Online class at www.parrottalk.com.

Harcourt-Brown, N. 2004. Development of the skeleton and feathers of dusky parrots (*Pionus fuscus*) in relation to their behavior. *Veterinary Record* 154: 42–48.

Holsen, R.R. 1986. Feeding neophobia: A possible explanation for the differential maze performance of rats reared in enriched or isolated environments. *Physiology and Behavior* 38:191–201.

Jenkins, T. 2000. "Feather picking in companion parrots." CPQ Conference paper.

Levine, S. 1960/1973. "Stimulation in infancy." In *Readings from Scientific American: The nature and nurture of behavior—Developmental psychology,* pp. 55–61. Scientific American Ltd.

Levine, S. 1962. "Psychophysiological effects of infantile stimulation." In *Roots of behavior: Genetics, instinct and socialization in animal behavior,* ed. E.L. Bliss, pp. 246–253. New York: Harper and Brothers.

Linden, P.G. 1999a. "Fledging and flight for avian companions." Proceedings of the Association of Avian Veterinarians, New Orleans, LA, pp. 61–76.

Linden, P.G. 1999b. Teaching psittacine birds to learn. *Seminars in Avian and Exotic Pet Medicine* 8 (4):154–164.

Linden, P.G. 1998. "Behavioral development of the companion psittacine bird." Proceedings of the Association of Avian Veterinarians, St Paul, MN, pp. 138–143.

McElroy, K. 1998. "Parent-rearing moluccan cockatoos and breeding cockatoos in outdoor aviaries in northern climates." Proceedings of the Midwest Avian Research Exposition, Toledo, OH, pp. 95–118.

Meehan, C.L., J.P. Garner, and J.A. Mench. 2003. Isosexual pair housing improves the welfare of young Amazon parrots. *Applied Animal Behavior Science* 81:73–88.

Meehan, C. L., and J.A. Mench. 2002. Environmental enrichment affects the fear and exploratory responses to novelty of young Amazon parrots. *Applied Animal Behavior Science* 79:75–88.

Meehan, C. L., J.R. Millam, and J.A. Mench. 2003. Foraging opportunity and increased physical complexity both prevent and reduce psychogenic feather picking by young amazon parrots. *Applied Animal Behavior Science* 80:71–85.

Nicol, C.J., & S.J. Pope. 1993. A comparison of the behavior of solitary and group-housed budgerigars. *Animal Welfare* 2:269–277.

Price, E.O. 1984. Behavioral aspects of animal domestication. *Q Rev Biol* 59:1–32.

Price, E.O. 1999. Behavioral development in animals undergoing domestication. *Applied Animal Behavior Science* 65:245–271.

Renner, M.J., and M.R. Rosenzweig, M.R. 1987. *Enriched and impoverished environments: Effects on brain and behavior.* New York: Springer-Verlag.

Ridley, M. 2003. *Nature via nurture: Genes, experience, and what makes us human.* New York: Harper Collins.

Rosenzweig, M.R. 1984. Experience, memory and the brain. *American Psychologist* 39:365–376.

Rosenzweig, M.R., and E.L. Bennett. 1996. Psychobiology of plasticity; effects of training and experience on brain and behavior. *Behavioral Brain Research* 78:57–65.

Sheehan, K.L. 2001. The effects of environmental enrichment and post-natal handling on the development, emotional reactivity and learning ability of juvenile nanday conures (*Nandayus nenday*). MS thesis. Purdue University.

Turner, C.A., M.C. Yang, and M.H. Lewis. 2002. Environmental enrichment: Effects on stereotyped behavior and regional neuronal metabolic activity. *Brain Research* 938:15–21.

van Hoek, C.S., and C.E. King. 1997. Causation and influence of environmental enrichment on feather picking of the crimson-bellied conure (*Pyrrhura perlata perlata*). *Zoo Biology* 16:161–172.

Winocur, G., and C.E. Greenwood. 1999. The effects of high fat diets and environmental influences on cognitive performance in rats. *Behavioral Brain Research* 101:153–161.

12

Handler Attitude and Chick Development

Brenda Cramton

INTRODUCTION

Avian Companions and the Human-Animal Bond

Human relationships with companion animals have existed for thousands of years (Lorenz 1953). Artifacts from ancient civilizations attest to our long-standing relationships with birds (Vriends 1984). Our relationships with birds continue to flourish. Today, there are millions of pet birds in the United States (Harris 1989).

Empirical studies have demonstrated conclusively that relationships with companion animals provide humans with valuable physical and psychosocial benefits (see, e.g., Mugford & M'Comisky, 1975; Beck & Katcher, 1989; Loughlin & Dowrick, 1993). Likewise, humans have been shown to influence the behavior of birds. Imprinting studies conducted early in this century by Lorenz are probably the most widely known experiments on the reactions of domestic avian species to interaction with human beings (Duncan 1992). Imprinting has been defined as a preprogrammed learned behavior (Alcock 1993). It allows the rapid establishment of a behavioral bond between an offspring and its parent. Lorenz (1952) found that baby Mallard ducks and Greylag goslings that he reared from hatching formed an immediate attachment to him either by sight (Greylags) or vocal expression (Mallards) and would maintain close proximity to him rather than their mother, another adult female of the same species, or another human.

Handling

More recently, studies have begun to focus on the long-term effects of other types of early experi-

ence on the human-animal bond. It has been shown that an animal's fear of humans can be reduced by habituation. One habituation technique is called "handling" (Duncan 1992). Although it is difficult to modify relationships between adult animals and humans (Murphy & Duncan 1978), young animals are responsive to learning experiences that include the formation of social attachments during a sensitive or critical period (Jones & Waddington 1993). Neonatal, or postnatal, handling has been shown to produce psychophysiological effects such as decreased fearfulness, decreased emotionality in open field tests (Denenberg & Zarrow 1971), and decreased novelty-induced fear (Bodnoff et al. 1987), as well as increased resistance to stress (Levine 1957, 1962). Many studies on mammals have shown that handled animals, such as puppies (Scott & Fuller 1965) and kittens (Karsh 1983), become closely attached to humans. Likewise, several studies have found similar effects in domestic poultry species (see, e.g., Jones & Faure 1981; Jones & Waddington 1993; Gross & Siegel 1979; Nicol 1992). Most neonatal handling studies have been conducted using mammals, primarily rats and mice. Levine initiated the classical infant-handling studies using rats to examine the effects of early experience on neural development and function under stress conditions (Smythe et al. 1994). He hypothesized from his results that "handling constitutes a stressful situation for the infant organism and that early experience with stress results in a greater ability of the organism to adapt to psychological and physiological stress in adulthood" (1957, p. 405). Meaney and his colleagues undertook studies to identify the mechanism that enables this adaptation to occur. Their findings suggest that the hypothalamic-pituitary-adrenal (HPA) axis is altered by early experiences such as postnatal handling.

The HPA Axis

The HPA axis is highly responsive to stress (Selye 1950). Any type of stress stimulates the neurons in the paraventricularis nucleus of the hypothalamus to secrete corticotropin-releasing hormone (CRH) into the portal system, which drains into the anterior lobe of the pituitary. CRH results in an increase in the release of adrenocorticotropin (ACTH) from the pituitary. The elevated level of ACTH stimulates an increase in the output of glucocorticoids from the adrenals. Elevated concentrations of glucocorticoids inhibit subsequent secretion of CRH from the hypothalamus and ACTH from the pituitary (Meaney et al. 1988). This negative feedback system involves the interaction of the hormones ACTH and CRH and a cytosolic glucocorticoid receptor in neural tissue (Meaney et al. 1985b).

Although glucocorticoids assist the organism under stressful conditions by increasing the availability of energy substrates, continued exposure to glucocorticoids may be detrimental to the organism after the termination of the stressor. Elevated glucocorticoid levels may lead to suppression of anabolic processes, muscle atrophy, hypertension, hyperlipidemia, arterial disease, impairment of growth and tissue repair, and immunosuppression (Meaney et al. 1996). Therefore, the capacity to effectively cope with these stimuli is adaptive. Gross and Siegel (1979) found that male Shaver Starcross chickens that were adapted to their handler produced more antibody to sheep, horse, or human erythrocytes; had more blood protein; gained more weight; and were more resistant to a *Mycoplasma gallisepticum* challenge than unadapted birds that were allowed minimal human contact.

Effect of Early Experience on the Maturation of the HPA Axis

In the rat, the pituitary-adrenal stress response and the stress-related, negative feedback system do not mature until after birth; therefore, the development of these systems is under way during the period when an animal is exposed to early environmental stimulation (Meaney et al. 1985b).

Meaney and his colleagues (1985a) suggest that the mechanism by which handling influences the development of the stress response involves the regulation of glucocorticoid receptor concentrations in the hippocampus and, perhaps, transcortin receptors in the pituitary. They found that handled rats showed an increase in hippocampal glucocorticoid receptor concentrations and a decrease in pituitary transcortin binding compared to non-handled animals. Since transcortin receptors bind circulating corticosterone, it is not able to inhibit the release of ACTH; therefore, higher transcortin levels in non-handled animals would lead to greater adrenocortical activity. The researchers hypothesize that early handling increases hippocampal glucocorticoid receptor concentration in one of two ways: (1) by increasing the number of receptor sites per cell, or (2) by stimulating postnatal neurogenesis in the hippocampus, which leads to an overall higher concentration of receptor sites. Their work also suggests that thyroid hormones have some role in the mediation of the development of glucocorticoid receptor concentrations in the hippocampus because their levels are known to be low from birth until about day 4, when they begin to increase, and peak at adult levels at the end of the second week of life; this pattern is identical to the developmental increase in glucocorticoid receptor concentrations in some brain regions (Meaney et al. 1987). Also, it is known that thyroid hormones are released during hypothermia, and handling is known to result in a transient period of mild hypothermia (Mitchell et al. 1990).

Increases in serotonin activity may also mediate the developmental changes in hippocampal glucocorticoid receptors and influence the effects of environmental events such as neonatal handling (Mitchell et al. 1990). Hippocampal concentrations of serotonin increase over the first two weeks of life and peak on day 14, which is similar to the developmental changes in hippocampal glucocorticoid receptor binding (Mitchell et al. 1990). Mitchell and his colleagues (1990) found that adult animals treated with a serotonin neurotoxin (5,7-dihydroxytryptamine) in the first few days of life had reduced hippocampal glucocorticoid receptor binding. In contrast, treatments that increased receptor binding capacity, such as neonatal handling or exogenous thyroid hormone treatment, increased hippocampal serotonin turnover. Furthermore, the effects of handling were blocked when the serotonin receptor antagonist, ketanserin, was administered concurrently (see also Smythe et al. 1994).

Postnatal Handling in Parrots

Since the interest in parrots as pets has grown in recent years, many species have become threatened due to capture for the pet trade. Habitat destruction and hunting for food have also contributed to the reduction in wild populations (Toft 1993). Every effort, therefore, must be made to alleviate collection from wild populations. Captive breeding is an alternative that can be employed to meet the demand for parrots for the pet trade market.

While many of the postnatal handling studies with rats and mice involve minimal amounts of handling (such as simple removal from the cage and placement in a container), the traditional aviculturalist's approach to taming chicks is at the opposite end of the handling spectrum: newly hatched chicks are permanently separated from parent birds and hand-fed by humans until weaning. This form of hand-raising may, however, introduce several sources of error. Inappropriate diets and thermal environments as well as the aspiration of food into the lungs may increase mortality rates of hand-raised chicks (Davis & Millam 1997). Furthermore, hand-raised chicks may lose their capacity to reproduce if they imprint on the humans that hand-rear them. These issues prompted Davis and Millam (1997) to ask whether a combination of hand-rearing and parent-rearing might alleviate some of these problems while at the same time producing tame parrots. A shared method of rearing tamed chicks would not only decrease the risk of chick mortality but also significantly decrease the amount of human labor necessary to produce tame birds. Davis and Millam demonstrated that tamed parrots could be produced by short, regular periods of handling by humans while parent birds provided the primary care for the chicks. In their study, chicks were handled daily for 15 to 30 minutes from day 12 until fledging. The researchers found that handled chicks scored high on a series of tameness tests. A follow-up study (Davis & Millam 1997) revealed that chicks that were handled later in life (handling began at 35 days of age) were more tame than the early handled birds

and the experimenters judged the birds to be as tame as hand-raised birds.

Collette et al. (2000) confirmed and extended Davis and Millam's findings. They found that postnatally handled chicks were more tame on all behavioral tests than non-handled chicks. They also examined the influence of taming on immune status. After fledging, birds were physically restrained for a period of ten minutes. For handled birds, the restraint consisted only of perching on a human hand; however, non-handled birds would not perch on a human hand so they were instead wrapped in a towel. After the period of restraint, immune status was assessed by responses to (1) humoral response to a killed Newcastle disease virus; (2) serum corticosterone levels; (3) heterophil:lymphocyte ratios; and (4) delayed-type hypersensitivity (DTH) test to a foreign protein (phytohemagglutinin). DTH responses are antigen-specific, cell-mediated immune reactions (Dhabhar 1998). Experiments have shown that acute stress administered immediately before the introduction of an antigenic challenge significantly enhances a cutaneous DTH response, whereas chronic stress suppresses cutaneous DTH (Dhabhar 1998). Collette found that handled chicks had a significantly greater humoral response to Newcastle disease virus and a significantly lower DTH response to a foreign protein than did non-handled chicks. According to current immunologic theory, antibody response is inversely related to DTH response (Hassig et al. 1996). Corticosterone levels were also lower in handled chicks, but the difference between the two groups was not statistically significant. Handled and non-handled chicks were indistinguishable with respect to heterophil:lymphocyte ratios.

Although Davis and Millam (1997) and Collette et al. (2000) found that postnatal handling resulted in tame chicks, both studies reported a considerable variation in degree of tameness. Since a high degree of tameness may be valued by individuals seeking parrots as companion animals, and tameness may reduce the degree of stress parrots experience in captive environments, it is important to consider what factor, or factors, may have led to the observed degrees of tameness in these studies.

Handler personality is one possibility. Seabrook (1972) examined the influence of the herdsman's personality on milk yields of dairy cows. He found that "good" herders' cows produced as much as 20% more milk than cows under the care of other herders at similar facilities under the same ownership. Seabrook defined a good herder as one with "knowledge of the behaviour of the individual cows in the herd and the ability to notice deviations from normal behaviour" (p. 376). He found that patient herdsmen that behaved consistently and showed consideration for their cows' needs had cows with the best milk yield. Other traits of the good herders included confidence, self-reliance, and introverted personalities. Other studies have found that pigs that are fearful of humans after intentional aversive handling experiences had depressed growth rates and reproductive performance (see, e.g., Hemsworth et al. 1981, 1986). This is probably due to a chronic stress response, since even after aversive handling ceased, and humans were no longer present, pigs continued to exhibit elevated levels of plasma-free corticosteroids.

Empathy

Although it is difficult to predict what factor, or factors, of human personality may influence an animal's fear response to a human, the ability to empathize might be one important trait. People who experience sympathy or empathy "are more likely to help, comfort, or share with other people or animals" (Eisenberg 1988, p. 16). Conversely, cruelty toward other people or animals is considered, by mental health professionals, to be the result of a distortion in the development of empathy (Ascione 1993).

Definitions of empathy are varied but similar. For example, it has been defined as "the capacity to feel what another is feeling" (Zahn-Waxler et al. 1985, p. 22), or "the power of understanding and imaginatively entering into another's feelings" (Fox 1985, p. 61), or "a vicariously induced emotional reaction based on the apprehension of another's state or condition that is similar to the other's emotional state or consistent with the other's situation" (Eisenberg 1988, p. 15).

Darwin described the empathy that developed between himself and his dog as an interaction whereby an animal and a human intuit the other's state from behavioral cues (cited in Buck and Ginsburg 1997). In animal handling, an empathic handler presumably makes accurate assessments

of an animal's fearfulness or timidity in certain situations. The empathic handler would then make adjustments in his or her behavior or the environment in order to lessen the animal's experience of fear or apprehension. In contrast, a handler that fails to take an animal's perspective and to recognize and correctly interpret the animal's cues may handle the animal inappropriately in relation to its internal state; if handled regularly by the same individual, the animal may become conditioned to fear humans and to experience them as stressful stimuli.

Purpose

This study was undertaken to address an aspect of emerging societal concern: human-animal interaction. The purpose of this study was to examine the relationship between the level of empathy of the handler, the attitude of the handler toward pets, and the degree of tameness and immune competence in handled parrots. It was hypothesized that parrots handled by more empathic handlers would exhibit a higher level of tameness and an increased ability to cope with stress than birds handled by less empathic handlers. Since genetic factors and quality of parrot parenting may also play a role in tameness and immune competence, these variables were also examined.

A better understanding of the human factors that increase tameness and the ability to respond effectively to stress is expected to (1) benefit aviculturists who wish to rear highly marketable parrots for the pet bird trade, (2) contribute to the overall welfare of parrots that must co-exist with humans in their captive environments, and (3) increase the knowledge of the effects that people have on the behavior of captive parrots.

PARTICIPANTS, ANIMALS, MATERIALS, AND METHODS

Human Participants

In order to examine the effect of handler empathy on parrot tameness, volunteer handlers that scored either high or low on the construct of empathy were solicited from the student population of the University of California, Davis. Potential participants were contacted by U.S. mail, electronic mail, posters, and classroom solicitations. In order to avoid any confounding sex differences, only female students were selected to participate in the study. The average age of the participants in this study was 21 years.

Procedure

Students interested in participating in the handling study were asked to call or e-mail the experimenter to request a personality test. Ninety-two students requested personality tests. Sixty-eight students returned completed personality tests. Seven students were selected to participate in the handling study. The number of participants selected was based on the number of chicks available to be handled. The ratio of handlers to chicks was 1:3.

Personality test scores were not revealed to any students. As compensation for the time required to complete the questionnaire, each student who returned a questionnaire was provided with a list of occupations engaged in by individuals with profiles similar to their own. These occupational profiles are often used by professionals in career counseling.

Selected participants were required to complete a health surveillance questionnaire and to discuss their responses with a nurse at Employee Health Services, University of California, Davis. Participants were also required by the Office of the Campus Veterinarian, University of California, Davis, to obtain tuberculosis clearance (via a tuberculin skin test) and to have a serum sample drawn for archival purposes. Both procedures were conducted by personnel at Employee Health Services. There was no cost to the participants for these medical procedures.

Instruments

16PF
The Sixteen Personality Factor Questionnaire (Institute for Personality and Ability Testing, Inc., Champaign, Illinois) is a psychological assessment instrument designed by Raymond B. Cattell. In the 1940s, Cattell used factor analysis to reduce 45 categories of words, commonly used in the English language to describe human personality, to 15 dimensions of personality (Karson & O'Dell 1976). Later, three less replicable factors were discarded and four factors that were considered important were added (Karson & O'Dell 1976). Currently, the test measures 16 normal dimensions of adult personality: warmth, reasoning ability, emotional stability, dominance, impulsiv-

ity, conformity, social boldness, sensitivity, vigilance, imagination, privateness, apprehension, openness to change, self-reliance, perfectionism, and tension. Since the first-order factors are correlated, or oblique factors, Cattell was able to conduct a second factor analysis and arrive at second-order factors. These factors summarize the relationships found among the 16 first-order factors. The test measures five second-order factors: extraversion, anxiety, tough-mindedness, independence, and self-control. The 16PF consists of a total of 187 questions.

The 16PF was employed in this study to measure the level of one second-order personality factor: tough-mindedness, a measure of empathy. An individual who scores *high* on tough-mindedness has *low* scores on four first-order factors: warmth, emotional sensitivity, imagination, and openness to change (Karson and O'Dell 1976). Karson and O'Dell (1976) explain that these people are much less likely to be controlled by their feelings than by their intellect. In contrast, a low tough-mindedness score is associated with high scores on the first-order factors of warmth, emotional sensitivity, imagination, and openness to change.

All tests were hand-scored. Females who scored high (7.7–10) or low (1.0–2.0) on tough-mindedness were selected to handle parrot chicks. Due to the fact that very few female test-takers scored on the high end of the tough-mindedness scale, a larger point spread was allowed in the high tough-mindedness handlers' scores than in the low tough-mindedness handlers' scores (2.3 versus 1.0 point spread).

PET ATTITUDE SCALE
Prior to the start of handling, the Pet Attitude Scale (PAS; Templer et al. 1981; see Appendix 12A) was administered to participants to measure favorableness of attitudes toward pets. The PAS was selected because it is one of few published scales with reliability information: Cronbach's alpha coefficient is 0.93, and two-week test-retest stability is 0.92 (Lago et al. 1988). The PAS consists of 18 7-point Likert format questions; therefore, 126 points are possible. A higher score represents a more favorable attitude toward pets. The items on the PAS represent three factorially derived scales: love and interaction, pets in the home, and joy of pet ownership.

Animals and Housing

The animals in this study were the offspring of wild-caught Orange-winged Amazon Parrots (*Amazona amazonica*). All chicks hatched in the animal colony at the University of California, Davis. Sixteen breeding pairs were housed in two adjacent rooms, one pair per cage, eight pairs per room. Pairs were housed in 1 m x 1 m x 2 m suspended, wire welded cages. Each cage had two 1 m x 4 cm x 8.5 cm wooden perches mounted with metal brackets to the 2 m lengths of the cage. One perch was mounted near the front of the cage (the cage door end) and the other near the rear (the nest box end) of the cage. Birds were maintained in accordance with the University of California, Davis, Animal Use and Care Provisions.

BREEDING CONDITIONS

Sixteen pairs of Orange-winged Amazons were stimulated to breed by exposure to long day-lengths and the provision of nest boxes. Nest boxes were presented to breeding pairs on May 21, 1997. Stainless steel sheet metal "grandfather clock" type (40 cm x 38 cm x 76 cm) nest boxes were installed at the rear of each cage on its exterior surface. A 14 cm x 18 cm opening in the wire of the cage provided access to the nest box hole. The nest box hole was surrounded with a wooden insert with a 9 cm diameter hole in it. The wooden insert enabled the birds to enlarge the hole and, in a sense, chew through it into the nest box. The nest box floors were lined with 8–12 cm of autoclaved, premium-grade pine shavings.

On the same day that nest boxes were presented, light schedules began to be increased from 10 hours light and 14 hours dark (10L:14D) to 14L:10D. Light was increased by 30-minute increments each day (15 minutes in the A.M. and 15 minutes in the P.M.) over a period of eight days.

Diet was changed from Roudybush maintenance pellets (provided during non-breeding periods) to Roudybush breeder pellets (Roudybush Inc., Sacramento, California) during breeding, laying, and rearing stages. Water was available ad libitum from nipple waterers.

CHICK FOSTERING

Due to the cannibalistic behavior of two breeding pairs (sire band #693 & dam band #458, and sire #187 & dam #338) in previous breeding seasons, all fertile eggs were removed from the nest boxes of these pairs. The eggs were placed either with another suitable breeding pair during the late incubation stage or in an incubator (RX2TT, serial no. MM, cat. no. 910-063, Lyon Electric Co., Chula Vista, California) during the early incubation stage and then transferred to another breeding pair during the late incubation stage. Incubator conditions were as follows: (1) average wet and dry bulb temperatures were 87 and 99 degrees Fahrenheit (30.6 and 37.2 Celsius), respectively; (2) relative humidity ranged from 60 to 65%; and (3) eggs were rotated by automatic turner once per hour.

Handling Procedure

Handling of chicks began between 28 and 35 days post-hatch. Each handler was assigned three chicks to handle for the duration of the study. Clutchmates were not assigned to the same handler. Within each clutch, chicks were randomly assigned to either a high or low tough-mindedness handler. When clutches consisted of an even number of chicks, equal numbers of chicks were assigned to high and low tough-mindedness handlers. A total of 20 chicks were included in the handling study: 11 chicks were assigned to low-empathy handlers and nine chicks were assigned to high-empathy handlers.

To allow for freedom of interaction between handlers and chicks, handlers were provided only basic instructions about the handling procedure. They were shown how to isolate the parent birds from the nest box by insertion of a metal plate between the lower one-third and upper two-thirds of the grandfather style next box, and how to remove the chicks from the nest box and place them in a shallow, towel-lined plastic tub. The handlers were instructed to handle each chick individually and to interact with the chick in any way they chose. Each chick was handled three times per week and handling sessions lasted for a period of 20 minutes. Handling continued until the time of testing.

All chicks were also handled briefly by the principal investigator during leg band placement, weekly weight measurements, and twice-weekly nest box cleaning. During nest box cleaning, the chicks in a clutch were placed in a towel-lined, plastic tub while the soiled pine shavings were replaced with clean shavings.

Tameness Tests

CHICKS

After fledging (approximately 56 days post-hatch), a series of tameness measures was made on each chick (see Chick Tameness Score Sheet, Appendix 12B). The tests consisted of both behavioral and physiological measures. The behavioral measures included (1) response to extended finger/hand; (2) response to touch on head, cheek, or back; (3) response to a food offering (Cheerios brand breakfast cereal, General Mills Inc., Minneapolis, Minnesota); (4) response to a novel object (a 4 cm length of plastic drinking straw); and (5) proximity seeking (i.e., did the bird seek closeness with a human or with another parrot of the same species?).

Two indirect measures of fear were made: respirations per minute and period of latency to defecation. These measures were selected because they were (1) non-invasive and (2) viewable at a distance by a second test administrator. Respirations per minute were measured after the bird was removed from the home cage and allowed to settle on the test perch for 60 seconds in full view of the test administrators. The latency to defecation test was limited to 300 seconds. A score of 300 was assigned to the bird if the latency period exceeded 300 seconds.

Five tameness test trials were made on each chick. The first trial was carried out by the bird's handler. Two succeeding trials were conducted by each of two individuals that the bird had never interacted with previously (i.e., a "stranger"). During each trial, the bird's behavior was recorded by two individuals: the person administering the tests to the bird and one additional individual. The latter also made timed measures of respiration rate and latency to defecation using a stopwatch. Test administrators were blind. When the two individuals recording the bird's behaviors disagreed about a behavioral tameness measure, the lower (i.e., less tame) score was awarded to the bird. The five scores from each of the five trials were averaged to obtain one overall tameness score. Likewise, the five measures of respiration rate and latency to defecation were averaged.

PARENT BIRDS

Behavioral and physiological measures of tameness were also made on the wild-caught parent birds in order to assess a possible genetic compo-
nent of fearfulness or tameness. The chick tameness tests were modified for use with the adult wild birds (see Appendix 12C). For example, most of the wild birds would not approach a human; therefore, a measure was made of whether or not the bird withdrew to the more distant perch when a human stood in front of the cage. Also, responses to the opening of the cage door and the extension of a hand into the cage were recorded. Respiration rate and latency to defecation were measured while the experimenter stood in front of the cage. Timing of latency to defecation began immediately after the experimenter stepped in front of the cage. As with the chicks, the latency test was limited to 300 seconds: a score of 300 was assigned to the bird when the latency period exceeded 300 seconds. Respiration rate was measured after the experimenter had been in full view of the birds for 60 seconds.

Quality of Parenting Measures

Two variables were selected to represent measures of quality of parenting: (1) chick rate of weight gain, and (2) chick plumage condition. Each chick was weighed every seven days beginning on day 7 post-hatch. Weekly rate of absolute weight gain over the first four weeks of life was averaged.

Since some breeding pairs had a history in prior breeding seasons of pulling out their chicks' feathers, this behavior was also recorded as a measure of quality of parenting. Chick plumage condition was scored either as feather-plucked or non-plucked.

Immunoresponse Test

Immune status was assessed by response to a DTH test to a foreign protein, phytohemagglutinin-M (USB Specialty Biochemicals, Cleveland, Ohio). This test was selected because Collette et al. (2000) found a significant DTH response in handled versus non-handled Amazon chicks. Following the completion of tameness measures, each chick was placed in an animal carrier (26 cm x 28 cm x 40 cm) to produce a condition of novel environment and mild immobilization stress. Chicks were retained in the carrier for a period of five minutes. Placement in an animal carrier was selected as a stressor because most captive animals will be transported in carriers during their lifetimes; therefore, it allowed the inducement of a stress that would occur under normal conditions in captivity.

Twenty-four hours after initial placement in the carrier (at 7 A.M.), each chick was again retained in the carrier for five minutes. After this, wing web thickness was measured with a micrometer and marked with a black marker dot. Phytohemagglutinin-M (0.25 mg dissolved in 0.05 ml sterile saline) was then injected subcutaneously to the marker dot in the wing web. After 12 hours (7 P.M.), the area was measured again for change in tissue thickness.

Statistics

SAS (1990) was employed to conduct all statistical analyses. The procedure used was PROC REG, version 6.12. Stepwise regression analysis was utilized to analyze the data. Regression analysis allowed the development of an equation that enabled the prediction of one variable from the knowledge of another variable.

At each stage in the stepwise regression procedure, the algorithm began with the calculation of F-statistics for each of the predictors that were currently selected for the regression model. If a predictor did not meet a specified significance level (0.100 in this study), it was removed from the equation. Next, an attempt was made to add a new predictor by calculating an F-statistic for each variable not currently in the equation. At each step in the model-building procedure, at most, one term was removed from or added to the model. If one or more terms were eligible to be removed, the one with the largest significance level (p-value) was removed. If one or more terms were eligible to be added to the model, the one with the smallest significance level was added. The stepwise regression procedure stopped when predictors were no longer added or deleted.

The procedure used to analyze the data in this study differed in that handler tough-mindedness was forced to be included in all regression models. This was done because the purpose of the study was to determine whether handler tough-mindedness had an impact on tameness; therefore, p-values were being sought regardless of whether they were or were not significant. Other predictors that were examined included handler attitude toward pets, whether or not chicks were feather-plucked, average rate of weight gain over

the first four weeks of life, and behavioral and physiological measures of tameness in parent birds.

RESULTS

Reproductive Response

Fourteen breeding pairs produced a total of 77 eggs. At least 44 of the 77 eggs were fertile. Thirty-four eggs hatched (hatch rate = ~77%). The average number of chicks reared by a breeding pair was 2.3 chicks. This number includes foster chicks (see the following section on chick fostering). Six fertile eggs suffered damage inflicted by the parent birds: one female (#352) fractured her five eggs by pecking them when the nest box door was opened; another pair (#369 and #172) punctured the shell of one of their eggs with a toenail. Although the holes and fractures were patched with tape, all of the damaged eggs failed to hatch.

Candling revealed that 27 eggs were infertile. The fertility status of six other artificially incubated eggs was indeterminable; either the embryos died early or the eggs were infertile.

Twelve chicks that hatched later died. Five hatchlings and one three-month-old chick (band #97-29) were killed by parent birds (sire #540 & dam #389, sire #436 & dam #602, and sire #183 & dam #374). Three hatchlings died due to parental neglect (sire #519 & dam #350, and sire #513 & dam #352). One six-week-old chick died from a respiratory infection (#97-22). The cause of death of two remaining hatchlings was unknown.

Six breeding pairs that experienced the loss of their first clutch produced a second clutch. Average size of second clutches was four eggs. Only one pair (sire #436 & dam #602) had a surviving chick from the first clutch. One pair (sire #433 & dam #504) failed to produce any fertile eggs in either the first or second clutch. Two pairs had the eggs in their first clutches removed to an incubator due a cannibalistic history by the pair (sire #693 & dam #458, and sire #187 & dam #338). One pair (sire #540 & dam #389) killed all of the chicks in the first clutch. Another pair (sire #513 & dam #352) fractured all of the eggs in the first clutch and, as a result, the embryos died.

One breeding pair failed to produce any eggs,

although a bowl was created in the nest box shavings. Another pair, later determined by genetic sexing to consist of two females, laid a total of five infertile eggs. Three other pairs produced only infertile eggs.

Of the surviving 23 chicks, 11 were assigned to low-empathy handlers and nine were assigned to the high-empathy handlers. Three chicks (#97-22, #97-23, and #97-24) were excluded from the study because they suffered from a chronic respiratory infection that required administration of twice-daily injectible and oral antibiotics; therefore, it was believed that tameness outcomes would be confounded by the frequent and aversive handling of these chicks.

Chick Fostering

Due to the cannibalistic behavior of two breeding pairs in previous breeding seasons (sire #187 & dam #338, and sire #693 & dam #458), their eggs were fostered to other possibly more suitable pairs. A third pair (sire #540 & dam #389) killed all of the chicks in their first clutch and the first chick in their second clutch during the current breeding season. The female of this pair had been treated for a respiratory infection during the incubation of her first clutch. The three remaining eggs in her second clutch were fostered to other pairs.

Four pairs were selected to foster eggs from the late incubation stage. During early incubation, some eggs remained with the biological parents and others were artificially incubated. Incubation in an incubator served a dual purpose: it provided an environment for the growth and development of embryos, and it also allowed the developing chicks to be photographed during the various stages of development without any disturbance to adult birds. The photographs of the embryos were used in another study. Four of ten artificially incubated eggs hatched. Two of these chicks were successfully reared by foster parent birds.

A total of 13 fertile eggs were fostered (four artificially incubated and nine naturally incubated). Eggs were fostered one week prior to the expected date of hatch. Ten chicks hatched and eight chicks survived. Two pairs successfully completed the incubation of foster eggs: chicks hatched and were successfully reared. One of these pairs (sire #368 & dam #407) completed the incubation of two eggs from the incubator. The other pair (sire #495 & dam #545) successfully completed the late incubation stage of three eggs that were previously incubated by the biological dam (#458). Neither foster pair had produced any fertile eggs of their own. Their infertile eggs were replaced with an equal number of fertile foster eggs.

Two other pairs successfully incubated foster eggs and chicks hatched; however, some chicks were killed or neglected (which resulted in death). One of these foster pairs (#379 & #646) produced no fertile eggs because both birds were later determined by genetic sexing to be females. The first hatchling in their care was found dead on day 2 post-hatch; therefore, the two remaining foster eggs were fostered to another pair (sire #183 & dam #374). The latter pair completed the incubation of the eggs and successfully reared the two chicks for three months before killing the younger chick. Another foster pair (sire #513 & dam #352) produced one hatchling of their own, but it was found dead on the same day that the first foster chick hatched. A second foster hatchling in their care survived only one week.

One chick hatched in the incubator five days prior to the expected date of hatch. This chick was fostered to a pair that was successfully raising four of their own chicks (sire #317 & dam #111). The pair's youngest chick was close in age to the fostered chick. The foster chick failed to thrive and expired after seven days. Whether this was due to a biological anomaly that may have been associated with the chick's early hatching or whether it was due to the possibly overworked parents' ability to provide for one additional chick is unknown.

Tameness

EMPATHY

The global factor "tough-mindedness" was utilized as a measure of handler empathy. The tough-mindedness scale ranges from 1 to 10. A lower tough-mindedness score is associated with a higher degree of empathy. Handler scores were 1.6, 1.9, 2.0, 7.7 (two handlers with this score), 8.7, and 9.3.

According to the stepwise regression models, handler tough-mindedness significantly predicted both physiological measures of tameness. Tough-mindedness predicted chick respiration rate,

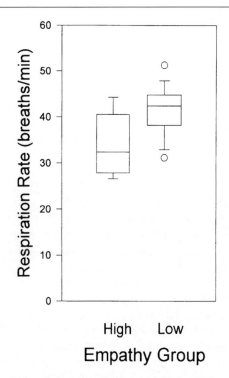

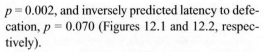

Figure 12.1. Chicks handled by low-empathy handlers had elevated respiration rates (p = 0.002 [coefficient = 1.282] by stepwise linear regression). Plots depict median (line), 25th, 75th percentiles (box), and 5th, 95th percentiles (circles).

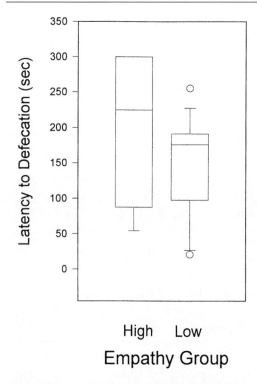

Figure 12.2. Chicks handled by low-empathy handlers had shorter latencies to defecation (p = 0.069 [coefficient = −9.713] by stepwise linear regression) (plot key as in Figure 12.1).

p = 0.002, and inversely predicted latency to defecation, p = 0.070 (Figures 12.1 and 12.2, respectively).

In contrast, handler tough-mindedness did not significantly predict the behavioral measure of tameness, p = 0.947. Birds handled either by high- or low-empathy handlers did not demonstrate appreciable differences in behavioral tameness. They perched on experimenters' hands, permitted human touch, and accepted food items and novel objects from experimenters.

ATTITUDE
Templer's PAS was employed to measure handler attitude toward pets. A higher score is associated with a more positive attitude toward pets. A total of 126 points are possible. Pet attitude scores of the handlers in this study were 108, 111, 112, 113, 117 (two handlers with this score), and 123.

According to the stepwise regression models,

handler attitude did not significantly predict behavioral tameness, p = 0.190, latency to defecation, p = 0.500, or respiration rate, p = 0.883. The correlation between pet attitude and tough-mindedness was weak, r = 0.101.

PARENTING VARIABLES
Quality of parenting was assessed by measures of two variables: (1) chick average rate of weekly weight gain over the first four weeks of life, and (2) chick plumage condition. Three breeding pairs (sire #513 & dam #352, sire #519 & dam #350, and sire #436 & dam #602) were responsible for feather plucking 25% of the chicks in the study.

A feather-plucked condition significantly predicted both physiological measures of tameness: respiration rate, p = 0.005, and latency to defecation, p = 0.048 (Figures 12.3 and 12.4, respectively). However, according to the sums of

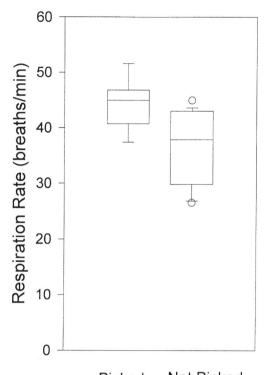

Figure 12.3. Feather-picked chicks had higher respiration rates than non-picked chicks ($p = 0.005$ [coefficient = -8.06] by stepwise linear regression) (plot key as in Figure 12.1).

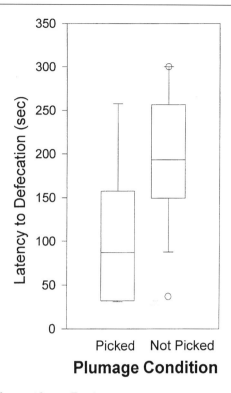

Figure 12.4. Feather-picked chicks had shorter latencies to defecation than non-picked chicks ($p = 0.048$ [coefficient = -78.5] by stepwise linear regression) (plot key as in Figure 12.1).

squares, handler tough-mindedness was a better predictor of respiration rate than was a feather-plucked condition (sum of squares = 329.7 versus 238.5, respectively). In contrast, a feather-plucked condition was a somewhat better predictor of latency to defecation than was handler tough-mindedness (sum of squares = 22,667 versus 18,632, respectively).

In contrast to the effect of handler tough-mindedness on behavioral tameness, a feather-plucked condition significantly and inversely predicted behavioral tameness, $p = 0.042$ (Figure 12.5).

Rate of weight gain did not significantly predict any measure of tameness. Mean weekly chick weight gain over the first four weeks of life was 84.55 grams/week ± 2.78 grams/week (mean ± SE).

PARENTAL TAMENESS

Paternal respiration rate inversely and significantly predicted latency to defecation in chicks, $p = 0.013$ (Figure 12.6). It was a more significant predictor of latency to defecation than either feather-plucked condition or handler tough-mindedness (sum of squares = 38,950 versus 22,667 and 18,632, respectively).

Maternal behavioral tameness inversely and significantly predicted chick tameness, $p = 0.007$ (Figure 12.7). Interestingly, the correlation between foster chick tameness and biological dam tameness was greater than the correlation between foster chick tameness and foster dam tameness, r = -0.400 versus r = -0.249, respectively.

Cell-Mediated Immunity

According to the stepwise regression model, handler empathy did not predict immune response, $p = 0.761$. Birds handled either by high- or low-empathy handlers did not demonstrate any dis-

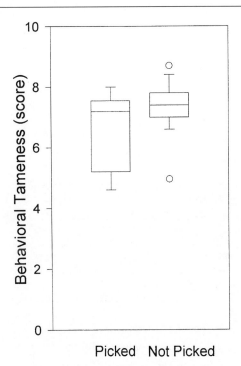

Plumage Condition

Figure 12.5. Feather-picked chicks were less tame than non-picked chicks (p = 0.042 [coefficient = 1.13] by stepwise linear regression) (plot key as in Figure 12.1).

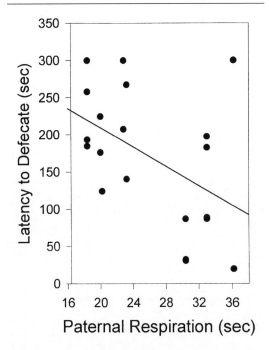

Figure 12.6. Paternal respiration rate inversely predicted chick latency to defecation (p = 0.013 [coefficient = -6.92] by stepwise linear regression).

cernible difference in change in wing thickness after the administration of PHA-M. Mean wing thickness change in birds handled by low-empathy handlers was 0.592 mm ±0.169 mm (n = 11) versus 0.579 mm ± 0.261 mm (n = 7) in birds handled by empathic handlers. Two birds handled by empathic handlers were omitted from the computations because one chick died before the test was conducted and an improper measuring technique led to an erroneous measure on a second chick.

DISCUSSION

Tameness

HANDLER EMPATHY

The results of this study support, in part, the hypothesis that degree of handler empathy affects parrot chick tameness. Level of handler empathy was found to significantly influence both physiological measures of fear examined in this study:

respiration rate and period of latency to defecation. In the presence of humans, chicks that had been handled by individuals with lower levels of empathy exhibited higher rates of respiration and shorter periods of latency to defecation than chicks that had been handled by high-empathy handlers.

The surprising finding in this study is that birds handled either by high- or low-empathy handlers exhibited overtly tame behaviors such as a willingness to perch on a human hand and permit human touch. However, although birds handled by low-empathy handlers exhibited tame behaviors, the results of this study suggest that these birds continued to experience fear on a physiological level when in the presence of humans. This outcome is consistent with Hennessy and Levine's (1979) finding that "some physiological responses may habituate more slowly than overt behavioral reactions" (qtd. in Levine et al. 1989, p. 344). Habituation is the process by which new stimuli or situations are compared with representations in the CNS of previous events (Sokolov,

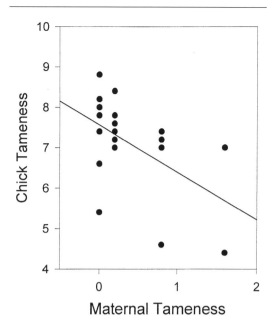

Figure 12.7. Maternal behavioral tameness inversely predicted chick behavioral tameness (p = 0.007 [coefficient = -1.39] by stepwise linear regression).

cited in Levine et al. 1989). Novelty, uncertainty, conflict, or fear may result in a mismatch upon which the animal experiences an alerting, or arousing, reaction that activates the neuroendocrine system.

The results of this study indicate that some factor, or factors, in the behavior of the low-empathy handlers led to the arousal of the birds, on a physiological level, to all humans in the study. As stated earlier, Beck and Katcher (1989) found that bird owners had to reduce their own state of activation in order to interact with their birds. Perhaps the low-empathy handlers in this study failed to reduce their state of activation; therefore, their behaviors were inconsistent with the handled birds' internal states. Consequently, these birds may have continued to experience fear, internal conflict, and/or uncertainty in the presence of any human. Also, unlike the "good" herders in Seabrook's (1972) study, perhaps the low-empathy handlers' behaviors were unpredictable; therefore, these birds continued to interpret each human encountered as a fear-inducing, novel, and/or uncertain stimulus.

HANDLER ATTITUDE

Handler attitude toward pets did not correlate with parrot chick tameness. Presumably, this is due to the fact that there was a cluster of high handler attitude scores. The small handler sample size (n = 7) may also have led to this negative result. It is not surprising that the participants scored high on a scale designed to measure attitude toward pets, since the sample was self-selected to participate in a research project involving the handling of neonatal parrots. Perhaps behavioral tameness, which was not predicted by tough-mindedness in this study, is more easily affected by handler attitude than handler tough-mindedness.

QUALITY OF PARENTING

At least one factor of parenting is an important predictor of chick tameness. Feather plucking of chicks by parent birds significantly predicted both measures of physiological tameness, but to a lesser degree than handler empathy.

Normal preening, or feather grooming, of chicks is a necessary parental bird behavior. In preening, each feather is drawn individually through the bird's beak; this process smooths the feather and removes debris. Hence, normal preening maintains good feather condition and is, therefore, essential to chick survival, especially in the wild.

Suchecki and her colleagues (1993) have found that some maternal behaviors in rats are necessary not only for the survival of the young but also for the regulation of the development of some physiological systems. The researchers found that maternal behaviors exert dual control over HPA axis regulation: (1) feeding keeps the adrenal glands insensitive to ACTH during the stress hyporesponsive period (SHRP) in the first two weeks of life, and (2) licking of the anogenital region to induce urination and defecation plays a role in inhibiting ACTH secretion. It is possible, therefore, that excessive parental behaviors, such as preening to the extent that it results in the removal of feathers, may perturb the normal ontogeny of the HPA axis and result in an oversensitization of the system to novel and/or stressful stimuli.

The degree to which feather plucking may occur in the wild is not known; however, it seems that extensive feather plucking would be maladaptive and selected against. The basis of feather plucking or "overgrooming" in captivity is not understood, but repeated human handling may be one contributing factor. It is interesting that the chicks in one feather-plucked clutch (not included in the study) required excessive, and intrinsically ungentle, human handling for treatment of a chronic respiratory infection. The chicks were frequently returned to the nest box or home cage with their plumage in disarray. If parental grooming of chicks is a response to soiled and/or malaligned feathers, overgrooming could conceivably develop from repeated human handling.

It is not surprising that parenting factors influence tameness. Since, in this study, chicks spent more than 99% of their time in the care of their parents, the opportunity for chick tameness to be influenced by parental factors was great. It is likely that numerous other parenting factors exist that may also affect chick tameness. The potential exists to select breeding pairs that exhibit specific parenting qualities that increase chick tameness. Work to identify important parenting variables has recently begun with the analysis of videotapes, made during the course of the present study, of parent and chick interaction in the nest box.

PARENTAL TAMENESS

One counterintuitive finding from this study is that maternal behavioral tameness inversely and significantly predicted chick behavioral tameness. This result may be due to either post-hatch environmental factors or genetic factors or some combination of the two. Perhaps an as-yet-unidentified difference in the maternal behaviors of more and less tame mothers accounts for the inverse relationship of maternal and chick behavioral tameness. The results indicate that there may be a genetic component, since foster chick tameness was more strongly correlated with biological dam tameness than with foster dam tameness.

Paternal respiration rate also significantly and inversely predicted chick latency to defecation: male parents with low respiration rates in the presence of humans had chicks with long periods of latency to defecation when humans were present. This outcome suggests that there may also be a genetic component to fearfulness. Taken together, these results suggest that chicks may inherit very different factors of tameness from each parent.

Immune Status

Neither degree of handler empathy nor attitude toward pets significantly predicted cell-mediated response to a foreign protein challenge. Chicks handled either by high- or low-empathy handlers showed similar changes in wing thickness. As stated earlier, Collette et al. (2000) found that handled parrot chicks had a lower cell-mediated response and a higher antibody response to a Newcastle disease virus challenge than did non-handled chicks. This inverse relationship between the two immune responses would be predicted if the birds had experienced handling as a stressful stimulus (Hassig et al. 1996). The results of the present study support Collette's finding that human handling is interpreted as stressful and activates the neuroendocrine system; however, the results here show that handling and human presence are interpreted as stressful only when postnatal handling has been carried out by a human handler with a low level of empathy.

CONCLUSION

Differences in empathy of humans providing neonatal handling of Amazon chicks produced differences in physiologic indices of stress, although no difference was detected in chick behavioral tameness or DTH response. Parental feather picking predicted differences in both physiologic and behavioral responses to handling but not DTH response to a foreign protein challenge. The results suggest that adaptability of wild animals to captivity might be improved by a better understanding of the basis for differences in the effects of quality of parenting and human handler personality on behavioral development of parrots.

REFERENCES

Alcock, J. 1993. Animal behavior. Sunderland, MA: Sinauer Associates, Inc.

Ascione, F.R. 1993. Children who are cruel to animals: A review of research and implications for developmental psychopathology. *Anthrozoos* 6:226–247.

Beck. A.M., and A.H. Katcher. 1989. Bird-human interaction. *Journal of the Association of Avian Veterinarians* 3:152–153.

Bodnoff, S.R., B. Suranyi-Cadotte, R. Quirion, and M.J. Meaney. 1987. Postnatal handling reduces novelty-induced fear and increases [^{3}H]flunitrazepam binding in rat brain. *European Journal of Pharmacology* 144:105–107.

Buck, R., and B. Ginsburg. 1997. "Communicative genes and the evolution of empathy." In *Empathic accuracy,* ed. W. Ickes, pp. 17–43. New York: Guilford Press.

Collette, J.C., J.R. Millam, K.C. Klasing, and P.S. Wakenell. 2000. Neonatal handling of Amazon parrots alters the stress response and immune function. *Applied Animal Behavior Science* 66:335–349.

Davis, W.L. (now Aengus), and J.R. Millam. 1997. Tameness produced by the neonatal handling of parent-raised orange-winged amazon chicks. Master's thesis, University of California, Davis.

Denenberg, V.H., and M.X. Zarrow. 1971. "Effect of handling in infancy upon adult behavior and adrenocortical activity: Suggestions for a neuroendocrine mechanism." In *Early childhood: The development of self regulatory mechanisms,* ed. D.H. Walcher and D.L. Peters, pp. 40–74. New York: Academic Press.

Dhabhar, F.S. 1998. Stress-induced enhancement of cell-mediated immunity. *Annals of the New York Academy of Sciences* 840:359–372.

Duncan, I.J.H. 1992. "The effect of the researcher on the behavior of poultry." In *The inevitable bond: Examining scientist-animal interactions,* ed. H. Davis and D. Balfour, pp. 285–294. Cambridge: Cambridge University Press.

Eisenberg, N. 1988. Empathy and sympathy: A brief review of the concepts and empirical literature. *Anthrozoos* 2:15–17.

Fox, M.W. 1985. "Empathy, humaneness and animal welfare." In *Advances in animal welfare science 1984,* ed. M.W. Fox and L.D. Mickley, pp. 61–73. Hingham, MA: Kluwer Academic Publishers.

Gross, W.B., and P.B. Siegel. 1979. Adaptation of chickens to their handler, and experimental results. *Avian Diseases* 23:708–714.

Harris, J.M. 1989. Avian companions and the human-animal bond. *Journal of the American Veterinary Medical Association* 195:1517–1518.

Hassig, A., L. Wen-Xi, and K. Stampfli. 1996. Stress-induced suppression of the cellular immune reactions: On the neuroendocrine control of the immune system. *Medical Hypotheses* 46:551–555.

Hemsworth, P.H., J.L. Barnett, and C. Hansen. 1981. The influence of handling by humans on the behaviour, reproduction and corticosteroids in the juvenile female pig. *Horm Behav* 15:396–403.

Hemsworth, P.H., J.L. Barnett, and C. Hansen. 1986. The influence of handling by humans on the behaviour, reproduction, and corticosteroids of male and female pigs. *Applied Animal Behavior Science* 15:303–314.

Hennessy, J.W., and S. Levine. 1979. Stress, arousal and the pituitary-adrenal system: A psychoendocrine model. *Progress in Psychobiology and Physiological Psychology* 8.

Jones, R.B., and J.M. Faure. 1981. The effects of regular handling on fear responses in the domestic chick. *Behavioral Processes* 6:135–143.

Jones, R.B., and D. Waddington. 1993. Attenuation of the domestic chick's fear of human beings via regular handling: In search of a sensitive period. *Applied Animal Behaviour Science* 36:185–195.

Karsh, E.B. 1983. "The effects of early handling on the development of social bonds between cats and people." In *New perspectives on our lives with companion animals,* ed. A.H. Katcher and A.M. Beck, pp. 22–28. Philadelphia: University of Pennsylvania Press.

Karson, S., and J.W. O'Dell. 1976. *Clinical use of the 16PF.* Champaign, IL: Institute for Personality and Ability Testing.

Lago, D., R. Kafer, M. Delaney, and C. Connell. 1988. Assessment of favorable attitudes toward pets: Development and preliminary validation of self-report pet relationship scales. *Anthrozoos* 1:240–254.

Levine, S. 1957. Infantile experience and resistance to physiological stress. *Science* 125:405.

Levine, S. 1962. Plasma-free corticosteroid response to electric shock in rats stimulated in infancy. *Science* 135:795–796.

Levine, S., C. Coe, and S.G. Wiener. 1989. "Psychoneuroendocrinology of stress: A psychobiological perspective." In *Psychoendocrinology,* ed. R.F. Brush and S. Levine, pp. 341–377. San Diego: Academic Press.

Lorenz, K. 1952. *King Solomon's ring.* New York: Signet.

Lorenz, K.Z. 1953. *Man meets dog.* Baltimore: Penguin.

Loughlin, C.A., and P.W. Dowrick. 1993. Psychological needs filled by avian companions. *Anthrozoos* 6:166–172.

Meaney, M.J., D.H. Aitken, S.R. Bodnoff, L.J. Iny, and R.M. Sapolsky. 1985a. The effects of postnatal handling on the development of the glucocorticoid receptor systems and stress recovery in the rat. *Progress in Neuro-Psychopharmacology & Biological Psychiatry* 9:731–734.

Meaney, M.J., D.H. Aitken, S.R. Bodnoff, L.J. Iny, J.E. Tatarewicz, and R.M. Sapolsky. 1985b. Early postnatal handling alters glucocorticoid receptor concentrations in selected brain regions. *Behavioral Neuroscience* 99:765–770.

Meaney, M.J., D.H. Aitken, and R.M. Sapolsky. 1987. Thyroid hormones influence the development of hippocampal glucocorticoid receptors in the rat: A mechanism for the effects of postnatal handling on the development of the adrenocortical stress response. *Neuroendocrinology* 45:278–283.

Meaney, M.J., D.H. Aitken, C. van Berkel, S. Bhatnagar, and R.M. Sapolsky. 1988. Effect of neonatal handling on age-related impairments associated with the hippocampus. *Science* 239:766–768.

Meaney, M.J., J. Diorio, D. Francis, J. Widdowson, P. LaPlante, C. Caldji, S. Sharma, J.R. Seckl, and P.M. Plotsky. 1996. Early environmental regulation of forebrain glucocorticoid receptor gene expression: Implications for adrenocortical responses to stress. *Developmental Neuroscience* 18:49–72.

Mitchell, J.B., L.J. Iny, and M.J. Meaney. 1990. The role of serotonin in the development and environmental regulation of type II corticosteroid receptor binding in rat hippocampus. *Developmental Brain Research* 55:231–235.

Mugford, R.A., and J.G. M'Comisky. 1975. "Some recent work on the psychotherapeutic value of cage birds with old people." In *Pet animals and society,* ed. R.S. Anderson, pp. 54–65. London: Bailliere Tindall.

Murphy, L.B., and I.J.H. Duncan. 1978. Attempts to modify the responses of domestic fowl towards human beings: II. The effect of early experience. *Applied Animal Ethology* 4:5–12.

Nicol, C.J. 1992. Effects of environmental enrichment and gentle handling on behaviour and fear responses of transported broilers. *Applied Animal Behaviour Science* 33:367–380.

Scott, J.P., and J.L. Fuller. 1965. *Genetics and the social behavior of the dog.* Chicago: University of Chicago Press.

Seabrook, M.F. 1972. A study to determine the influence of the herdsman's personality on milk yields. *J Agric Labour Sci* 1:45–59.

Selye, H. 1950. *The physiology and pathology of exposure to stress.* Montreal: Acta.

Smythe, J.W., W.B. Rowe, and M.J. Meaney. 1994. Neonatal handling alters serotonin (5-HT) turnover and 5-HT2 receptor binding in selected brain regions: Relationship to the handling effect on glucocorticoid receptor expression. *Developmental Brain Research* 80:183–189.

Statistical Analysis Systems Institute, Inc. 1990. *SAS/STAT user's guide: Version 6,* 4th ed. SAS Institute Inc., Cary, NC.

Suchecki, D., P. Rosenfeld, and S. Levine. 1993. Maternal regulation of the hypothalamic-pituitary-adrenal axis in the infant rat: The roles of feeding and stroking. *Developmental Brain Research* 75:185–192.

Templer, D.I., C.A. Salter, S. Dickey, R. Baldwin, and D.M. Veleber. 1981. The construction of a pet attitude scale. *Psychological Record* 31:343–348.

Toft, C.A. 1993. *Genetics of captive propagation for conservation: A manual for aviculturists.* Special publication No. 1, Psittacine Research Project, Dept. of Avian Sciences, University of California, Davis.

Vriends. M.M. 1984. *Pet birds.* New York: Simon and Schuster.

Zahn-Waxler, C., B. Hollenbeck, and M.R. Radke-Yarrow. 1985. "The origins of empathy and altruism." In *Advances in animal welfare science 1984,* ed. M.W. Fox and L.D. Mickley, pp. 21–41. Hingham, MA: Kluwer Academic Publishers.

Appendix 12A

Pet Attitude Scale

1. I really like seeing pets enjoy their food. (+)
2. My pet means more to me than any of my friends. (+)
3. I would like a pet in my home. (+)
4. Having pets is a waste of money. (−)
5. Housepets add happiness to my life (or would if I had one). (+)
6. I feel that pets should always be kept outside. (−)
7. I spend time every day playing with my pet (or I would if I had one). (+)
8. I have occasionally communicated with a pet and understood what it was trying to express. (+)
9. The world would be a better place if people would stop spending so much time caring for their pets and started caring more for other human beings instead. (−)
10. I like to feed animals out of my hand. (+)
11. I love pets. (+)
12. Animals belong in the wild or in zoos, but not in the home. (−)
13. If you keep pets in the house you can expect a lot of damage to furniture. (−)
14. I like housepets. (+)
15. Pets are fun but it's not worth the trouble of owning one. (−)
16. I frequently talk to my pet. (+)
17. I hate animals. (−)
18. You should treat your housepets with as much respect as you would a human member of your family. (+)

Plus and minus signs denote the direction in which the question is to be scored.

Note: From "The Construction of a Pet Attitude Scale," by D.I. Templer, C.A. Salter, S. Dickey, R. Baldwin, and D.M. Veleber, 1981, *The Psychological Record*, 31, p. 344. Reprinted with permission.

Appendix 12B

Chick Tameness Score Sheet

Chick Band # _____/Cage # _____

Test Administrator _____/

Date _____

I. Behavioral Data

  A. Response to extended finger/hand

    _____ approach/perch: _____ latency in seconds

    _____ no response

    _____ withdraws/aggressive display/bites: _____ latency in seconds

  B. Response to touch on head (cheek or back)

    _____ permits

    _____ permits with flinch or vocalization

    _____ withdraws/aggressive display/bites

  C. Response to food offering (Cheerios cereal)

    _____ accepts: _____ latency in seconds

    _____ no response/turns away: _____ latency in seconds

    _____ withdraws/aggressive display/bites: _____ latency in seconds

  D. Response to novel object (piece of a drinking straw)

    _____ accepts: _____ latency in seconds

    _____ no response/turns head away: _____ latency in seconds

    _____ withdraws/aggressive display/bites: _____ latency in seconds

  E. Proximity seeking to

    administrator____ parrot ____ ambivalent____ no response ____

II. Physiological Data

  A. Respiration rate

    _____ rpm

  B. Latency to defecation

    _____ seconds

Appendix 12C

Parent Tameness Score Sheet

Bird Band # _____

Sex _____

Cage # _____

Test Administrator _____

Test Trial #_____

I. Behavioral Data

  A. Response to person in front of cage

    _____ approach (non-aggressive)

    _____ no response

    _____ aggressive display

    _____ withdrawal

  B. Response to opening of cage door

    _____ approach (non-aggressive)

    _____ no response

    _____ aggressive display

    _____ withdrawal

  C. Response to extended (empty) hand

    _____ approach (non-aggressive)

    _____ no response

    _____ aggressive display

    _____ withdrawal

  D. Response to food offering (fruit)

    _____ acceptance

    _____ no response

    _____ aggressive display

    _____ withdrawal

II. Physiological Data

  A. Respiration rate

    _____ rpm

  B. Latency to defecation

    _____ seconds

13
Grey Parrot Cognition and Communication

Irene M. Pepperberg

For over 25 years, I have used the modeling technique described in this chapter to teach Grey Parrots (*Psittacus erithacus*) to use elements of English speech meaningfully and then used this communication code to examine their cognitive capacities. My oldest subject, Alex, exhibits abilities comparable to those of marine mammals and apes, and sometimes to those of four- to six-year-old children (Pepperberg 1999). These abilities are not, however, inferred from Alex's responses to various types of operant behavior tasks, as is common in animal research (Zentall 1993) but, because he uses human speech, are determined from his *direct vocal* answers to *direct vocal* questions, much as we study young children. Thus he demonstrates intriguing communicative and cognitive parallels with humans, despite his phylogenetic distance. I doubt I taught Alex and the other parrots these abilities de novo; rather, their achievements likely derive from existent cognitive and neurological architectures used in nature. This point is critical in discussing my research involving the importance of direct interspecies communication as an investigative tool, the capacities this communication form enables us to unveil, and the centrality of birds for studying the evolution of communication and cognition.

THE IMPORTANCE OF INTERSPECIES COMMUNICATION

Parrots' vocal plasticity enables *direct interspecies communication* (Pepperberg 1981). But why use this code rather than their natural system to examine how communication and cognition evolved and the extent to which their abilities match those of other creatures? The answer lies in the just-mentioned existent cognitive architecture. I believe parrots acquire elements of human communication that can be mapped or adapted to their code. By observing what they do and do not learn, we determine what is held in common with humans and thus more about the avian system. I do not believe parrots could, for example, learn aspects of reference (e.g., labels for specific classes of objects such as apples, or for colors such as green or red) unless their own natural code has such referentiality. Although determining referentiality in this manner is inferential, direct determination also has difficulties (see Cheney & Seyfarth 1992). I also believe that stressing the avian system to see what aspects of input are needed for exceptional learning—that which does not necessarily occur during normal development (Bandura 1971; e.g., acquiring another species' code)—provides a detailed understanding of the learning process. Because richer input is needed to learn another species' code (allospecific learning) than to learn one's own species' code (conspecific learning; Pepperberg 1985), we can determine how and whether "nurture" modifies "nature" (i.e., the innate predispositions that facilitate conspecific learning and may initially block allospecific learning), and thus uncover additional mechanisms for, and the full extent of, communicative learning. Again, these mechanisms must be part of the existent cognitive architecture and not something taught de novo, and are mechanisms that could be missed without proper experimentation. And only by elucidating such mechanisms can we understand the complexity of the parrot system.

Interspecies communication also has practical applications for studying cognition. It (1) directly states the content of our queries—animals needn't determine both the answer *and* nature of a question via trial and error; (2) incorporates research showing that social animals may respond more readily and accurately within an ecologically valid social context (see Menzel & Juno 1982); (3) allows facile data comparisons among species, including humans; (4) allows rigorous testing of the acquired communication code that avoids expectation cuing (i.e., subjects choose responses from their *entire* repertoire rather than from a subset relevant only to a particular topic); and, most importantly, (5) is an open, arbitrary, creative code with enormous signal variety, enabling animals to respond in novel, possibly innovative ways that demonstrate greater competence than do operant paradigms' required responses, and (6) thereby allows examination of the nature *and* extent of information animals perceive. Interspecies communication thus facilely demonstrates non-humans' inherent capacities and may enable more complex learning (see Pepperberg 1981, 1999).

HOW GREYS LEARN: PARALLELS WITH HUMANS

My Greys' learning sometimes parallels human processes and suggests insights into how acquisition of complex communication may have evolved. Input that is referential, demonstrates functionality (i.e., is contextually applicable), and is socially rich allows parrots, like young children (e.g., Hollich et al. 2000), to acquire communication skills effectively (Pepperberg 1981, 1985, 1990a, 1994b, 1999; Pepperberg & McLaughlin 1996; Pepperberg et al. 1998, 1999). Reference is generally defined as an utterance's meaning—the relationship between labels and the objects to which they refer—and is exemplified by our use of referential rewards (the bird receives the objects it labels). Context/functionality involves the particular situation in which an utterance is used and effects of its use; initial use of a label to request objects gives the bird a reason to learn the unique, unfamiliar sounds of English labels. Social interaction signals which environmental components should be noted, emphasizes common attributes—and possible underlying rules—of diverse actions, and allows input to be contin-

uously adjusted to the learner's level. Interaction also engages the subject directly, provides contextual explanations of the reasons for the actions, and demonstrates actions' consequences. I describe the primary technique for training our birds, our results, and experiments to determine which input elements are both necessary and sufficient to engender learning.

The primary training technique, the *model/rival* (M/R) system (Pepperberg 1981), is based on that of Todt (1975), who examined parrots' social learning, and Bandura's (1971) studies of how social modeling affects human learning. The M/R procedure involves three-way interactions among two human speakers and the avian student; it uses *social interaction* to demonstrate targeted vocal behavior. M/R training introduces new labels and concepts and aids in shaping pronunciation

During M/R training, humans demonstrate interactive responses to be learned. Sessions begin with a parrot observing two humans handling one or more items in which the bird has shown an interest. The bird watches as one human "trains" the other. The trainer presents and asks questions about the item(s) (e.g., "What's here?" "What color?"), and gives the human model praise and the object(s) in question to reward correct answers referentially. Multiple exemplars of the object are used to help the bird generalize the label beyond a specific stimulus. Incorrect responses (like those the bird may make at the time) are punished by scolding and temporarily removing the item(s) from sight. Thus the second human is not only a model for the parrot's responses and a rival for the trainer's attention but also illustrates the effects of an error: The model is asked to try again or talk more clearly if the response was (deliberately) incorrect or garbled, thereby allowing a bird to observe corrective feedback (see Pepperberg 1999). A bird is included in interactions and rewarded for successive approximations to a correct response; thus training is adjusted to its level.

Unlike Todt's procedure (and that of others; see Pepperberg & Sherman 2000), our protocol also involves *reversing* roles of human trainer and model, and includes the parrot in interactions. Thus one person is not always the questioner and the other the respondent, and we show how the procedure effects environmental change (Pepperberg 1981). Inclusion of role reversal in M/R training counteracts drawbacks associated with Todt's method: His birds, whose trainers always maintained their respective roles, responded only to the human posing the questions. In contrast, our birds respond to, interact with, and learn from all trainers.

Importantly, M/R training exclusively uses *intrinsic reinforcers*. That is, the bird's reward for producing a label ("X") is the object (X) to which the label or concept refers. This procedure ensures the closest possible correlation of label or concept to be learned and the object or task to which it refers. Earlier unsuccessful programs for teaching psittacids to communicate with humans (e.g., Mowrer 1950) used *extrinsic* rewards. Thus, on the few occasions when those subjects correctly labeled food or non-food items, or made appropriate responses to various specific commands, they received a single, favored food that neither directly related to, nor varied with, the label or concept being taught. Extrinsic rewards, however, delay label/concept acquisition by confounding the label of the exemplar or concept to be learned with that of the food (see Miles 1983; Pepperberg 1981; Pepperberg & Sherman 2000). My birds never receive extrinsic rewards. Too, use of intrinsic rewards demonstrates label *functionality*: Initially, label use results in acquisition of desired objects, and thus provides a reason for the bird to acquire that label.

Occasionally, Alex receives a more general reward: Because he sometimes will not focus on objects used to train a particular concept, we taught him "I want X" (i.e., to separate labeling and requesting; Pepperberg 1988b) so his reward is the right to request vocally something more desirable than what he identified. This protocol provides flexibility but maintains referentiality: Alex never, for example, automatically receives nuts for identifying a cork. He must state "I want nut," and trainers will not respond to requests until the appropriate prior task is completed. Thus birds learn the label as a true identifier, not merely on an emotional level. Training "want" provides two additional advantages: First, trainers can distinguish incorrect labeling from appeals for other items; that is, during a test birds unable to use "want" might not be making errors but could be asking for treats, and test scores might decline for reasons unrelated to competence. Second, birds can be tested for a simple form of intentionality.

For example, if Alex asks for a certain object, he is rarely satisfied with a replacement and continues to request the desired item (Pepperberg 1999).

RESULTS (FROM PEPPERBERG 2002b)

Labeling and Basic Requests, Overview

Through M/R training, Alex learned tasks that were once thought beyond the capability of all but humans or, possibly, certain non-human primates (Premack 1978). He can label over 50 objects. He has functional use of "no" and phrases such as "come here," "I want X," and "Wanna go Y," where X and Y are appropriate labels for objects or locations (Pepperberg 1981, 1999). Trainers' incorrect responses to his requests (e.g., substitution of something other than what he requested) generally result in his saying "No" and repeating the request (Pepperberg 1987c, 1988b). He labels seven colors and identifies five shapes (as "two-," "three-," "four-," "five-," or "six-corner"; Pepperberg 1983). He uses the labels "two," "three," "four," "five," and "six" to distinguish quantities of objects, including collections made of novel items and randomly placed and heterogeneous sets of items (Pepperberg 1987b, 1994a). He combines vocal labels to identify proficiently, request, refuse, categorize, and quantify over 100 objects, including those varying somewhat from training exemplars. His accuracy averages ~80% when tested on these abilities (Pepperberg 1981, 1983, 1987b, 1987c, 1988a, 1994a, 1999).

Concepts of Category

Alex comprehends the concept of "category." He learned not only to label different hues and shapes, but also to categorize objects having both color and shape with respect to either category by responding to "What color?" or "What shape?" (Pepperberg 1983). He understands that "green," for example, is a particular instance of the category "color," and that, for objects with both color *and* shape, specific instances of these attributes (e.g., "green," "three-corner") represent *different* categories. Thus, he learned that a set of responses exists—color labels—that forms the class "color" and another set—shape labels—that forms the class "shape" (Pepperberg 1996). His success shows understanding of higher-order class concepts, because color labels have no intrinsic connection to the label "color" nor do shape labels to the label "shape". Our protocol requires Alex to categorize the same exemplar with respect to shape at one time and color at another, and thus involves flexibility in changing the basis for classification. Such capacity for *re*classification is thought to indicate "abstract aptitude" (Hayes & Nissen 1956/1971).

Same/Different and Absence

In the 1970s, comprehension of same/different was singled out as requiring abilities not typically attributable to non-primates and specifically not to birds (Premack 1978, 1983; Mackintosh et al. 1985). Researchers argued that understanding the same/different concept is more complex than learning to respond to match-to-sample and nonmatch-to-sample or oddity-from-sample, or homogeneity and non-homogeneity. The first requires use of arbitrary *symbols* to represent *relationships* of sameness and difference between sets of objects *and* the ability to denote the attribute that is same/different (Premack 1983). Specifically, Premack (1983) claims animals need symbolic representation—some elementary form of language—to succeed. The other tasks, in contrast, require only that subjects show savings in the number of trials needed to respond to B and B as a match (or as a homogeneous field) after learning to respond to A and A as a match (and likewise by showing a savings in trials involving C and D after learning to respond appropriately to A and B as non-matching or non-homogeneous). Subjects in match-to-sample and nonmatch-to-sample studies might even be responding based on "old" versus "new" or "familiar" versus "unfamiliar," that is, on the relative number of times they experience A versus the number of times they see different Bs (Premack 1983). Subjects that understand same/different, however, not only know that two non-identical red objects are related in the same way as are two non-identical blue objects—by color—but also know the red objects are related to each other differently than are two non-identical square objects, and, moreover, can transfer this understanding to *any* attribute of an item (Premack 1978, 1983). Subjects likewise have to understand the concept of difference.

Alex learned abstract concepts of "same" and "different" and to respond to the *absence* of information about these concepts if nothing is same or different. Thus, given two objects that are identical or that vary with respect to some or all of the attributes of color, shape, and material, Alex responds with the appropriate *category* label as to which attribute is "same" or "different" for any combination (Pepperberg 1987a), or "none" if nothing is same or different (Pepperberg 1988a). He responds accurately for novel objects, colors, shapes, and materials, including those he cannot label. Furthermore, Alex responds to the specific questions, not merely on the basis of his training and physical attributes of the objects: He was still above chance when, for example, we asked "What's same?" for a green wooden triangle and a blue wooden triangle. If he had ignored the question and responded based on prior training, he would have determined, and responded with the label for, the one anomalous attribute (in this case, "color"). Instead, he produced one of the two appropriate answers (i.e., "shape" or "mahmah" [matter]; Pepperberg 1987a).

Alex's use of "none" is important because understanding and commenting upon non-existence, or even the slightly more basic notion of absence, although seemingly simple, denotes a relatively advanced stage in cognitive and linguistic development (Brown 1973). Organisms react to absence only after acquiring knowledge about the expected *presence* of events, objects, or other information in their environment, that is, only when discrepancy exists between the expected and actual state of affairs (e.g., Skinner 1957; de Villiers & de Villiers 1979; Hearst 1984). (Such behavior is, however, qualitatively different from learning what stimulus leads to absence of reward—e.g., Astley & Wasserman 1992—where subjects simply learn what to avoid.) Non-humans have been tested on absence using Piagetian object permanence, and some do react to the disappearance or non-existence of specific items they expect to be present (e.g., Funk 1996; Pepperberg et al. 1997). Evidence also exists in nature. Some songbirds, for example, react to absence of signs of territorial defense (e.g., song) from conspecific neighbors with positive acts of territorial invasion (Peek 1972; Krebs 1977; Smith 1979). Bloom (1970), however, suggests that not only comprehension but also verbal production of terms relating to non-existence is necessary before an organism is thought to have the *concept* of non-existence. Experimentally demonstrating this concept thus is difficult, even in humans, and Alex's capacities are therefore notable.

Numerical Concepts

I then asked whether Alex could form a new categorical class of labels for quantity, that is, learn a concept of number. Could he now learn, for example, to reclassify a group of wooden objects known as "wood" or "green wood" as "five wood"? To succeed, he would have to understand that a new set of labels, "one," "two," "three," "four," "five," and "six," represented a novel class: a means to categorize objects based on a combination of physical similarity within a group and the group's quantity, rather than only physical characteristics of group members. He would also have to generalize this new class of numerical labels to novel items, objects in random arrays, and heterogeneous collections. Note that Koehler (1943, 1950, 1953) and colleagues (Braun 1952; Lögler 1959) had already demonstrated Greys' sensitivity to quantity and basic concepts of numerosity/numerousness; Koehler's birds could open boxes randomly containing zero, one, or two baits until they obtained a fixed number (e.g., four). The number of boxes to be opened to obtain the precise number of baits varied across trials, and the number sought depended upon independent visual cues: black box lids denoted two baits, green lids three, and so forth; Koehler's birds supposedly solved four different problems of this kind. He did not state, however, if different colored lids were presented randomly in a single series, and thus whether colors indeed "represented" particular quantities (see Pepperberg 1987b). Lögler (1959) transferred such behavior to light flashes and flute notes, thus going from simultaneous visual representations to sequential auditory ones. But could Alex, like Matsuzawa's (1985) chimpanzee, go beyond these tasks and use number as a categorical label?

Although Alex's numerical understanding is simpler than that of human children (Fuson 1988), he does comprehend some concept of quantity. We have yet to show conclusively that Alex can, for example, without training, transfer from enumerating simultaneous visual displays to enumerating sequential auditory ones (e.g., transfer to count sequential metronome clicks to state he has heard "three"), but he can label quantities of physical objects up to and including six

(Pepperberg 1987b). The object sets need not be familiar, nor be in any particular pattern, such as a square or triangle. Furthermore, shown a heterogeneous collection—of Xs and Ys—he can respond appropriately to either "How many X?" or "How many Y?" (Pepperberg 1987b). This ability is beyond what might be considered subitizing in young children, who are generally given only homogeneous sets (e.g., Starkey & Cooper 1995), and who, if asked about subsets, generally label the total number of objects in a heterogeneous set if, like Alex, they have been trained on homogeneous sets exclusively (see Greeno et al. 1984). Shown a "confounded number set" (collections of four groups of items that vary in two colors and two object categories—e.g., blue and red wood and blue and red wool), Alex can label the number of items uniquely defined by the combination of one color and one object category (e.g., "How many blue wood?"). Although Alex's mechanisms may not be identical to those of humans, his accuracy (Pepperberg 1994a) replicates that of humans (Trick & Pylyshyn 1989); thus a nonprimate, non-mammal shows competence that, in a chimpanzee, would be taken to indicate a human level of intelligence (Pepperberg 1999).

Relative Size

All research discussed until now involves formation of categorical classes based at least indirectly on absolute physical criteria, not relative concepts. Color and shape labels are symbolic and thus abstract, but refer to concrete entities (Pepperberg 1996). Demonstrating that animals, and birds in particular, can respond to relative concepts is difficult: Previous studies suggested that response on an absolute basis was always used in preference to response on a relative basis; the latter response was apparent only if the former was blocked (e.g., Page et al. 1989; Hulse et al. 1990; cf. Weisman & Ratcliffe 1989; Hurly et al. 1990). Might Alex's categorical class training enable him to respond on a relative basis (e.g., bigger/smaller)? Such data would provide direct comparisons with research on marine mammals (Schusterman & Krieger 1986).

After M/R training on "What color bigger/smaller?" with a limited set of colors and objects (yellow, blue, green; cups, woolen felt circles, Play-Doh rods), we tested Alex on a variety of familiar and unfamiliar items. Alex could indeed classify objects with respect to relative size; overall test scores were 78.7% (Pepperberg & Brezinsky 1991). Although we did not examine whether he could (or would) transfer this concept to a different modality (e.g., amount of sound), whether acquisition of this concept might help him learn a different relationship (e.g., relative darkness), or how close in size two objects must be before he could not discriminate a difference, Alex demonstrated an understanding at least equivalent to that of certain marine mammals (e.g., Schusterman & Krieger 1986). He transposed size relationships to stimuli outside the training domain (Pepperberg & Brezinsky 1991) and, because he responded with the label for an attribute other than size (i.e., color), we could remove many absolute stimulus cues by using entirely novel objects (see Pepperberg 1987a, 1987b, 1990a): unfamiliar shapes, materials, sizes, and colors, often ones he could not label (e.g., hand-dyed styrofoam stars; Pepperberg & Brezinsky 1991). Most interesting was that he could also, *without any training*, indicate when exemplars did not differ in size by responding "none" and answer questions based on object material rather than color (Pepperberg & Brezinsky 1991). Thus he was not limited to responding within a single dimension, he was attending to our questions, and he transferred information learned in one domain (the same/different study) to another. Such ability to transfer is, as just noted, a mark of complex cognitive processing (Rozin 1976).

Comprehension via Recursive and Conjunctive Tasks

We next compared Alex's comprehension abilities with those of marine mammals trained in interspecies communication (e.g., Herman 1987; Schusterman & Gisiner 1988). Most work with cetaceans and pinnipeds uses the comprehension mode; that is, researchers demonstrate how well animals understand the communication code by acting appropriately upon various commands. In contrast, most work with non-human primates up until the early 1990s and all prior work with Alex, although clearly involving comprehension (e.g., the difference between queries of "How many?" "What's same/different?" "What color bigger/ smaller?" etc. with respect to any two objects), emphasized how accurately subjects *produce* the

code (Gardner & Gardner 1969; Pepperberg 1981; Miles 1983; Savage-Rumbaugh 1984; cf. Savage-Rumbaugh et al. 1993). To maintain our vocal paradigm but provide the necessary comparisons, students and I trained and tested Alex on a recursive task like that used with other animals (Pepperberg 1990b; also Granier-Deferre & Kodratoff 1986). In a recursive task, subjects are presented with several different objects and one of several different possible questions or commands concerning the attributes of these objects. Each question or command contains several parts, the combination of which uniquely specifies which object is targeted and what action is to be performed. Question complexity is determined by context (number of different possible objects from which to choose) and the number of its parts (e.g., number of attributes used to specify the target and number of actions from which to choose). Subjects must divide the question into these parts and (recursively) understand each part to answer correctly. Subjects demonstrate competence by reporting on only a single aspect (e.g., color, shape, or material) of, or performing one of several possible actions (fetching, touching) on, an object that is one of several differently colored and shaped exemplars of various materials. Alex was shown many unique combinations of seven exemplars and asked, "What color is object-X?" "What shape is object-Y?" "What object is color-A?" or "What object is shape-B?" His accuracy, above 80% (Pepperberg 1990b), was comparable to that of marine mammals and non-human primates.

Students and I took this work one step further, by adding a conjunctive condition to the recursive task (Pepperberg 1992). Here Alex was again shown seven-member collections but was now asked to provide information about the specific instance of one category of an item uniquely defined by the conjunction of two other categories; for example, "What object is color-A *and* shape-B?". Other objects on the tray exemplified one, but not both, of these defining categories. Alex's accuracy was 76.5%, indicating he understood all elements in the question. Again, his data was comparable to that of marine mammals.

FURTHER STUDIES ON ACQUISITION

M/R training successfully demonstrated what input elements enabled acquisition of some level of allospecific communicative competence but did not elucidate which were *necessary and sufficient*. What happens if input lacks some elements? Answering that question required additional parrots, because Alex might have ceased learning simply because circumstances had changed, not because of the quality of the change. New, untrained subjects would be uninfluenced by prior experience. With three new Greys, Kyaaro, Alo, and Griffin, students and I began testing the relative importance of three major input elements of M/R training: reference, context/function, and social interaction.

Initial Studies Eliminating Aspects of Input

I first gave Alo and Kyaaro three types of input: (1) audiotapes of Alex's sessions, which were non-referential, not contextually applicable, and non-interactive; (2) videotapes of Alex's sessions, which were referential, minimally contextually applicable, and non-interactive; and (3) usual M/R training that was referential, contextually applicable, and interactive. In the first two experiments, birds listened to or watched tapes in social isolation. The first condition paralleled earlier studies on allospecific song acquisition (Marler 1970; Baptista & Petrinovich 1984, 1986; speech is not a natural parrot vocalization), and the second involved still-unresolved issues about avian vision and video (e.g., Ikebuchi & Okanoya 1999; Lea & Dittrich 1999). I counterbalanced labels across birds and ensured equivalent training time across sessions. Like songbirds, neither parrot learned anything substantive from audio, nor from videotapes. Both, however, learned to comprehend and produce M/R-trained labels (Pepperberg 1994b). But such studies were just the first steps in determining strictures for allospecific acquisition.

Further Studies on Elements of Input

We then completed five more experiments to tease out effects of input. In the first, juveniles' video sessions were repeated with "co-viewers" who merely ensured birds attended to the monitor (Pepperberg et al. 1998). Trainers provided social approbation for viewing and pointed to the screen, making comments like "Look what Alex has!" but did not repeat new labels, ask questions, or relate content to other training. The procedure was based on data from young children that sug-

gested that video learning (e.g., from *Sesame Street*) increased when children watched with interactive co-viewers (Corder-Bolz & O'Bryant 1978; Lemish & Rice 1986; Lesser 1974; Salomon 1977; Watkins et al. 1980; but see Rice et al. 1990). For this experiment, any attempt to produce the label would be rewarded with vocal praise, not the object. Thus social interaction was limited and functional meaning was the same as in basic videotape sessions. In the second study, we increased the amount of interaction, so the trainer now repeated the new labels and asked questions (Pepperberg et al. 1999); the rationale was additional data for children showing that extent of interaction might affect video learning (St. Peters et al. 1989). In the third study, we ensured that lack of reward for an attempted targeted vocalization did not prevent learning from video (Pepperberg et al. 1998): Using the basic videotape protocol, we included a reward system that enabled a socially-isolated parrot to receive the item if it attempted to produce its label. The system was controlled by a student in another room who monitored the parrot's utterances through headphones. In the fourth study, the M/R procedure was amended to eliminate some functionality and as much social interaction as possible (Pepperberg & McLaughlin 1996). Here we replicated studies with children that demonstrated the effect of an adult jointly focusing (with the child) on the object being labeled: For children, lack of joint attention prevented label acquisition (e.g., Baldwin 1995). In our study, a single trainer sat with her back to the bird, who was seated on a perch within reach of an object (e.g., key). The trainer repeated various phrases about the object (e.g., "Look, a shiny *key*!" "Do you want the *key*?" etc.; sentence frames; Pepperberg 1981) but did not make eye contact with the parrot, nor did she present the object to the bird. Any attempt at the targeted label received vocal praise. In the fifth study, we tested whether the bird might have become habituated to the single tape we used. Although the tape contained many interactions and all the different responses that Alex and the trainers made, the bird might have ignored the material after several sessions. We therefore replicated the study using live video input from Alex's sessions (Pepperberg et al. 1999). In none of these experiments did parrots learn referential use of labels, but they did learn simultaneously presented

M/R-trained labels. Although we are currently replicating video studies using a liquid crystal monitor to determine whether flicker-fusion of the standard cathode ray tube affects video learning (Ikebuchi & Okanoya, 1999), our results so far emphasize the importance of training that involves reference, demonstration of contextual use/functionality, and social interaction if a parrot is to communicate and not simply mimic human speech.

Nevertheless, at least one set of conditions remained to be tested: What would happen if we eliminated just the modeling aspect, that is, if only a single student labeled the object, queried the bird, jointly attended to the object, and thus interacted fully with the bird and the object? Griffin did not learn labels trained in this manner after 50 sessions (Pepperberg et al. 2000). When we switched to M/R training, however, he produced labels with complete clarity after two or three sessions. Apparently, latent learning had occurred: Griffin had acquired the label but did not know how to use it until he saw its use modeled. In other instances of similar switching (e.g., after 50 video sessions to M/R training), birds needed ~20 sessions before producing the label clearly (Pepperberg et al. 2000). Thus specific demonstration of label functionality is also a vital aspect of the training.

Mutual Exclusivity: A More Subtle Form of Input

In yet another study, students and I found that context-dependent input engenders a form of mutual exclusivity (ME) during label learning by Grey Parrots, much like that of young children (Pepperberg & Wilcox 2000). For children, ME refers to their assumption during early word learning that an object has one, and only one, label (e.g., Liittschwager & Markman 1991, 1994; Merriman 1991). Along with the whole object assumption (that a label likely refers to the entire object, not some attribute; Macnamara 1982; Soja et al. 1985; Markman & Wachtel 1988), ME supposedly guides children in initial label acquisition. ME may later help children overcome the whole object assumption by helping them interpret a novel word as something other than an object label (Markman 1990), but for very young children, any second label for an object can initially be more difficult to acquire than the first,

because the second label is viewed as an alternative (Liittschwager & Markman 1991, 1994). But ME depends upon input: Children (Gottfried & Tonks 1996) and parrots like Alex, who receive inclusivity data (X is a kind of Y; color labels taught as additional, not alternative, labels for an item, i.e., "Here's a key; it's a green key"), tend to accept multiple labels for items and form hierarchical relations. Thus Alex responds to "What color?" "What shape?" "What matter?" *and* "What toy?" for a wooden block (Pepperberg 1990a, 1990b). If, however, subjects are given color or shape labels as alternative labels (i.e., "Here's a key; it's green"), they resist using these modifiers for a previously labeled item. Griffin, trained in the latter manner, thus responded to "What color?" with previously learned object labels in over 50 training sessions (Pepperberg & Wilcox 2000). Results were not confined to modifiers. If, for example, he lacked an object label—cup—he used its color label even if asked "What toy?" and had difficulty learning "cup" (Pepperberg & Wilcox 2000). Thus even small changes in input (e.g., "It's a green key" versus "It's green") affect label acquisition in parrots in a way that matches young children.

Combinatory Learning

On the basis of primarily behavioral data, researchers (e.g., Greenfield 1991) argue that (1) parallel development of communicative and physical object (manual) combinatorial abilities exists in young children, (2) these abilities initially have a common neural substrate, (3) a homologous great ape substrate allows for similar, if limited, co-emergence of these two abilities, and (4) such abilities indicate a shared evolutionary history for communicative and physical behavior (Johnson-Pynn et al. 1999). Interestingly, we found comparable, if limited, parallel combinatorial development in a Grey Parrot (Pepperberg & Shive 2001).

Our juvenile Griffin spontaneously combined physical objects in similar proportions to spontaneous label combinations. His two-label combinations (e.g., "want X," "color + object"; Pepperberg & Wilcox 2000) preceded our study; we were thus unable to see if the two behavior patterns co-emerged. We did, however, track systematic initiation of both three-item and three-label combinations. Both began in early 2000, though Griffin's first—and then for several months only—successful three-object combination occurred in June 1999. Interestingly (1) percentages of physical and vocal combinations were roughly equal; (2) despite several months of training on x-corner wood/paper, vocal three-item combinations emerged only when he more frequently began to combine three objects; (3) such vocal combinations were not exclusively those trained; and (4) combinations were performed with his beak rather than his feet. Our data imply that a particular mammalian brain structure is not uniquely responsible for such behavior and that co-occurrent combinations need not arise manually.

Unlike the *Cebus* studied (Johnson-Pynn et al. 1999), Griffin was not trained on item-based tasks; we wanted to see if, as his vocalizations developed complexity, spontaneous manipulative behavior co-emerged. He rarely combined more than two items, possibly because of difficulty simultaneously grasping more than two items: Failed attempts at multiple combinations occurred because he lacked physical dexterity, not because he tried to form impossible combinations. However, the frequency with which he picked up and manipulated paired caps/lids, and his manipulations of other items, could be examples of intermediate or transitory stages leading to more difficult combinations. And, by limiting training on three-label combinations, we provided only an example; we then could document spontaneous utterances. Although we trained "x-corner wood/paper" (x = 2, 5), "2-corner wood" was only one of 14 recorded three-label combinations.

We do not argue that Griffin's behavior—or even that of our most advanced subject, Alex (e.g., Pepperberg 1999)—constitutes anything comparable to human language or the complex combinatory behavior of two- to three-year-old humans. We have, however, documented co-occurrence of vocal and physical-object combinatorial behavior not previously described in birds. We suggest that (1) our Greys' behavior patterns compare to some of those of non-human primates, (2) parallel communicatory and physical development is not restricted to primates, and (3) neural structures involved in such behavior are not unique to primates. Although avian neuroanatomy and its relation to the mammalian line is not yet well enough understood to determine specific parallels among oscine, psittacine, and mammalian structures, the responsible substrates are likely analogous and arose independently under similar evolutionary pressures (e.g., Deacon 1997); nevertheless, recent arguments (e.g., Jarvis & Mello 2000; Medina & Reiner 2000) suggest that additional study is needed before definite conclusions are made. Given the evolutionary distance between parrots and primates, we suggest that the search for and arguments concerning responsible substrates and common behavior should be approached with care and not be restricted to the primate line.

PARALLEL EVOLUTION OF AVIAN AND MAMMALIAN ABILITIES?

In sum, I am not claiming isomorphism for human language and any animal communication system, or for human and non-human cognition, but do argue that we must look across species for information on evolutionary pressures that helped shaped existent systems (Pepperberg 1999). Such pressures were exerted on more than primates and the existence of complex analogous communication systems and cognitive abilities demonstrate the need to accept their bases in analogous neural architectures. Moreover, complex communicative systems apparently require or at least co-evolve with complex cognition: Communication is a social function, but its complexity is based on the complexity of information that must be communicated, processed, and received (Smith 1997); thus contingencies that shape intelligence (social, ecological, etc.) also likely shape communication. Humphrey (1976), among others, looking at primates, proposed that intelligence (and presumably the need for cognitive processing) is a correlate of a complicated social system and a long life, that is, that intelligence resulted from selection favoring animals that could remember and act upon knowledge of detailed social relations among group members; more generally, Rozin (1976) defined intelligence as flexibility in transferring skills acquired in one domain to another. How these two patterns might also drive parrot cognitive skills and vocal behavior seems obvious: Long-lived birds existing in complex social systems, not unlike those of some primates, use abilities honed for social gains to direct other forms of information processing and vocal learning. Add the need for categorical classes (e.g., to distinguish neutral stimuli from predators, poisonous from healthful foods, etc.), abilities both to recognize and remember environmental regularities and adapt to unpredictable environmental changes over an extensive lifetime, and a communication system that is primarily vocal, the capacities of parrots are not surprising. In fact, Marler (1996) proposed some similar parallels between birds and primates, although not specifically for parrots. I believe we must look for parallels—essential commonalities—across many species to develop theories about those behavioral elements that are essential to, and the evolutionary pressures that have shaped, complex communication (Pepperberg 1999). Whether avian communication and human language (and avian and human cognition) demonstrate convergent evolution—where similar adaptive responses have independently evolved in remotely associated taxa in association with similar environmental pressures (Ball & Hulse 1998)—is unclear, but a common core of skills likely underlies complex cognitive and communicative behavior in many species, even if specific skills have different manifestations in each species.

ACKNOWLEDGMENTS

This chapter was based on articles published previously (Pepperberg 2002a, 2002b) that summarized other cited material. Writing of this article was supported by the MIT School of Architecture and Planning and a grant from The American Foundation. Research was supported by NSF (IBN 96-03803) and REU supplements, the John Simon Guggenheim Foundation, the Kenneth A. Scott Charitable Trust, the Pet Care Trust, the University of Arizona Undergraduate Biology Research Program, and many, many donors to the Alex Foundation.

REFERENCES

Astley, S.L., and E.A. Wasserman. 1992. Categorical discrimination and generalization in pigeons: All negative stimuli are not created equal. *Journal of Experimental Psychology: Animal Behavior Processes* 18:193–207.

Baldwin, D.A. 1995. "Understanding the link between joint attention and language." In *Joint attention: Its origin and role in development*, ed. C. Moore and P.J. Dunham, pp. 131–158. Hillsdale, NJ: Erlbaum.

Ball, G.F., and S.H. Hulse. 1998. Birdsong. *American Psychologist* 53:37–58.

Bandura, A. 1971. "Analysis of social modeling processes." In *Psychological modeling*, ed. A. Bandura, pp. 1–62. Chicago: Aldine-Atherton.

Baptista, L.F., and L. Petrinovich. 1984. Social interaction, sensitive phases, and the song template hypothesis in the white-crowned sparrows. *Animal Behaviour* 32:172–181.

Baptista, L.F., and L. Petrinovich. 1986. Song development in the white-crowned sparrow: Social factors and sex differences. *Animal Behaviour* 34:1359–1371.

Bloom, L. 1970. *Language development: Form and function in emerging grammars.* Cambridge, MA: MIT Press.

Braun, H. 1952. Uber das Unterscheidungsvermögen unbenannter Anzahlen bei Papageien. *Zeitschrift für Tierpsychologie* 9:40–91. [Concerning the ability of parrots to distinguish unnamed numbers.]

Brown, R. 1973. *A first language: The early stages.* Cambridge, MA: Harvard University Press.

Cheney, D.L., and R.M. Seyfarth. 1992. Precis of "How monkeys see the world." *Behavioral and Brain Sciences* 15:135–182.

Corder-Bolz, C.R., and S. O'Bryant. 1978. Teacher vs. program. *Journal of Communication* 28:97–103.

Deacon, T.W. 1997. *The symbolic species: The co-evolution of language and the brain.* New York: Norton.

de Villiers, P.A., and J.G. de Villiers. 1979. *Early language.* Cambridge, MA: Harvard University Press.

Funk, M.S. 1996. Development of object permanence in the New Zealand parakeet (*Cyanoramphus auriceps*). *Animal Learning & Behavior* 24:375–383.

Fuson, K.C. 1988. *Children's counting and concepts of number.* New York: Springer-Verlag.

Gardner, R.A., and B.T. Gardner. 1969. Teaching sign language to a chimpanzee. *Science* 187:644–672.

Gottfried, G.M., and J.M. Tonks. 1996. Specifying the relation between novel and known: Input affects the acquisition of novel color terms. *Child Development* 67:850–866.

Granier-Deferre, C., and Y. Kodratoff. 1986. Iterative and recursive behaviors in chimpanzees during problem solving: A new descriptive model inspired from the artificial intelligence approach. *Cahiers de Psychologie Cognitive* 6:483–500.

Greenfield, P.M. 1991. Language, tools and brain: The ontogeny and phylogeny of hierarchically organized sequential behavior. *Behavioral & Brain Sciences* 14:531–595.

Greeno, J.G., M.S. Riley, and R. Gelman. 1984. Conceptual competence and children's counting. *Cognitive Psychology* 16:94–143.

Hayes, K.J., and C.H. Nissen. 1956/1971. "Higher mental functions of a home-raised chimpanzee." In *Behavior of non-human primates, Volume 4*, ed.

A.M. Schrier and F. Stollnitz, pp. 57–115. New York: Academic Press.

Hearst, E. 1984. "Absence as information: Some implications for learning, performance, and representational processes." In *Animal cognition*, ed. H.L. Roitblat, T.G. Bever, and H.S. Terrace, pp. 311–332. Hillsdale, NJ: Erlbaum.

Herman, L.M. 1987. "Receptive competencies of language-trained animals." In *Advances in the study of behavior, Volume 17*, ed. J.S. Rosenblatt, C. Beer, M-C. Busnel, and P.J.B. Slater, pp. 1–60, New York: Academic Press.

Hollich, G.J., K. Hirsh-Pasek, and R.M. Golinkoff. 2000. Breaking the language barrier: An emergentist coalition model for the origins of word learning. *Monographs of the Society for Research in Child Development* 262:1–138.

Hulse, S.H., S.C. Page, and R.F. Braaten. 1990. Frequency range size and the frequency range constraint in auditory perception by European starlings (*Sturnus vulgaris*). *Animal Learning & Behavior* 18:238–245.

Humphrey, N.K. 1976. "The social function of intellect." In *Growing points in ethology*, ed. P.P.G. Bateson and R.A. Hinde, pp. 303–317. Cambridge, UK: Cambridge University Press.

Hurly, T.A., L. Ratcliffe, and R. Weisman. 1990. Relative pitch recognition in white-throated sparrows, *Zonotrichia albicollis*. *Animal Behaviour* 40:176–181.

Ikebuchi, M., and K. Okanoya. 1999. Male zebra finches and Bengalese finches emit directed songs to the video images of conspecific females projected onto a TFT display. *Zoological Science* 16:63–70.

Jarvis, E.D., and C.V. Mello. 2000. Molecular mapping of brain areas involved in parrot vocal communication. *Journal of Comparative Neurology* 419:1–31.

Johnson-Pynn, J., D.M. Fragaszy, E.M. Hirsh, K.E. Brakke, and P.M. Greenfield. 1999. Strategies used to combine seriated cups by chimpanzees (*Pan troglodytes*), bonobos (*Pan paniscus*), and capuchins (*Cebus apella*). *Journal of Comparative Psychology* 113:137–148.

Koehler, O. 1943. "Zähl"-Versuche an einem Kolkraben und Vergleichsversuche an Menschen. *Zeitschrift für Tierpsychologie* 5:575–712. ["Number" ability in a raven and comparative research with people.]

Koehler, O. 1950. The ability of birds to "count." *Bulletin of the Animal Behavior Society* 9:41–45.

Koehler, O. 1953. "Thinking without words." Proceedings of the XIVth International Congress of Zoology, pp. 75–88.

Krebs, J. 1977. "Song and territory in the great tit." In *Evolutionary ecology*, ed. B. Stonehouse and C. Perrins, pp. 47–62. New York: Macmillan.

Lea, S.E.G., and W.H. Dittrich. 1999. What do birds see in moving video images? *Cahiers de Psychologie Cognitive/Current Psychology of Cognition* 18:765–803.

Lemish, D., and M.L. Rice. 1986. Television as a talking picture book: A prop for language acquisition. *Journal of Child Language* 13:251–274.

Lesser, G.S. 1974. *Children and television: Lessons from Sesame Street*. New York: Random House.

Liittschwager, J.C., and E.M. Markman. 1991. Mutual exclusivity as a default assumption in second label learning. Paper read at the biennial meetings of the Society for Research in Child Development, April, Seattle, OR.

Liittschwager, J.C., and E.M. Markman. 1994. Sixteen- and 24-month olds' use of mutual exclusivity as a default assumption in second-label learning. *Developmental Psychology* 30:955–968.

Lögler, P. 1959. Versuche zur Frage des "Zähl"-Vermögens an einem Graupapagei und Vergleichsversuche an Menschen. *Zeitschrift für Tierpsychologie* 16:179–217. [Studies on the question of "number" sense in a grey parrot and comparative studies on humans.]

Mackintosh, N.J., B. Wilson, and R.A. Boakes. 1985. Differences in mechanism of intelligence among vertebrates. *Philosophical Transactions of the Royal Society, London, Series B* 308:53–65.

Macnamara, J. 1982. *Names for things: A study of human learning*. Cambridge, MA: MIT Press.

Markman, E.M. 1990. Constraints children place on word meaning. *Cognitive Science* 14:57–77.

Markman, E.M., and G.F. Wachtel. 1988. Children's use of mutual exclusivity to constrain the meanings of words. *Cognitive Psychology* 20:121–157.

Marler, P. 1970. A comparative approach to vocal learning: Song development in white-crowned sparrows. *Journal of Comparative and Physiological Psychology* 71:1–25.

Marler, P. 1996. "Social cognition: Are primates smarter than birds?" In *Current ornithology, Volume 13*, ed. V. Nolan Jr. and E.D. Ketterson, pp. 1–32. New York: Plenum Press.

Matsuzawa, T. 1985. Use of numbers by a chimpanzee. *Nature* 315:57–59.

Medina, L., and A. Reiner. 2000. Do birds possess homologues of mammalian primary visual, somatosensory, and motor cortices? *Trends in Neurosciences* 23:1–12.

Menzel, E.W., Jr., and C. Juno. 1982. Marmosets (*Saguinus fuscicollis*): Are learning sets learned? *Science* 217:750–752.

Merriman, W.E. 1991. The mutual exclusivity bias in children's word learning: A reply to Woodward and Markman. *Developmental Review* 11:164–191.

Miles, H.L. 1983. "Apes and language." In *Language in primates*, ed. J. de Luce and H.T. Wilder, pp. 43–61, New York: Springer-Verlag.

Mowrer, O.H. 1950. *Learning theory and personality dynamics.* New York: Ronald Press.

Page, S.C., S.H. Hulse, and J. Cynx. 1989. Relative pitch perception in the European starling (*Sturnus vulgaris*): Further evidence for an elusive phenomenon. *Journal of Experimental Psychology: Animal Behavior Processes* 15:137–146.

Peek, F.W. 1972. An experimental study of the territorial function of vocal and visual displays in the male red-winged blackbird (*Agelaius phoeniceus*). *Animal Behaviour* 20:112–118.

Pepperberg, I.M. 1981. Functional vocalizations by an African grey parrot (*Psittacus erithacus*). *Zeitschrift für Tierpsychologie* 55:139–160.

Pepperberg, I.M. 1983. Cognition in the African grey parrot: Preliminary evidence for auditory/vocal comprehension of the class concept. *Animal Learning & Behavior* 11:179–185.

Pepperberg, I.M. 1985. Social modeling theory: A possible framework for avian vocal learning. *Auk* 102:854–864.

Pepperberg, I.M. 1987a. Acquisition of the same/different concept by an African grey parrot (*Psittacus erithacus*): Learning with respect to categories of color, shape, and material. *Animal Learning & Behavior* 15:423–432.

Pepperberg, I.M. 1987b. Evidence for conceptual quantitative abilities in the African grey parrot: Labeling of cardinal sets. *Ethology* 75:37–61.

Pepperberg, I.M. 1987c. "Interspecies communication: A tool for assessing conceptual abilities in the grey parrot (*Psittacus erithacus*)." In *Language, cognition, and consciousness: Integrative levels*, ed. G. Greenberg and E. Tobach, pp. 31–56. Hillsdale, NJ: Erlbaum.

Pepperberg, I.M. 1988a. Acquisition of the concept of absence by an African grey parrot: Learning with respect to questions of same/different. *Journal of the Experimental Analysis of Behavior* 50:553–564.

Pepperberg, I.M. 1988b. An interactive modeling technique for acquisition of communication skills: Separation of "labeling" and "requesting" in a psittacine subject. *Applied Psycholinguistics* 9:59–76.

Pepperberg, I.M. 1990a. "An investigation into the cognitive capacities of an African grey parrot (*Psittacus erithacus*)." In *Advances in study of behavior*, ed. P.J.B. Slater, J.S. Rosenblatt, and C. Beer, pp. 357–409. New York: Academic Press.

Pepperberg, I.M. 1990b. Cognition in an African grey parrot (*Psittacus erithacus*): Further evidence for comprehension of categories and labels. *Journal of Comparative Psychology* 104:41–52.

Pepperberg, I.M. 1992. Proficient performance of a conjunctive, recursive task by an African grey parrot (*Psittacus erithacus*). *Journal of Comparative Psychology* 106:295–305.

Pepperberg, I.M. 1994a. Evidence for numerical competence in an African grey parrot (*Psittacus erithacus*). *Journal of Comparative Psychology* 108:36–44.

Pepperberg, I.M. 1994b. Vocal learning in African grey parrots: Effects of social interaction. *Auk* 111:300–313.

Pepperberg, I.M. 1996. "Categorical class formation by an African grey parrot (*Psittacus erithacus*)." In *Stimulus class formation in humans and animals*, ed. T.R. Zentall and P.R. Smeets, pp. 71–90. Amsterdam: Elsevier.

Pepperberg, I.M. 1999. *The Alex studies.* Cambridge, MA: Harvard University Press.

Pepperberg, I.M. 2002a. Cognitive and communicative abilities of grey parrots. *Current Directions in Psychological Science* 11:83–87.

Pepperberg, I.M. 2002b. In search of King Solomon's ring: Cognition and communication in grey parrots. *Brain, Behavior & Evolution* 59:54–67.

Pepperberg, I.M., and M.V. Brezinsky. 1991. Relational learning by an African grey parrot (*Psittacus erithacus*): Discriminations based on relative size. *Journal of Comparative Psychology* 105:286–294.

Pepperberg, I.M., L.I. Gardiner, and L.J. Luttrell. 1999. Limited contextual vocal learning in the grey parrot (*Psittacus erithacus*): The effect of co-viewers on videotaped instruction. *Journal of Comparative Psychology* 113:158–172.

Pepperberg, I.M., and M.A. McLaughlin. 1996. Effect of avian-human joint attention on allospecific vocal learning by grey parrots (*Psittacus erithacus*). *Journal of Comparative Psychology* 110:286–297.

Pepperberg, I.M., J.R. Naughton, and P.A. Banta. 1998. Allospecific vocal learning by grey parrots (*Psittacus erithacus*): A failure of videotaped instruction under certain conditions. *Behavioural Processes* 42:139–158.

Pepperberg, I.M., R.M. Sandefer, D. Noel, and C.P. Ellsworth. 2000. Vocal learning in the grey parrot (*Psittacus erithacus*): Effect of species identity and number of trainers. *Journal of Comparative Psychology* 114:371–380.

Pepperberg, I.M., and D. Sherman. 2000. Proposed use of two-part interactive modeling as a means to increase functional skills in children with a variety of disabilities. *Teaching and Learning in Medicine* 12:213–220.

Pepperberg, I.M., and H.A. Shive. 2001. Hierarchical combinations by a grey parrot (*Psittacus erithacus*): Bottle caps, lids, and labels. *Journal of Comparative Psychology* 115:376–384.

Pepperberg, I.M., and Wilcox, S.E. 2000. Evidence for a form of mutual exclusivity during label acquisition by grey parrots (*Psittacus erithacus*)? *Journal of Comparative Psychology* 114:219–231.

Pepperberg, I.M., M.R. Willner, and L.B. Gravitz. 1997. Development of Piagetian object permanence in a grey parrot (*Psittacus erithacus*). *Journal of Comparative Psychology* 111:63–75.

Premack, D. 1978. "On the abstractness of human concepts: Why it would be difficult to talk to a pigeon." In *Cognitive processes in animal behavior*, ed. S.H. Hulse, H. Fowler, and W.K. Honig, pp. 421–451. Hillsdale, NJ: Erlbaum.

Premack, D. 1983. The codes of man and beast. *Behavioral and Brain Sciences* 6:125–167.

Rice, M.L., A.C. Huston, R. Truglio, and J. Wright. 1990. Words from *Sesame Street*: Learning vocabulary while viewing. *Developmental Psychology* 26:421–428.

Rozin, P. 1976. "The evolution of intelligence and access to the cognitive unconscious." In *Progress in psychobiology and physiological psychology*, *Volume 6*, ed. J.M. Sprague and A.N. Epstein, pp. 245–280. New York: Academic Press.

Salomon, G. 1977. Effects of encouraging Israeli mothers to co-observe *Sesame Street* with their five-year olds. *Child Development* 48:1146–1151.

Savage-Rumbaugh, E.S. 1984. "Acquisition of functional symbol use in apes and children." In *Animal cognition*, ed. H.L. Roitblat, T.G. Bever, and H.S. Terrace, pp. 291–310. Hillsdale, NJ: Erlbaum.

Savage-Rumbaugh, S., J. Murphy, R.A. Sevcik, K.E. Brakke, S.L. Williams, and D.M. Rumbaugh. 1993. Language comprehension in ape and child. *Monographs of the Society for Research in Child Development* 233:1–258.

Schusterman, R.J., and R.C. Gisiner. 1988. Artificial language comprehension in dolphins and sea lions: The essential cognitive skills. *Psychological Record* 38:311–348.

Schusterman, R.J., and K. Krieger. 1986. Artificial language comprehension and size transposition by a California sea lion (*Zalophus californianus*). *Journal of Comparative Psychology* 100:348–355.

Skinner, B.F. 1957. *Verbal behavior.* New York: Appleton-Century-Crofts.

Smith, D.G. 1979. Male singing ability and territorial integrity in red-winged blackbirds (*Agelaius phoeniceus*). *Behaviour* 68:191–206.

Smith, W.J. 1997. "The behavior of communicating, after twenty years." In *Perspectives in ethology, Volume 12*, ed. D.H. Owings, M.D. Beecher, and N.S. Thompson, pp. 7–53. New York: Plenum Press.

Soja, N., S. Carey, and E. Spelke. 1985. Constraints on word learning. Paper read at the biennial convention of the Society for Research in Child Development, April, Toronto, CA.

Starkey, P., and R.G. Cooper. 1995. The development of subitizing in young children. *British Journal of Developmental Psychology* 13:399–420.

St. Peters, M., A.C. Huston, and J.C. Wright. 1989. Television and families: Parental coviewing and young children's language development, social behavior, and television processing. Paper presented at the Society for Research in Child Development, April, Kansas City, KS.

Todt, D. 1975. Social learning of vocal patterns and models of their applications in grey parrots. *Zeitschrift für Tierpsychologie* 39:178–188.

Trick, L., and Z. Pylyshyn. 1989. Subitizing and the FNST spatial index model. University of Ontario, COGMEM #44. [Based on paper presented at the 30th Psychonomic Society Meeting, Atlanta, GA.]

Watkins, B., S. Calvert, A. Huston-Stein, and J.C. Wright. 1980. Children's recall of television material: Effects of presentation mode and adult labeling. *Developmental Psychology* 16:672–674.

Weisman, R., and L. Ratcliffe. 1989. Absolute and relative pitch processing in black-capped chickadees, *Parus atricapillus*. *Animal Behaviour* 38:685–692.

Zentall, T.R., ed. 1993. *Animal cognition: A tribute to Donald A. Riley.* Hillsdale, NJ: Erlbaum.

14
Behavior Analysis and Parrot Learning

S.G. Friedman, Steve Martin, and Bobbi Brinker

Some parrots behave in friendly, sociable ways while others are flat-out unapproachable. Some parrots entertain themselves for hours in their cages while others scream incessantly. Observing this kind of behavioral variability leads many of us to ask some very important questions, such as, Why do parrots behave the way they do? How should we expect them to behave? Can they learn to behave as pets? Knowing the answers to these questions can make the difference between life-long success and failure to thrive for parrots in captivity, particularly in our homes. However, to understand, predict, and change behavior we first need to know how it works.

BEHAVIOR ANALYSIS

Learning and behavior have been studied as a natural science within the field of psychology for well over a century. This science has come to be known as behavior analysis. Pierce and Cheney (2004, p. 420) provide the following contemporary definition: "Behavior analysis is a comprehensive experimental approach to the study of the behavior of organisms. Its primary objectives are the discovery of principles and laws that govern behavior, the extension of these principles over species, and the development of an applied technology."

Behavior can be investigated at many different levels of analysis, as with genetics, neurology, and pharmacology. The focus of behavior analysis is the environmental determinants of behavior, from which behavioral learning theory has been formulated and continues to be refined. (The term "theory" is used technically to mean an established explanation accounting for known facts or

phenomena, as opposed to the non-technical usage, which means an unproven guess or personal opinion. Other theories of learning and behavior are named according to their particular focuses, such as cognitive theory and psychodynamic theory.)

Behavioral learning theory explains a second kind of selection by consequences first recognized in natural selection (Skinner 1981). Whereas natural selection is the process of functional genomic adaptation of an entire species across generations, learning is the process of functional behavioral adaptation of a single individual within its lifetime. The two keystones of learning theory are (1) learning is largely determined by external environmental influences, and (2) the laws of learning are general in nature, transcending species and situations. In its simplest terms, according to each individual's experience interacting with his or her environment, behaviors that "work" are repeated and behaviors that don't work are modified or suppressed.

Over the last 60 years, the applied branch of behavior analysis has matured into a highly effective technology to solve practical, real-world behavior problems. Its widespread applicability continues to expand, having already been demonstrated across seemingly diverse areas such as special education, industrial safety, and animal management. Other names such as operant conditioning, behavior modification, and behavior therapy refer to the same basic intervention strategies; however, applied behavior analysis includes a more rigorous and comprehensive course of action involving the scientific procedures of hypothesis generation (functional assessment), testing (functional analysis), and evaluation (measurement). Intervening to change behavior in this systematic way allows us to solve behavior problems with a high degree of precision, replicability, and accountability. In this chapter the tools and techniques of applied behavior analysis are discussed in reference to the care and management of captive parrots, particularly those kept as pets.

THE ABCs OF BEHAVIOR

The fundamental unit of behavior analysis is the three-term contingency, described by Skinner (as cited in Chance 1998, p. 38): "An adequate formulation of the interaction between an organism and its environment must always specify three things: (1) the occasion upon which a response occurs, (2) the response itself, and (3) the . . . consequences."

These three terms comprise the behavior ABCs: antecedent, behavior, and consequence. Behavior does not occur independently of the environmental events that surround it, therefore there is never just behavior. The smallest element of behavior that can be meaningfully analyzed is an ABC unit, described further in the following sections.

Antecedents

Antecedents are the stimuli, events, and conditions that immediately precede a behavior. They are functionally related to the behavior that follows if the appearance of the behavior depends on the presence of the antecedent stimuli. Antecedents set the occasion for behavior rather than cause it. For example, an open hand presented to a parrot can be an antecedent for either stepping up or running away, depending on the consequences the parrot experienced for doing so in the past. Thus, we can increase the probability that a particular behavior will occur by carefully arranging antecedents, but ultimately the animal makes a choice to behave as we have planned or in some other way. By definition, operant (i.e., voluntary) behavior acknowledges the individual's power to operate on his or her environment.

Behavior

In applied behavior analysis, behavior is what an organism *does* that can be measured. The main focus is overt behaviors that can be operationally defined and unambiguously observed. Birds *do* jump off perches, hang upside down, rouse their feathers, bite hands, ring bells, pin their eyes, and flare their tails. These behaviors can be unambiguously observed and measured according to different dimensions of interest such as frequency, rate, duration, and intensity. Covert behaviors, including thinking and feeling, are private events that can only be observed and measured by the individual engaging in it. This makes parrots' covert behaviors impractical, if not impossible, behavior-changing targets at this time.

Psychological constructs, such as intelligence, neurosis, and confidence, are not behaviors. Gall et al. (2003, p. 621) define constructs in this way: "A concept that is inferred from commonalities among observed phenomena that can be used to explain these phenomena. In theory development, a concept that refers to a structure or process that is hypothesized to underlie particular observed phenomena."

Thus, constructs are what we think may be occurring inside an organism that explains why it is acting in particular ways. We don't really perceive intelligence, neurosis, or confidence with our senses. What we perceive are overt behaviors such as talking in context, plucking feathers, and going to strangers without hesitation. Constructs are best thought of as placeholders for internal processes as yet unknown involving nerves, brains, hormones, and muscles (Manning & Stamp Dawkins, 1992). Unfortunately, constructs all too easily come to be thought of as real entities residing somewhere in the brain. This leads to what Gould (1981) calls the fallacy of reification and explanatory fictions. The fact remains that even when the underlying physiological processes that support behavior are understood, no account of behavior can be complete without the behavior-environment factor.

Vague labels, such as sweet, spoiled, and jealous, are also not behavior. Labels typically describe what people think a bird is rather than what it does. For example, the label "is sweet" tells us nothing about the behavior we want to train or maintain. We can't train a bird to *do* sweet but we can train a bird to step up for all family members. To improve our ability to understand, predict, and change parrots' behavior, the focus should be on observable, measurable behaviors, not constructs or vague labels.

Consequences

Consequences are the stimuli, events, and conditions that occur after a behavior and influence the probability that the behavior will occur again. There is a functional relation between a specific behavior and a consequence if the appearance of the consequence depends on the behavior occurring first. Social attention, items and activities, sensory feedback and escape from aversive events are all consequences that affect parrot behavior. Consequences are nature's feedback about the effectiveness of an individual's behavior. In this way, past consequences affect motivation for future behavior. This is the law of effect that states, "In any given situation, the probability of a behavior occurring is a function of the consequences that behavior has had in that situation in the past" (Chance 2003, p. 137).

Thus, parrots, like all animals, don't just "suffer the consequences"—they learn from the consequences how to behave in the future, given similar antecedent circumstances. Learning by consequences is a natural process that accounts for behavior in both the free range and captivity. Even innate behavior (elicited automatically, without prior learning) is flexible according to consequences. For example, although nest building tends to be stereotypical within many species, we expect that birds improve in their abilities to build nests with experience.

FUNCTIONAL ASSESSMENT/ANALYSIS

The ABCs form the basis of an important tool called functional assessment, the hypothesis-generating phase of changing behavior. After carefully observing and operationally defining the target behavior (the one we want to understand, change, or both), functional assessment is the next step in any behavior change program. By hypothesizing the antecedents that set the occasion for a behavior and the consequences that give the behavior function, the chance of successfully changing behavior is greatly increased. For example, consider the following common scenario: Sam Parrot has started refusing to step onto Grace's hand from the top of his cage. Grace worries that Sam is trying to dominate her from his high perch, and she wonders if she should force him down with a towel to show him who's boss. It was suggested to her that she cut off the

cage legs so as not to trigger this innate response again.

A functional assessment of Sam's prior step-up behavior reveals a convincing alternative hypothesis to that posed by Grace: Sam refuses to step up to avoid being locked in his cage, as indicated by the following.

Setting: Sam Parrot is playing with his bell on top of his cage.
A: Grace offers her hand.
B: Sam steps up.
C: Grace returns Sam to his cage.
Prediction: Sam will step up less often in the future.

The hypothesis that Sam no longer steps up from his cage top to avoid being locked in his cage can be tested by changing the antecedents, the consequences, or both, and observing any concomitant changes in the frequency of Sam's step-up behavior. It is at this point that functional assessment turns into functional analysis. One possible antecedent solution is to allow Sam access to the cage top only when there is sufficient time for him to tire of being there. One possible consequence change is to offer a special treat as Sam steps up and to have a special item in the cage to be discovered once he's inside it.

The process of functional assessment allows us to generate highly specific and testable hypotheses about behavior-environment relations. The question addressed with functional assessment is not why does the bird behave this way, but rather what valued consequence does the bird get by behaving this way; in other words, what's the function of the behavior? It is through changing antecedents and consequences that behavior changes. Since the environment in which captive parrots live is largely controlled by their caregivers, changing parrot behavior is usually the result of changing human behavior first.

THE PROBLEMS WITH DOMINANCE

With this foundation in place, we can better evaluate two common misconceptions about behavior that have caused particular problems for parrots and their owners. The first is that parrots are strongly motivated by an innate drive or character trait to dominate their human caregivers. The second is that caregivers must establish and enforce superior rank over parrots to control them. These two misconceptions, and many others like them, come to have a life of their own, independent of sound scientific information about behavior. They appeal to conventional wisdom and our penchant for quick fixes, but in the long run they pose serious obstacles to appropriate learning solutions and the behavioral health of captive parrots. The important implications of these two fallacies are discussed separately in the following sections.

Parrots and Dominance

Giving commands, following orders, and jockeying for position within linear social hierarchies are common activities for most humans. These behaviors are well supported by our educational, religious, sports, military, and corporate organizations throughout our lives. We are also prone to observe, or think we observe, in other species that which we most expect to see. This problem, known as observer-expectancy bias, is well documented even among those who watch birds (see for example, Balph & Balph 1983.) Perhaps this accounts for the widely held and persistent belief among parrot enthusiasts that parrots' dominant nature impels them to refuse to step off cage tops (height dominance), to chase and bite humans and other animals while on the floor (floor dominance), to scream when the telephone is in use (phone dominance), and to lunge at feed doors (cage dominance). In the companion parrot arena, the different supposed forms of dominance that parrots use to subjugate their caregivers goes on, ad infinitum.

In fact, even among scientists the term "dominance" is ambiguous and varies significantly from report to report (an inherent problem with constructs). In technical usage, dominance generally describes some aspect of an animal's priority access to resources such as food, location, and mates, which is often achieved through agonistic control of another animal. However, in Barrow's *Animal Behavior Desk Reference* (2001) there are seven different definitions of social dominance, including four subcategories, one of which has two subtypes. As reported by Barrow, "Hand (1986, p. 202) indicates that there is no agreement regarding how to define, or measure, social dominance."

To further complicate matters, Barnett (1981) suggests that "Dominance should be distinguished from an animal's superiority resulting from its being in its own *territory*. Dominance should also be distinguished from being a *leader*" (p. 633). Moreover, a critical omission in many discussions of dominance is variables such as changing motivations, contexts, and prior learning history (see, e.g., the influence of context, Cloutier et al. 1995). This lack of scientific consensus about what dominance is should call into question its usefulness for understanding and managing companion parrot behavior (as is currently being done regarding the behavior of wolves and dogs; see Mech 1999, 2000, and Van Kerkhove 2004).

Although some people support the validity of the dominance model applied to pet parrots based on free-range behavior, social hierarchies among wild parrots have not been well documented. Other people support the validity of the dominance model based on the unnatural demands of the captive environment. No studies could be located on dominance relationships between parrots and humans. One study, of a flock of 12 group-housed Cockatiels (*Nymphicus hollandicus*), lends support to the hypothesis that males tend to hold higher dominance ranks than females, based on well-operationalized definitions of aggression, submission, and rank (Seibert & Crowell-Davis 2001). These findings are consistent with those reported by Weinhold with aviary-kept Blue-fronted Amazon Parrots (*Amazona aestiva*) (as cited in Seibert & Crowell-Davis 2001). Seibert and Crowell-Davis discussed several limitations of their study that restrict the extent to which these conclusions can be generalized to other flock-housed Cockatiels: Only one flock of 12 Cockatiels was investigated; the genetic relatedness of the birds was unknown; and the data were collected during mate selection and breeding season. Further research is needed to assess the extent to which these findings generalize to parrots kept as pets and to parrot-human interactions. The implications, if any, to companion parrot behavior management appear to be remote.

The ubiquitous dominance interpretation of companion parrot behavior has other problems as well. First, the expectation that pet parrots are motivated to win superior rank over their caregivers in some pecking order can serve as a self-fulfilling prophecy. As mentioned previously, when people have expectations about another individual's behavior, they act differently and tend to get what they expect. Second, since dominance is thought to be an invisible drive or character trait inside the bird, a dominance problem is a bad bird problem. This provides a convenient excuse for getting rid of the bird rather than taking responsibility for the circumstances (antecedents and consequences) under which these behaviors arise. Third, the dominance explanation predisposes many caregivers to use forceful management strategies in order to counterdominate their birds and win the struggle for alpha organism. Fourth, the dominance explanation ends the search for proximal, environmental causes and solutions. The very process of labeling a problem provides a false sense of closure when in fact it has only provided a name. Thus, the essential processes of functional assessment and solution building are prematurely terminated and the known and remediable relations between behavior and environment remain unexplored (Chance 1998).

THE CASE FOR EMPOWERMENT

When the dominance construct is extended into parrot management practices it takes the form of "show them who's boss" and "never let them make any important decisions." These suggestions are ubiquitous in both popular magazines and professional veterinary literature. However, much to the contrary, scientific evidence indicates that animals tend to thrive in environments in which they are not subjugated but rather have control over significant life events (Schwartz et al. 2002). Given knowledge of how behavior works and sound training skills, parrots can be empowered instead of overpowered, without altering our standards for good companion behavior.

One important demonstration of the emotional gain that comes from having control over one's environment is experiments conducted by Watson with two groups of human babies only three months old (as cited in Schwartz et al. 2002). Under the pillows of the first group was a switch that operated a mobile whenever the infants turned their heads. The babies in the second group had no control over their mobiles, although their mobiles automatically moved as much as the first group's did. As expected according to the law of effect, the frequency of head movements in only the first group increased since doing so was reinforced by the mobiles' movement (i.e., the mobiles' movement depended on what the babies

did). However, other differences were observed in the two groups of babies that were very surprising. Initially, both groups of babies responded to the moving mobiles by cooing and smiling, a reasonable measure of well-being. These happy responses continued throughout the experiment for those babies who controlled their mobiles but for the babies who did not control their mobiles, the cooing and smiling quickly stopped. Apparently, controlling one's consequences explains, at least in part, what makes them reinforcing.

Another relevant line of research is the free food phenomenon, also known as contrafreeloading. With contrafreeloading, animals choose to perform a learned response to obtain reinforcers even when the same reinforcers are freely available. For example, given a choice between working for food and obtaining food for free, animals tend to choose to work, often quite hard, with a bowl of free food placed right next to them. This phenomenon has been replicated with rats, mice, chickens, pigeons, crows, cats, gerbils, Siamese fighting fish, and humans (Osborne 1977); starlings (Inglis & Ferguson 1986); Abyssinian Ground Hornbills and Bare-faced Curassows (Gilbert-Norton, 2003); and captive parrots (Coulton et al. 1997). There are several interesting hypotheses explaining why this phenomenon occurs. Contrafreeloading behavior may be motivated by innate foraging behaviors that are otherwise frustrated in captivity; animals may be engaging in information-seeking behaviors as they work to predict the location of optimal food sources; or they may be responding to the additional reinforcement provided by stimulus changes when one works for food, such as the sound of a hopper. Nonetheless, animals' preference to behave in ways that impact their environment is demonstrated once again. Animals are built to behave, not to be passive.

A third area of scientific inquiry called learned helplessness adds additional support to the theory that personal control over significant environmental events is necessary for animals to behave healthfully. This phenomenon further demonstrates that a lack of control can have pathological effects including depression, learning disabilities, emotional problems (Maier & Seligman 1976), and suppressed immune system activity (Laudenslager et al. 1983). Learned helplessness occurs when an animal with no prior escape history is

Table 14-1 A simple model of behavioral support

	Not enough behavior	Too much behavior
Goal	Increase/maintain current frequency	Decrease/suppress current frequency
Antecedent changes	Setting events	Setting events
	Establishing operations	Establishing operations
	Adding a cue	Removing a cue
Consequence changes	Reinforcement	Punishment

prevented from escaping severe, aversive stimuli. Under this condition, the animal eventually gives up attempting to escape and remains passive. Later when escape is made blatantly possible the animal does not make the expected escape response, as if helpless. This research has been replicated with cockroaches (Brown et al. 1988), dogs, cats, monkeys, children, and adults (Overmier & Seligman 1967). Further, Seligman's (1990) research suggests that we can "immunize" learners from the effects of lack of control by providing them with experiences in which their behavior is effective, that is, in which they control their own outcomes. In this way, the effects of exposure to uncontrollable aversive stimuli, which is inevitable in all our lives to some degree, can be minimized.

Based on these three related research areas, it is very possible that a lack of control explains some, if not many, of the pathological behaviors we see in parrots such as self-mutilation, mate killing, and phobias. To the greatest extent possible, parrots should be empowered to make important decisions, such as when to exit or enter their cages or go on and off their caregiver's hands. Parrots so empowered will likely experience greater behavioral and emotional health in captivity.

TOOLS AND TECHNIQUES FOR BEHAVIOR CHANGE

Although a parrot's biological history often takes center stage, much of the time behavior problems are the result of its learning history in captivity, which is composed of all the environmental events that have affected the parrot's behavior up to the present. When one stops to think about it, behavior problems can be reduced to two simple categories: not doing something enough (e.g., stepping up, staying put, and eating pellets) and doing something too much (e.g., screaming, biting, and chewing woodwork). Our responsibility is to suc-

cessfully increase desirable behavior and decrease problem behavior using the most positive, least intrusive methods possible. Table 14-1 describes this simple behavior support model, after which the major strategies that compose the teaching technology of behavior analysis are discussed.

Changing Behavior with Antecedent Strategies

There are three general categories of antecedents that precede behavior: discriminative stimuli, setting events, and establishing operations. A discriminative stimulus (S^D, pronounced ess-dee), or "cue", belongs to a special class of antecedents that signal that a certain response will be reinforced (among all possible responses). A stimulus or event becomes an S^D by being repeatedly present when a response is reinforced. For example, when the doorbell rings, we open the door rather than pick up the phone, hurry to the exits, or gather up our school books. We do so because in the past, the doorbell has been consistently paired with reinforcement for opening the door and not for those other behaviors. The strength of a stimulus to cue a behavior is related to the strength of the reinforcer that follows the behavior. For some birds a perching stick comes to signal that stepping up will be reinforced with activities outside the cage. A ringing phone signals that saying "hello" will be reinforced with gales of laughter, and a person approaching a cage with a bowl in hand signals that coming to the feed door will be reinforced with food.

Problem behaviors are cued by discriminative stimuli as well. The very same cues just described can just as easily signal that biting will be reinforced if we remove the perching stick, return the phone to its base, or hastily install the food bowl and retreat fast. Cues don't only come from people. The setting sun, cage covers, and microwaves can function as cues for particular behavior too. The approach of one of the author's (Friedman)

Shih Tzu pups cued (antecedent) her Umbrella Cockatoo to call raucously (behavior), which was then reinforced by the Shih Tzu's howling (consequence); thus, the frequency of the bird's raucous calling increased. (Turning the raucous parrot call into a cue for the dog to return to its owner for a biscuit took care of the problem.)

Setting events also influence behavior. They are the context, conditions, or situational influences that affect the contingencies that follow. Hands held too low, noisy environments, cage arrangements, and the number of people in the room are all potential setting events that can affect the way in which a bird responds to an offered hand. The relation between setting events and problem behavior should be considered carefully, as the setting is often one of the easiest things to change.

Establishing operations (Michael 1982) temporarily alter the effectiveness of consequences. As further explained by Kazdin (2001), "Motivational states, emotions, and environmental events are establishing operations because they momentarily alter the effectiveness of the consequence that may follow behavior and influence the frequency of the behavior" (p. 454). The effectiveness of a consequence to increase the frequency of a behavior is often related to its availability

(i.e., excess or deficit). For example, hunger and satiation alter the reinforcing strength of food treats in opposite ways: A few sunflower seeds may be a highly motivating consequence to a bird that rarely has access to them but not motivating at all to a bird that has unlimited access to them every day.

Establishing operations can be used to alter the strength of other non-food reinforcers as well. For example, a bird may be more motivated to stay on a play gym after some quality time with a favorite caregiver. Chasing the family cat may be less reinforcing after an energetic training session, and stepping onto a hand may be more reinforcing when the bird is on the floor. Table 14-2 lists additional examples of the many ways antecedents can be carefully arranged to decrease the occurrence of problem behaviors and increase desirable behaviors.

Changing Behavior with Consequence Strategies

At the heart of good training is two-way communication that results from the planned arrangement of contingencies. Contingencies are the if/then dependencies between behavior and its consequences. For example, to increase the frequency of quiet vocalizations we can offer the fol-

Table 14-2   Examples of antecedent behavior change strategies

Type of antecedent event	Antecedent technique	Problem behavior	Application
Discriminative stimulus	Add a cue for the right behavior.	Lunges when cage is serviced.	Cue bird to go to a far perch before servicing cage.
	Remove a cue for the problem behavior.	Bites shirt buttons.	Don t-shirt before handling bird.
Setting events	Decrease the response effort for the right behavior.	Refuses to go to others from preferred person's shoulder.	Set bird on counter before offering non-preferred hand.
	Increase the response effort for the problem behavior.	Chews door frame.	Move play tree to center of room.
Establishing operations	Increase reinforcer strength for the right behavior.	Resists returning to cage.	Remove treat from diet except when bird enters cage.
	Decrease reinforcer strength for the problem behavior.	Jumps off T-stand.	Offer undivided attention for 10 minutes before T-stand.

lowing contingencies: *if* the parrot vocalizes quietly, *then* a preferred person approaches, but *if* the parrot vocalizes loudly, *then* no attention follows. Unfortunately, the opposite contingencies are often provided (i.e., if the parrot vocalizes loudly, then a preferred person approaches), inadvertently giving function to problem behaviors like excessive screaming.

Contingencies empower learners to choose how to operate on their environment. When a person offers a hand to a parrot, it chooses to step up or not depending on past consequences. If the parrot runs away, it communicates clearly that past consequences for stepping up are not sufficiently motivating at that moment to repeat the behavior. Rather than force the bird to comply, this is the time to consider ways to alter the antecedents and consequences to change the behavior. The question to ask before making any request of a parrot is, "Why should he"? and the answer lies in the consequences we consistently provide.

There are two broad categories of consequence techniques: Reinforcement strengthens behavior and punishment weakens it. Although the terms mean many different things in common usage, they have specific, technical meaning in the science of behavior that maximizes their usefulness. Behavioral strength can refer to different response dimensions such as frequency, rate, duration, intensity, topography (form, e.g., a foot barely lifted off a perch versus a foot raised high in the air), and latency (the time lag between the cue and the onset of the behavior). To simplify the discussion, frequency of behavior, the most often used measure of behavioral strength, is discussed throughout this section.

REINFORCEMENT

When a behavior doesn't occur often enough we can increase its frequency with reinforcement. Reinforcement is the procedure of contingently providing consequences for a behavior that increase or maintain the frequency of that behavior. Positive reinforcement, sometimes called reward training, is a reinforcement procedure in which a behavior is followed by the *presentation* of a stimulus. Negative reinforcement, sometimes called escape training, is a reinforcement procedure in which a behavior is followed by the *removal* of a stimulus. Technically, the terms "positive" and "negative" refer only to the operation of presenting (+) or removing (−) a stimulus that, in the case of reinforcement, functions to increase or maintain the behavior it follows. However, it is generally accurate and often easier to assume that positive reinforcers have "positive" value to the learner (something it works to get) and negative reinforcers have "negative" value (something it works to escape). Examples of positive and negative reinforcement are in Table 14-3.

Although both positive and negative reinforcements increase or maintain behavior, they can affect the manner in which a learner engages in training quite differently: To get positive reinforcers, learners often enthusiastically exceed the minimum effort necessary to gain them. Alternatively, to escape negative reinforcers, learners tend to offer only the minimum behavior neces-

Table 14-3 Examples of positive and negative reinforcement

	Antecedent	Behavior	Consequence	Future behavior
Positive reinforcement (reward)	Grace asks Sam to go to the back perch	Sam hops onto perch	Grace adds food bowl through feed door	Sam goes to perch more
	Grace is working on her computer	Sam nips her hand	Grace scratches Sam's head	Sam nips hand more
Negative reinforcement (escape)	Grace offers left hand with towel in right hand	Sam steps up	Grace puts down towel	Sam steps up more
	Grace offers perch while holding Sam's toes with her thumb	Sam pulls back foot to step on perch	Grace removes thumb as Sam steps down	Sam steps on perch more

sary to avoid the aversive stimuli. Moreover, the use of aversive procedures has been repeatedly demonstrated to increase learners' escape behaviors, aggression, apathy, and generalized fear (Azrin & Holz 1966). These side effects are detrimental and are discussed further in the section on punishment. As a result, positive reinforcement is the gold standard of behavior-change procedures. It is powerful, effective, and is not associated with aversive fallout (Sulzer-Azaroff & Mayer 1991).

Factors Affecting Reinforcement

Several important factors affect reinforcement. The first is contingency, the degree to which delivery of the reinforcer depends on the behavior occurring first. Consistent pairing of the behavior and the reinforcer clearly communicates the contingency between a behavior and a reinforcer. Without consistency, it's difficult for a parrot to make the connection between the two events, which slows down learning and produces inconsistent behavior.

Contiguity refers to the temporal closeness of the behavior and the reinforcer. Reinforcers that are delivered immediately after the behavior communicate the contingency most clearly. Lattal (1995) demonstrated the importance of timing to effective reinforcement with pigeons learning to peck a disk. With just a ten-second delay before delivering the food reinforcer, the pigeons never learned to peck the disk after 40 days of one-hour training sessions. When the delay was reduced to one second, the pigeons learned to peck the disk in less than 20 minutes.

Certain characteristics of the reinforcers such as type and magnitude also affect reinforcement. Simmons (1924) found that rats reinforced at the end of a maze with bread and milk ran significantly faster than those reinforced with sunflower seeds. In two studies comparing frequency and magnitude, Schneider (1973) and Todorov et al. (1984) found that small, frequent reinforcers tended to be more effective than large, occasional ones. Research continues on the many other factors that affect reinforcement such as task characteristics, task difficulty, relative availability, and learning history.

Amid these general factors, individual differences should be carefully considered when arranging contingencies for desirable behavior. A consequence that is reinforcing to one parrot may be neutral or aversive to another. Regardless of the teacher's intentions, the proof of reinforcement is in the strength of the resulting behavior. Only by watching the data, the parrot's behavior, can we know the extent to which it has been reinforced. To determine an individual parrot's reinforcers, one can observe the bird's favorite items, foods, activities, people, sounds, and locations. Establishing new reinforcers, a process discussed in the next section, keeps the list growing throughout a learner's lifetime.

Establishing New Reinforcers

The enormous degree of behavioral flexibility inherent in many species is related to the capriciousness of the environments in which they live. Indeed, if the environment remained constant, and therefore predictable, all the behavior we would ever need to survive could be genetically transmitted and elicited reflexively by particular triggering stimuli. Instead, for parrots, as with humans, learning is the rapid-adaptation system that allows them to meet the demands of an unpredictable environment in constant change. This extraordinary behavioral flexibility includes the process by which neutral stimuli become reinforcers, called secondary or conditioned reinforcers.

Secondary reinforcers, such as praise, favorite perches, and the sound of a clicker or whistle, are previously neutral stimuli that acquire their reinforcing value by repeated pairing with existing reinforcers. Primary, or unconditioned, reinforcers, such as food, water, and relief from heat or cold, are automatically reinforcing; that is, they require no prior pairing or experience to function as behavior increasing consequences. Primary reinforcers are related to basic survival functions, which makes them a good starting point for conditioning secondary reinforcers.

Primary and secondary reinforcers have different advantages and disadvantages in the context of training (Chance 2003). On one hand, primary reinforcers are generally quite powerful and they are not dependent on their association with other reinforcers; but, they are few in number and more susceptible to a temporary loss of effectiveness due to satiation. For most parrots, the first few sunflower seeds will be more motivating (a stronger reinforcer) than the last few. On the other hand, secondary reinforcers tend to hold their value longer (satiate slower) and they can be delivered with less disruption, better contiguity, at a greater distance, and in a wider variety of situations. However, secondary reinforcers tend to be somewhat weaker than primary reinforcers and their effectiveness relies on being paired with other reinforcers, at least some of the time. Both kinds of reinforcers, in the greatest possible number, add power to a trainer's toolbox and increase the quality of life for companion parrots.

Schedules of Reinforcement

Schedules of reinforcement are the rules that determine which particular instance of behavior will be reinforced. Although it can be a complicated topic and beyond the scope of this chapter, the three simple schedules that are most important to understanding and managing parrot behavior are discussed briefly here. They are continuous, intermittent, and extinction schedules.

A continuous reinforcement (CRF) schedule is one in which each and every instance of the behavior is reinforced (1:1). Given this perfect consistency, CRF provides the clearest communication to the learner about what behavior is being reinforced. As a result, the CRF schedule produces rapid learning and is recommended for stabilizing and increasing existing behaviors and teaching new behaviors (Sulzer-Azaroff & Mayer 1991).

At the other end of the spectrum is extinction (EXT), in which no instances of the behavior are reinforced (1:0). As the name suggests, when the reinforcer that previously maintained a behavior is withheld, the rate of that behavior predictably decreases to pre-reinforcement levels (not necessarily total suppression).

Another category of simple schedules of reinforcement is intermittent schedules. With intermittent schedules only some instances of the behavior are reinforced, as opposed to all (CRF) or none (EXT). Once a behavior is learned, an intermittent schedule produces persistent behavior in the sense that it takes longer to extinguish than behaviors maintained on a continuous reinforcement schedule. Perhaps the clearest example of this partial reinforcement effect is the different patterns of responding that occur at vending machines versus slot machines. Given a continuous reinforcement history interacting with vending machines, most people stop dropping coins into the slot after the first or second instance that

nothing comes out. But, given an intermittent reinforcement history with slot machines, most people continue dropping coins into a slot persistently although rarely does anything ever come out.

The partial reinforcement effect explains many of the persistent misbehaviors we see in companion parrots. The occasional time a lunge to the feed door results in an escape to the top of the cage or a top decibel scream produces an expletive from a caregiver is often enough to produce enduring problem behaviors, due to the intermittent reinforcement schedule on which these behaviors are maintained. The solution to each of these problems is not to ignore the behaviors better but to consider antecedent and consequence changes to prevent them from happening in the first place and to reward alternative positive behaviors instead.

All things considered, our birds benefit most from our ability to catch them being good with the highest possible rate of reinforcement. One important benefit of this approach is that the people who deliver dense schedules of reinforcement are more likely to become valued secondary reinforcers themselves. A common axiom is, "You get what you reinforce." Where problem behaviors are concerned, what you get when you reinforce intermittently is persistent problems.

Implementing Reinforcement Effectively

Sulzer-Azaroff and Mayer (1991) present several guidelines for maximizing the effectiveness of reinforcement procedures that, when overlooked, account for ineffective behavior change programs with children. As these guidelines apply to all learners and situations, they should be accounted for carefully in our work with parrots. An adapted list of guidelines follows.

- Reinforce immediately until the behavior is occurring at a high steady rate, then gradually introduce delay.
- Reinforce every response initially until the behavior is well established, and then gradually introduce intermittent reinforcement.
- Specify the conditions under which reinforcers will be delivered (i.e., the cue and criterion for reinforcement) and incorporate other antecedent conditions (e.g., setting events and establishing operations).

- Deliver a quantity of reinforcers sufficient to maintain the behavior without causing rapid satiation.
- Select reinforcers appropriate to the individual.
- Use a variety of reinforcers and reinforcing situations.
- Provide opportunities to experience new reinforcers.
- Eliminate, reduce, or override competing contingencies.

Shaping New Behaviors

A behavior can't be reinforced until it occurs, which could present a problem when one needs to teach a new behavior to a parrot. Waiting for the behavior to occur by happenstance and capturing it with reinforcement might be an option, but some behaviors occur too infrequently or not at all. The solution to this problem is known as shaping, technically called differential reinforcement of successive approximations. Shaping is the procedure of reinforcing a graduated sequence of subtle changes toward the final behavior, starting with the closest response the bird already does. The following are two examples of shaping plans for teaching independent toy play and bathing.

Shaping Plan 1: Playing with Toys
1. Final behavior: Independent toy play.
2. Closest behavior bird already does: Looks at toy.
3. Reinforcer for each approximation that meets the criterion: Safflower seeds and praise.
4. Tentative approximations:
   a. Look at toy
   b. Move toward toy
   c. Touch beak to toy
   d. Pick up toy with beak
   e. Touch foot to toy
   f. Hold toy with foot while manipulated with beak
   g. Repeat previous approximation for longer durations

Shaping Plan 2: Triggering the Bathing Response
1. Final behavior: Step into shallow water dish.
2. Initial behavior: Looks at water dish.
3. Reinforcers for each approximation that meets criterion: Applause and praise.
4. Tentative steps:
   a. Look at dish
   b. Face dish
   c. Take a step toward dish
   d. Take two steps toward dish
   e. Walk up to dish
   f. Look at water in dish
   g. Lift foot next to dish
   h. Touch water in dish with foot
   i. Step into dish with one foot
   j. Step into dish with both feet
   k. Walk around in dish

Implementing a shaping procedure requires noticing the subtle, natural variation in the way behaviors are performed within a response class (called an operant class). For example, a parrot naturally lifts its foot a little differently every time (left or right, high or low, fast or slow, with toe movement or without, etc.). Typically this variation is unimportant and it is simply classified as one behavior, or operant class, called lifting a foot. However, this subtle variation is exactly what allows us to shape a parrot to "wave" with a foot lifted fast, held high, and toes open and closed.

Shaping starts by reinforcing the first approximation every time it is offered, until it is performed without hesitation. Next, an even closer approximation is reinforced, at which time reinforcement for the first approximation is withheld. Once the second approximation is performed without hesitation, an even closer approximation is reinforced while withholding reinforcement for all previous approximations. In this way, the criterion for reinforcement is gradually shifted (graduated) closer and closer to the target behavior. Finally, every instance of the target behavior is reinforced.

If the learner experiences difficulty at any criterion, the trainer backs up and repeats the previous successful step, or reinforces smaller approximations. Once an approximation is performed without hesitation, more variability can be generated from which to select the next approximation by switching from continuous reinforcement to intermittent reinforcement (see the discussion of extinction bursts later). Ultimately, it is the parrot who determines the exact sequence and pace of the shaping plan. This is where sensitivity and experience is required on the part of the trainer to observe the nuances of behavior.

With shaping toy play and bathing, the toys and water dish are the antecedents that set the occasion for the respective behaviors. For other behaviors, a cue from the trainer (discriminative stimulus) can be added to signal the behavior. To add a cue, start by introducing it while the behavior is occurring. Next, gradually deliver the cue earlier and earlier until it is signaled *before* the behavior. Last, reinforce only cued instances of the behavior and ignore all others. This will establish the relationship between the cue and behavior, called stimulus control. When a behavior is said to be under stimulus control, it is emitted after the cue and rarely or not at all when the cue is absent.

With shaping we can theoretically train any behavior within the biological constraints of the learner. Husbandry, medical, and enrichment behaviors can be shaped to reduce stress and increase physical and mental stimulation. Birds can learn such behaviors as raising each foot for nail trims, going in and out of crates, staying calm wrapped in towels, flying to designated perches, and playing basketball. Shaping can also be used to change different dimensions of existing behaviors such as duration, rate, intensity, topography, and response time.

Not surprisingly, problem behaviors are often unwittingly shaped as well. We inadvertently teach our birds to bite harder, scream louder, and chase faster through the subtle mechanisms of shaping. For better and for worse, shaping is endlessly applicable to teaching captive parrots, making targeting the sharpest of all training tools. Its uses are limited only by one's imagination and commitment to learning how to use it well.

Shaping Touch-to-Target

Regarding cats, Catherine Crawmer (2001) describes the technique known as targeting this way: "If we could get a cat to touch his nose to a stick on cue what could we do with that behavior? The answer is a question: What couldn't we do with it?" (p. 57).

Targeting is the behavior of touching a body part (e.g., beak, wing, or foot) to a designated object or mark and it is taught easily to parrots with shaping. By teaching birds how to target the end of a wooden dowel with their beaks, caretakers can predict and control the birds' movements. For example, an untamed bird can be taught to target a stick while inside its cage, enabling the caretaker to safely increase interaction with the bird, deliver positive reinforcement, and establish two-

way communication. A bird that refuses to come off the top of its cage can be targeted to a perch inside it; a wary bird can be targeted into a travel crate for veterinary visits; and an aggressive bird can be quickly redirected to the target to distract it from biting. Also, enrichment behaviors can be taught with targeting such as turning in a circle, climbing up and down ladders, and ringing a bell. Target training is an important basic skill for all companion parrots, as it opens the door to all sorts of positive reinforcement and management opportunities.

Differential Reinforcement of Alternative Behaviors

Differential reinforcement is any training procedure in which certain kinds of behavior are systematically reinforced and others are not. Shaping is one example of differential reinforcement; at any point in the shaping sequence reinforcement is delivered for one approximation and withheld for all earlier ones. The process of withholding reinforcers that previously maintained a behavior is called extinction and it results in an overall reduction in the frequency of the behavior. Thus, differential reinforcement is technically two procedures, positive reinforcement and extinction, the combined effect of which is to increase the reinforced behavior and extinguish (decrease) the unreinforced one.

The relevance of differential reinforcement procedures to companion parrot behavior is enormous, specifically as an alternative to punishment. Punishment procedures focus solely on decreasing or suppressing behavior, teaching what *not to do*, which necessarily reduces the amount of positive reinforcement available to the bird. Instead, differential reinforcement of alternative behavior focuses on reinforcing appropriate replacement behaviors, teaching what *to do*, while at the same time the undesired behavior is ignored. When properly implemented, the result is a high rate of positive reinforcement for the bird, and a low rate of the problem behavior for the teacher.

There are three things to consider when selecting an alternative behavior for a differential reinforcement procedure (Alberto & Troutman 2003). First, although the behavior targeted for reduction is a problem to people, it serves a legitimate function to the parrot or it would not continue to exhibit the behavior. The function is either to gain something of value (positive reinforcement, e.g., social attention, items or activities, sensory reinforcement) or to remove something aversive (negative reinforcement, e.g., escape), as when screaming gains attention from caregivers and lunging removes intruding hands. An alternative behavior should be selected that replaces the function served by the problem behavior but in a more appropriate way. If the alternative behavior is incompatible with the problem behavior (i.e., if both behaviors can't physically be performed at the same time), the behavior change program will be that much more powerful. For example, talking is incompatible with screaming, and waiting on a far perch is incompatible with lunging at the feed door.

Second, the alternative behavior must result in the same amount of or more reinforcement than the problem behavior, in order to successfully compete with and replace it. This is predicted by the matching law, which states "that the distribution of behavior between alternative sources of reinforcement is equal to the distribution of reinforcement for these alternatives" (Pierce & Cheney 2004, p. 434). Thus, given a choice between two alternatives, parrots will exhibit the behavior that results in the greater reinforcement. Third, the alternative behavior should be one the bird already knows how to do; a well-established behavior is more likely to be performed than one that is newly acquired.

When alternative behaviors are strengthened and maintained, differential reinforcement can provide long-lasting results. As this method relies on positive reinforcement to reduce problem behaviors by teaching birds what to do, it offers a positive, constructive, and practical approach to managing parrots in captivity.

PUNISHMENT

As discussed previously, even with the most proficient and proactive behavior management skills, the time will likely come when the frequency of some behavior needs to be decreased. Although the following behavior reduction procedures may be useful adjuncts to positive reinforcement, they should not be used alone (Kazdin 2001). Overall, punishment is used too frequently and less effectively than it should be, partly because it is such an ambiguous concept. In behavior analysis it has a specific, technical meaning: Punishment is the procedure of contingently providing consequences for a behavior that decreases or suppresses the frequency of that behavior. Positive punishment is a behavior reduction procedure in which a behavior is followed by the presentation (+) of an aversive stimulus. Negative punishment is a behavior reduction procedure in which a behavior is followed by the removal (−) of positive reinforcers. Examples of positive and negative punishment are listed in Table 14-4. As can be seen in the table, the frequency of the target behaviors is decreased in each example as that defines punishment.

Like reinforcement, punishment is defined solely by its effect on behavior. Punishment can be said to have occurred only if the frequency of the target behavior decreases. Statements like "I've sprayed him a million times, punishment doesn't work with parrots!" are nonsensical. There is no such thing as failed punishment (or reinforcement). When an attempt to reduce the

Table 14-4   Examples of positive and negative punishment

	Antecedent	Behavior	Consequence	Future behavior
Positive punishment	Grace passes Sam's cage	Sam charges again bars	Grace sprays water at Sam	Sam charges bars less
	Grace is on the telephone	Sam bites her hand	Grace drops Sam to the floor	Sam bites less
Negative punishment	Grace offers hand	Sam hangs on cage door	Time out—Grace walks away for a few minutes	Sam hangs on cage door less
	Grace enters home	Sam whistles shrilly	Extinction—Grace remains silently out of sight	Sam whistles shrilly less

frequency of a behavior produces no immediate change whatsoever, punishment has not occurred and different strategies should be implemented (Chance 2003). Although both positive and negative punishment decrease or suppress behavior, positive punishment is associated with particularly adverse side effects discussed in the next section. It seems logical that having something of value taken away (negative punishment) is ultimately less aversive, although not necessarily less effective, than having something noxious administered (positive punishment). This makes negative punishment the preferred strategy after antecedent arrangements and differential reinforcement of alternative behaviors.

Like reinforcement, punishing stimuli can be classified as primary (automatic) or secondary (learned by association with existing punishers), and the effectiveness of punishment procedures depends on clear contingency, close contiguity, type, magnitude, and schedule of delivery, as well as other factors.

The Problems with Positive Punishment

Positive punishment, such as shaking perches, banging cages, spraying, hitting, laddering, flashing lights, and plucking out feathers, is problematic for parrots and their relationship with humans for several reasons. Like all learned behaviors, problem responses continue because they are reinforced. When we implement punishment we not only fail to teach what to do, we necessarily reduce the amount of reinforcement previously available to the learner for misbehaving—a double negative of sorts, as punishment is added and reinforcement is subtracted. This makes it vitally important to use punishment in conjunction with positive reinforcement procedures to strengthen desirable behaviors and maintain a reinforcing environment. This guideline is called the fair pair rule (White & Haring 1976).

Another problem with punishment is the severity required to produce lasting effects. Research has shown (e.g. Azrin & Holz 1966) that high-intensity punishment is more effective than either low-intensity punishment or escalating levels of punishment. The intensity required to suppress parrots' problem behaviors is often greater than that which meets acceptable standards of ethical practice or is comfortably administered by caregivers.

With negative reinforcement an aversive stimulus is present in the antecedent environment, the removal of which reinforces the escape behavior. With positive punishment the aversive stimulus is administered without escape, which sets the stage for the detrimental side effects frequently observed with positive punishment. They are escape behaviors; aggression and other emotional reactions; generalization of emotional reactions to unrelated people, settings, and items; apathy (a general reduction of all behavior); and behavioral contrast (the increase of the target behavior in other settings). These side effects are well established, having been broadly investigated for many decades with countless species of animals (e.g., Azrin et al. 1965; Sidman 1989); and they are startlingly common among captive parrots, many of which show extreme aggression, apathy, and fear.

It is the narrow view that effectiveness is the sole criterion for choosing behavior-change procedures that perhaps keeps so many people using punishment. Unfortunately, every time a problem behavior is successfully decreased with positive punishment, the person delivering the punishment is negatively reinforced for having used it. Of course, this will result in an increased probability that positive punishment will be used more. Yet based on the nature of parrots' problem behaviors in captivity, the known detrimental side effects of positive punishment, and the power of reinforcement-based alternatives, there can be little justification for using positive punishment with captive parrots.

Negative Punishment

The two negative punishment procedures relevant to parrot behavior are time out from positive reinforcement (time out) and extinction. Time out is the contingent, temporary removal of access to all positive reinforcers and extinction is the contingent, permanent removal of the specific reinforcer(s) maintaining the problem behavior. Both procedures can be very effective when used correctly but they are frequently misunderstood and very poorly implemented.

The effectiveness of time out is undermined by unclear contingency, slow contiguity (timing), and inadvertent reinforcement, also known as "bootleg" reinforcement (Chance 1998, p. 458). For example, chasing the bird, scolding, and marching to distant cages can provide bootleg reinforcement that renders time out ineffective. Under these conditions, the parrot has little chance of perceiving clearly the contingent withdrawal of positive reinforcers, thereby obscuring the association between the offending behavior and being returned to its cage. Time out is more effective when using the following guidelines:

- Plan the time out location ahead of time to ensure that it can be managed with clear contingency and immediacy. For many tame parrots, simply turning away or being set down for a short time is an effective time out from positive reinforcement.
- Increase the salience of the contingency between the behavior and the consequence by keeping the time out interval short (approximately 30 seconds to a few minutes). Watch the clock or count out the seconds to track the time systematically.
- Immediately after the time out interval, give the bird the opportunity to practice the appropriate behavior and reinforce it amply every time it is exhibited.
- Allow time out to do all the work in decreasing the problem behavior. There is no need for other consequences or emotional displays from the caregiver, which may provide bootleg reinforcement for the problem behavior.

Extinction used in combination with positive reinforcement has already been discussed as it applies to shaping and differential reinforcement of alternative behavior. To implement extinction as a single behavior reduction procedure, the reinforcer that maintains the problem behavior should be identified first by conducting a functional assessment (ABCs). In the case where the maintaining reinforcer is human attention, extinction is tantamount to inviolate ignoring—the total and permanent withholding of attention. Unfortunately, for some parrot behaviors like excessive screaming, biting, and chewing unapproved items, ignoring is easier to prescribe than to implement effectively.

As discussed by Alberto and Troutman (2003), careful consideration should be given to the following points before using extinction to decrease a problem behavior. First, extinction tends to be a slow procedure. Once the maintaining reinforcer is withheld, the behavior continues for an indeter-

minate amount of time. As discussed previously, behaviors with an intermittent reinforcement history are the slowest to change, the most resistant to extinction. Second, the frequency, intensity, and/or duration of the behavior may sharply increase before a significant decrease in the problem behavior occurs. This phenomenon is known as an extinction burst. This predictable escalation is often beyond toleration for caregivers. As a result, they abandon the program by providing attention, and the behavior is unintentionally reinforced at the new level of intensity. Third, behaviors associated with frustration, such as aggression, are commonly induced by extinction. For parrots, this may mean an increase in the frequency and intensity of already severe biting. Fourth, as with time out, bootleg reinforcement can be a problem. Reinforcement can be delivered by other pets, children, or even an echo in the room. Further, some behaviors appear to be automatically reinforcing. When the maintaining reinforcer is not in the control of the trainer, extinction cannot be effective.

The fifth point to consider is spontaneous recovery, also known as resurgence (Sulzer-Azaroff & Mayer 1991). Resurgence is the reappearance of the extinguished behavior after an extended period of time. Forewarned, the immediate reimplementation of strict extinction conditions will return the behavior to its pre-recovery frequency. Sixth, the problem behaviors that caregivers ignore can be imitated by other parrots. This produces additional behavior problems for caregivers to solve and increases the probability of bootleg reinforcement: One parrot's imitative behavior can reinforce another parrot's problem behavior.

On the whole, ignoring is most effective as a preventative strategy rather than a problem solution. It offers a window of opportunity to avoid giving the problem behavior function by withholding reinforcement the very first time it is exhibited. Once a problem behavior is well established, differential reinforcement of alternative behaviors is usually the better strategy.

CONCLUSION

The allure of companion parrots is often outweighed by the collateral challenges of keeping them in captivity. This is especially true when the welfare of the animals is kept in the foreground. A basic understanding of how behavior works combined with a practical, humane teaching technology will help stem the tide of parrots advertised for resale in newspapers and relinquished to shelters and sanctuaries.

There are currently several popular belief systems regarding how best to manage parrot behavior. When opinions differ, emotions are strong, and the stakes are high, science should hold a higher value than conventional wisdom and personal recipes about behavior. Science demonstrates an important association between behavioral health and empowerment; that is, the personal power to control significant environmental events. Overpowering parrots with forceful and coercive training methods should be understood as stealing behavior that could be given to us instead with facilitative antecedents and positive reinforcement. Empowering captive parrots to the greatest extent possible, within the context of appropriate training objectives, may mitigate the behavioral pathologies so prevalent among them.

Given a choice between different behavioral interventions, selecting the most positive, least intrusive, effective strategy meets the highest standard of ethical practice. Antecedent changes and positive reinforcement procedures should always be tried before implementing negative punishment (removing positive reinforcers) or negative reinforcement (escape training). Positive punishment procedures, in which aversive stimuli are applied, should be used rarely, if ever. Finally, all three procedures—negative reinforcement, negative punishment, and positive punishment—should only be used as an adjunct to positive reinforcement strategies.

Taking full responsibility for parrots' learning and behavior is the first and most important step to supporting their behavioral health. Companion parrots offer their caregivers the opportunity to educate themselves about behavior and significantly improve the quality of life for parrots in captivity.

REFERENCES

Alberto, P.A., and A.C. Troutman. 2003. *Applied behavior analysis for teachers,* 6th ed. Upper Saddle River, NJ: Merrill Prentice Hall.

Azrin, N.H., and W.C. Holz. 1966. "Punishment." In *Operant behavior: Areas of research and application,* ed. W.K. Honig, pp. 380–447. New York: Appleton-Century-Crofts.

Azrin, N.H., R.R. Hutchinson, and R. McLaughlin. 1965. The opportunity for aggression as an operant reinforcer during aversive stimulation. *Journal of the Experimental Analysis of Behavior,* 8:171–180.

Balph, D.F., and M.H. Balph. 1983. On the psychology of watching birds: The problem of observer-expectancy bias. *Auk* 100:755–757.

Barnett, S.A. 1981. *Modern ethology.* New York: Oxford University Press.

Barrow, E.M. 2001. *Animal behavior desk reference: A dictionary of animal behavior, ecology, and evolution,* 2nd ed. Boca Raton, FL: CRC Press.

Brown, G.E., G.D. Hughs, and A.A. Jones. 1988. Effects of shock controllability on subsequent aggressive and defensive behaviors in the cockroach (*Periplaneta americana*). *Psychological Reports* 63:563–569.

Chance, P. 1998. *First course in applied behavior analysis.* Pacific Grove, CA: Brooks/Cole Publishing Company.

Chance, P. 2003. *Learning and behavior,* 5th ed. Belmont, CA: Wadsworth/Thomson Learning.

Cloutier, S., J.P. Beaugrand, and P.C. Lague. 1995. The effect of prior victory or defeat in the same site as that of subsequent encounter on the determination of dyadic dominance in the domestic hen. *Behavioral Processes* 35:293–298.

Coulton, L.E., N.K. Warren, and R.J. Young. 1997. Effects of foraging enrichment on the behavior of parrots. *Animal Welfare* 6:357–363.

Crawmer, C. 2001. *Here kitty, kitty: Catherine Crawmer on training cats.* Sand Lake, NY: Author.

Gall, M.D., J.P. Gall, and W.R. Borg. 2003. *Educational research,* 7th ed. Boston: Allyn and Bacon.

Gilbert-Norton, L. 2003. Captive birds and freeloading: The choice to work [Electronic version]. *Research News* 4.

Gould, S.J. 1981. *The mismeasure of man.* New York: W.W. Norton & Company.

Inglis I.R., and N.J.K. Ferguson. 1986. Starlings search for food rather than eat freely available food. *Animal Behaviour* 34:614–616.

Kazdin, A.E. 2001. *Behavior modification in applied settings,* 6th ed. Belmont, CA: Wadsworth/Thomson.

Lattal, K.A. 1995. Contingency and behavior analysis. *Behavior Analyst* 24:147–161.

Laudenslager, M.L., S.M. Ryan, R.C. Drugan, and R.L. Hyson. 1983. Coping and immunosuppression: Inescapable but not escapable shock suppresses lymphocyte proliferation. *Science* 221:568–570.

Maier, S.F., and M.E.P. Seligman. 1976. Learned helplessness: Theory and evidence. *Journal of Experimental Psychology: General* 105:3–46.

Manning, A., and M. Stamp Dawkins. 1992. *An introduction to animal behavior,* 4th ed. Cambridge: Cambridge University Press.

Mech, L.D. 1999. Alpha status, dominance, and division of labor in wolf packs. *Canadian Journal of Zoology* 77:1196–1203.

Mech, L.D. 2000. Leadership in wolf, *Canis lupus*, packs. *Canadian Field-Naturalist* 114:259–263.

Michael, J. 1982. Distinguishing between discriminative and motivational functions of stimuli. *Journal of Analysis of Behavior* 37:149–155.

Osborne, S.R. 1977. The free food (contrafreeloading) phenomenon: A review and analysis. *Animal Learning & Behavior* 5:221–235.

Overmier, J.B., and M.E.P. Seligman. 1967. Effects of inescapable shock upon subsequent escape and avoidance responding. *Journal of Comparative and Physiological Psychology* 63:28–33.

Pierce, W.D., and C.D. Cheney. 2004. *Behavior analysis and learning,* 4th ed. Mahwah, NJ: Lawrence Erlbaum Associates, Inc.

Schneider, J.W. 1973. Reinforcer effectiveness as a function or reinforcer rate and magnitude: A comparison of concurrent performance. *Journal of Experimental Analysis of Behavior* 20:461–471.

Schwartz, B., E.A. Wasserman, and S.J. Robbins. 2002. *Psychology of learning and behavior,* 5th ed. New York: W.W. Norton & Company, Inc.

Seibert, L.M., and S.L. Crowell-Davis. 2001. Gender effects on aggression, dominance rank, and affiliative behaviors in a flock of captive cockatiels. *Applied Animal Behavior Science* 71:155–170.

Seligman, M.E.P. 1990. *Learned optimism.* New York: Knopf.

Sidman, M. 1989. *Coercion and its fallout.* Boston: Authors Cooperative.

Simmons, R. 1924. The relative effectiveness of certain incentives in animal learning. *Comparative Psychology Monographs* 7.

Skinner, B.F. 1981. Selection by consequences. *Science* 213:501–504.

Sulzer-Azaroff, B., and G.R. Mayer. 1991. *Behavior analysis for lasting change.* Orlando, FL: Harcourt, Brace, Jovanovich.

Todorov, J.C., E.S. Hanna, and M.C.N. Bittencourt de Sa'. 1984. Frequency versus magnitude or reinforcement: New data with a different procedure. *Journal of the Experimental Analysis of Behavior* 4:157–167.

Van Kerkhove, W. 2004. A fresh look at the wolf-pack theory of pet dog social behavior. *Journal of Applied Animal Welfare Science* 4:279–285.

White, O.R., and N.G. Haring. 1976. *Exceptional teaching.* Upper Saddle River, NJ: Merrill/Prentice Hall.

15

Behavior Classes in the Veterinary Hospital: Preventing Problems Before They Start

Kenneth R. Welle

INTRODUCTION

Behavior problems are well recognized as a leading cause of euthanasia or abandonment for dogs and cats.[1, 2] People become disillusioned with a pet that does not meet their expectations. Pet birds are not exempt from this type of problem. Behavior problems such as biting, screaming, and feather picking are very common among pet birds. In fact, since they are still essentially unchanged from the wild state, these behavioral problems may be even more common. Euthanasia is still a very uncommon request in pet birds. Owners and veterinarians alike are hesitant to end a bird's life for their own convenience. As a result, these birds are often bounced from one home to another, frequently ending up as breeding birds. It is not difficult to find even very expensive birds given away because of behavioral problems. The author owns five psittacids with a combined value of over $4,000 that were given up because of various behavioral problems. The birds that are sold or given to a new home are the lucky ones. Others are ignored or neglected because the owners are afraid of them, or they are put into basements or other isolated areas because they are too noisy. While the idea of placing these birds in breeding programs may have merit in some instances, over many generations, we may be selectively breeding for the least desirable behavioral traits. The author has seen at least one African Grey Parrot pair whose offspring start feather picking before they ever leave the pet store. Obviously, this could be due to the early practices of the breeder or many other factors. However, like many other traits, behavior can have genetic and environmental influences. If only those pets that develop undesirable behaviors are brought into breeding programs, this situation may become increasingly common.

Wild parrots are usually hatched in clutches of two to six, and the mother and father tend them constantly. Following fledging and weaning, parrots continue to learn from their parents and other flock members. They follow the parent birds around the environment and learn what to fear, what not to fear, what to eat, how to find food, where to sleep, and how to interact with other members of the flock. In captivity, neonatal parrots often are poorly socialized during the hand-feeding process. They are often housed in individual brooders and their only interaction is when they are fed. Once weaned, many are immediately sold or placed into new homes. Very infrequently are they "educated" regarding coping with the captive environment.

Behavior classes for owners and birds are one measure to both prevent and rehabilitate problem parrots. When a dog trainer began to offer obedience training in the author's practice, the idea of a similar forum for addressing avian behavior issues was formed. By offering a class where several clients could be educated at the same time, a greater amount of information could be transferred. The owners are given information that they can use at home to work with the bird. In addition to the benefit of improving the relationship between bird and owners, a behavior class can afford an opportunity for introducing the bird to novel situations. Many pet birds live their entire lives in one room of a house. These birds often become very intolerant of small changes in their lives and will be easily stressed by inevitable events.[3, 4] An organized class, with birds included, allows for socialization of birds, owners, and the veterinary staff in a much less intimidating setting than the clinical examination.

Many of today's bird owners are hungry for information of any kind, and behavior is a hot topic. Even those owners who know quite a bit about avian behavior are anxious for more. The information regarding avian behavior is scattered in many places. In addition, there is considerable disagreement among "authorities" on bird behavior. This can lead to confusion and inappropriate handling of birds. Advice about bird behavior is often taken from untrained pet store personnel. In many areas, the avian veterinarian may be the only authoritative resource for bird owners. Of course, not every avian veterinarian is qualified to teach such a class. The veterinarian wishing to start behavior training must thoroughly familiarize him- or herself with pet birds, their behavior, and their relationships with owners. The instructor of such a class must be very confident handling birds. Some veterinarians restrain birds regularly but have little experience handling them in an interactive setting. Counseling pet owners on behavior is an art that must be studied prior to starting.[5] It is often helpful to directly observe the interactions between a bird and its owner. This can reveal a wealth of information about the relationship that an owner may be unable or unwilling to recognize.

COURSE DESCRIPTION

The author's behavior class was started in 1996. Since this time the course has evolved and changed to adopt the changing opinions regarding the best ways of preventing and treating common behavior problems. Because of the popularity of obedience training for dogs, the term "avian obedience training" was originally adopted. Since this time the term "bird socialization class" has been used in place of obedience training. The course is five weeks long; the first week is for owners only, while the following four weeks are for birds and owners. Each session is about one

hour long. During the first session, a videotape, *Parrots: Look Who's Talking* (*Nature,* Thirteen-WNET, and PBS, New York) is shown. This tape is very entertaining and informative and introduces some of the concepts discussed in the class. The remainder of the first session is used to begin discussion of the course topics. Wild parrot behavior, psittacine social structure, and environmental factors for pet birds are some of the first topics covered.[6–11] In the sessions where birds are present, discussions and bird exercises are mixed to keep up the interest of both the birds and owners. Ten minutes of talking followed by ten minutes of exercises appears to work well. Table 15-1 lists the topics and exercises covered in each of the sessions. To complement the class, a written handout is given to the class members. At the completion of the course, each bird is given a diploma, which is easily generated on a personal computer. Clinics wishing to begin these classes can start with this format and then modify it to suit their own practice. The author's original class handout is available through the Association of Avian Veterinarians publication office.

CAVEATS

One concern with a class such as this is the transmission of infectious diseases. While this is not entirely preventable, requiring that all applicable infectious diseases be screened for in all registrants can minimize the risk. The type of client who is interested in such a class generally will agree to this requirement. In the author's practice, the requirements include an examination, a complete blood count, and chlamydophila screening within the past year. Old world parrots are required to have a negative screening for circovirus at some point. Any birds with problem behaviors should be worked up for medical causes of these problems before assuming that it is solely behavioral. Some types of behavioral problems are more suitable for individual counseling than a group setting. Clients should bring their own towels and carriers. The perches are made of polyvinyl chloride pipes and covered with disposable self-adhesive elastic bandage so that they can be sanitized in between uses. Alternately, owners can be required to provide their own perches. Preweaned babies are not permitted, as they are very susceptible to bacterial infections. This is not a program that should be used for aviculture birds.

Table 15-1   Sample outline for in-clinic avian behavior classes

Session	Topic	Exercises
1	Environment Psittacine socialization Communication	Step up Step down Stay
2	Development and learning Independence and confidence	Step up Step down Stay Hooding
3	Interactive games	Step up Step down Stay Hooding Carrier
4	Bonding	Step up Step down Stay Hooding Carrier Towel play
5	Motivation and reinforcement	Step up Step down Stay Hooding Carrier Towel play Tricks

It is intended for pet birds where the need for protecting them must be tempered by the need to improve the quality of life. If more than one bird is in the household, the class participant should be considered a "new bird" again after the completion of the class and all applicable quarantine procedures should be followed.

The other concern with this program is the liability. During the course of the sessions, owners may be bitten by their birds. As with clinical examinations, the liability for such bites is with the practice owner. However, having a technician handle the bird for the owner defeats the purpose. A waiver, indicating that owners are aware of the risk of being bitten, provides some protection in the event of a severe bite. If younger family members participate, a parent should give consent. Bird to bird aggression could also result in liability claims. While this has never occurred in the author's practice, it could easily ruin an otherwise pleasant class. To minimize risks, all birds are re-

quired to have trimmed wings and owners are not allowed to bring more than one bird for each handler. The room should allow the birds enough space that they do not feel threatened by the proximity of other birds or handlers.

COURSE CONTENT

Psittacine Socialization

During the class, it is emphasized that parrots are altricial and that they have very long behavioral development.[3, 6] Hand-raised parrots do not have the instincts needed to be well-adjusted pets. The owner's family must take on the role of the flock and guide the development of the chick. While some owners feel that teaching obedience to a bird is cruel and unnatural, the opposite is true; it is cruel and unnatural to let them try to figure things out for themselves.[3] It is emphasized that pet parrots must be "educated" to properly adapt to human habitats. Parrots and their relatives are highly social and intelligent birds. There are 332 species of psittacine birds and the social structure of each of these is somewhat different. These facts make it inherently difficult to provide an appropriate social setting for these birds in the captive environment. When social needs are not met, companion birds often develop behaviors that are self-destructive or make them undesirable as pets.

A common misconception is that social behavior evolved because of a need for companionship. In reality the congregation of groups of animals within a species serves a much more utilitarian purpose. Aptly put by Christine Davis, "In the wild, the flock is primarily a protective unit, and affiliation with others is essential to the survival of each individual. The need for social interaction, although extremely important, is secondary to the instinct for survival."[12] The presence of conspecifics makes it much more difficult for a predator to successfully stalk and kill a given individual. Even with a less altruistic perspective, the presence of other potential prey items in the vicinity makes it mathematically less likely for an individual to be preyed upon. Behaviors necessary for relatively conflict-free interaction between individuals of a group evolved as a secondary requirement. This fact makes social interaction even more critical. Not only is a bird lonely when alone, it feels vulnerable to attack. A close analogy would be to compare the situation to a person walking at night. Generally people feel more secure and safe when with a group of people than when walking alone.

While descriptions of natural psittacine social behavior abound, most of these are based more on television, magazines, captive observations, and conjecture rather than scientific observation of parrots in the wild. Both the descriptions of parrot behavior and their interpretation vary to some extent. Nonetheless, these descriptions currently provide the best basis for determining what the healthiest social environment will be for captive birds.

Most parrots pair bond. Keas are polygamous. Asiatic Parakeets and Eclectus bond only for breeding season. Most parrots separate in pairs during breeding, while some, such as Quakers, Brown-throated Conures, and Patagonian Conures, are colony nesters. Outside breeding season, parrots live in small to very large flocks (A.U.

Luescher, unpublished data, March 1999). In order for any animal society to function, communication and conflict-resolution mechanisms must be developed. For most social animals a form of hierarchy develops to prevent true combat situations. According to some, most parrot flocks function under a hierarchic arrangement.[12] Young parrots learn to submit to the leader. If they try to share resources, they are bitten and chased away.[6] Others argue that while within pairs there appears to be a dominance relationship, in flock situations no dominance has been described (A.U. Luescher, unpublished data, March 1999). Because of their intelligence, parrot social structure may not be a linear dominance hierarchy. There may be a matter of creating alliances more than of dominance. Also, dominance in one situation may not apply to another.[13] Whether it comprises a true dominance hierarchy system or not, it certainly appears that parrots avoid violent conflict by ritualized posturing and positioning.

Vertical placement or height is frequently referred to in avian behavior literature. It has been said that the dominance order can often be determined by seeing dominant individuals in higher positions.[12] Others claim that the apparent relationship of height to dominance may be related to the high spot being the most desirable perch rather than the height itself.[13] Others still maintain that the notion of a flock leader and dominant birds sitting higher than submissive birds is a myth entirely (A.U. Luescher, unpublished data, March 1999).

Most parrots are noisy and communicate vocally. They learn a flock dialect. They also communicate visually with body language and color (A.U. Luescher, unpublished data, March 1999). Different vocalizations are used by parrots to signal danger or food or to greet another bird.[13, 14] Vocalization is critical for keeping flocks together, especially in dense rain forest habitats. Calls are used to bring the flock together at the end of the day.[14] According to Davis, "Screaming, especially at daybreak and dusk, is a normal activity in the wild, essential in keeping track of companions at those particular times and at various intervals throughout the day."[12] Pairs engage in social grooming and mutual feeding to maintain their bonds. These interactions are uncommon between other members of the flock (A.U. Luescher, unpublished data, March 1999). Various behaviors are used for communication with less intimate flock mates.[14]

- Beak clicking: greeting or warning
- Beak grinding: contentment
- Eye pinning: excitement, either good or bad
- Facial feather twitching: startled or intrigued
- Fluffing: prelude to preening or tension releaser
- Foot tapping: territorial defense
- Tail fanning: courtship or aggressive display

Development and Learning

For many altricial species, including most of the psittacine family, behaviors tend to be learned. This is true whether the bird is in the wild or in captivity. Birds learn various skills more efficiently at certain stages of development, known as sensitive periods or critical periods.[13] One such behavior is imprinting, either filial imprinting (forming social attachments) or sexual (forming an image of a desirable mate).[13] This can lead to conflict when birds are raised by humans. As stated by Harrison in *Avian Medicine: Principles and Applications,* "Birds raised by human foster parents will imprint as people, not birds. As they mature, their natural instincts to choose a mate may cause objectionable behaviors. . . . An imprinted bird will spend all of its time attempting to drive unwanted individuals, other pets or objects out of its territory, while trying to find one chosen person with whom to mate."[6] This species confusion is compounded when the human caretaker fails to continue the bird's education to include necessary skills for coping with the artificial environment.

Once the bird fledges, it becomes versed in the "flock experience."[6] Early learning can be extremely critical for the long-term development of the bird. Any synapses that are not stimulated by early sensory experiences may be "pruned" by the brain and eliminated.[15] Play is used frequently to learn the environment and reaffirm flock position.[14] When normal play behaviors of White-fronted Amazons were studied, behaviors included play solicitation, play biting, or play fighting, or those associated with pair bonding, such as allopreening and bill nibbling.[6] In captivity, playing with a bird can provide an effective means of teaching necessary skills to pet birds.

Structured training or play sessions can allow owner and pet to interact in an entertaining but structured manner.[16] The objectives are to teach both behaviors required for companionability and behaviors that assure comfort, health, and happiness.[15] Play should focus on behaviors the animal likes to do and encourage those that are desirable.[16]

Developing a Healthy Social Environment for Pet Birds

A healthy human-avian bond requires each side to behave in a manner that promotes this bond. Necessary components of a well-adjusted and well-behaved pet bird include respect and trust of the owner and other humans, independence, and a platonic bond.

As wild animals, parrots have no concept of the human-animal bond and can only interact with human companions as flock members.[12] Initially this may be the role of a parent bird. In *Guide to the Quaker Parrot,* Athan writes, "A successful relationship between human and companion bird casts the human in the role of loving parent. Because parrots have a strong instinct to understand what is expected of them, a loving, authority-based relationship is probably the best way to maintain a long-term relationship between human and parrot."[17] This relationship is relatively easy to accomplish. It is important to set rules for an authority-based relationship, in which the bird understands that the humans are the boss.[11] One of the rules pertains to height. Whether because of dominance, site-related aggression, or other unknown reasons, birds are more aggressive when placed in high positions.[12] Pet birds should be kept below the eye level and in front of the handler. Shoulders are particularly bad locations because they prevent the person from keeping eye contact, from placing hands properly for handling, and because bites from this position can be particularly dangerous. The next aspect of maintaining the authority-based relationship is teaching some basic commands and using them frequently. Steady hands impart confidence on the part of the handler and also give steady footing to the bird. Birds often become infuriated when someone offers a hand to a bird only to pull it back when they reach out with their beak to test it. The step-up drill is one that every pet bird should know. In this drill the command "step up" is given and the bird is coaxed to step up onto the hand. Each time this exercise is performed, respect and trust are built. It is not enough that the bird knows what the command means. Practice must be maintained to maintain that mutual trust and respect. Once trust and respect are established, other skills can be taught. Important social skills can include interaction with other birds, playing with water, exploring foods, meeting strangers, and many others.[15] These behaviors are learned through imitation. In the home, parrots imitate their companions, whether avian or mammal. If they cannot copy behaviors, they improvise. If the improvised behaviors are reinforced, the behavior can become a pattern. Likewise, desirable behaviors can be encouraged by modeling those behaviors in front of the bird. The motivation to copy behaviors can be enhanced by providing a competitive situation in which the bird learns. The method is known as the model-rival technique and has been pioneered in birds by Dr. Irene Pepperberg.[11]

Independence and Confidence

Contrary to popular opinion, behavioral disorders are not always a result of inadequate interaction with a pet bird. Very often, the interactions are excessive or inappropriate and the bird never develops the ability to be comfortable by itself. Birds that have not been taught independence are much more likely to develop stress-related behaviors. Most of the strategies a parrot uses to get along in life are learned. Linden describes four distinct behavioral stages, each with skills that must be learned in order to move to the next. Neonates need comfort, "neophytes" develop curiosity, fledglings develop coordination, and "thinklings" acquire decision-making capabilities.[18] Communicating, eating, and learning how to play and what to be afraid of all must be learned for the bird to develop independence. While many types of parrots are independent by nature, others must learn this from caregivers. When they meet a new situation they look for cues as to how they should react to the situation. If the caregiver is happy, the bird will not be afraid.[19] Parrots must be taught to be adventurous. Owners should model playing with the toys or add another bird or person to play, providing a model-rival.[19] These skills are critical for the development of independent behavior in pet birds. Many pet bird owners fear spoiling a bird by responding to cries. With juvenile birds displaying baby behaviors such as crying, responding to the bird will not "spoil" the bird but make it more secure.[19] Particularly in very young birds, withholding food, attention, or other necessities can make them doubt the safety of their situation. The common advice of ignoring a vocalizing bird can contribute to a nuisance-screaming problem. A bird that is ignored will continue to scream until something happens. Acknowledging the bird and maintaining some auditory contact can minimize the begging and vocalizations. Vocal cues can be used to calm birds. The key is to plan ahead and consistently use particular words and expressions in the same situations. This way the association between the word and the situation is clearly patterned. These words can then be used in a threatening situation to give a sense of security.[20] Vocal games can also promote independence. Some games that are recommended to owners in the author's practice include the following. These were devised from many suggestions and sources and are not necessarily original. They are written in the same way that they are presented in client education materials.

HOUSE TOUR

Theory: In the wild, fledgling birds follow parents and flock mates around their environment. By seeing the response of the adult birds to various stimuli, they learn what to eat, what to fear, what to avoid, and so forth. This game is intended to do the same thing.

How to play: The bird must be tame and must know the basic step-up command. Carry the bird on the hand and walk around the house. Point out everything you see and say its name. Most importantly, be very calm. By seeing that you are not upset, the bird will learn not to be. Don't forget to introduce all of the human and animal household members. Also, do not neglect sounds. Take the bird near the source of some sounds and do the same exercise. The bonus of this game is that talking birds often learn how to identify people and things in the house.

COLOR GAME

Theory: Parrots are very visually oriented and intelligent creatures. This game helps stimulate their curiosity.

How to play: Take pieces of colored construction paper. Say the color to the bird. Repeat for all of the other colors. Keep in mind that the bird sees colors slightly differently than you do but can still distinguish them well. More advanced lessons will ask the bird what color. For even better results, do this game with another person in front of the bird. When the person gets the answer correct, he/she is lavishly praised.

WHISTLE WHILE YOU WORK

Theory: In the wild, parrots vocalize to maintain audio contact with members of their flock. Being alone puts birds at greatly increased risk of predation. Survival depends on maintaining contact. If they cannot hear the response of the group, they think they have lost contact, then they call louder. It is often said to never respond to a bird's vocalization. Imagine the following scenario. You are at home alone and you hear someone come in the door. You think it is your spouse so you call out his/her name but you get no response. You call again and still no response. At this point you start to panic and get ready to call 911! This is what we are doing to the bird when we ignore its calls.

How to play: In order to take the flock contact initiative away from the bird, announce where you are as you move about the house. This is especially true if you are out of sight. Try whistling, humming, singing, or talking as you go.

TRICK TRAINING

Theory: Parrots are highly intelligent birds. Mental challenges can occupy some of the time they may otherwise use for self-destructive behaviors. Additionally, trick training provides ammunition for counterconditioning. Tricks can and should be relatively natural behaviors that the bird learns to do on request.

How to play: Watch your bird for certain behaviors that are interesting. Then start to give a cue, try to get the bird to do the behavior, and reward even mild attempts at performing it. As time goes on, require a little better performance to receive a reward. Rewards can be verbal or food treats. Ideas that may be useful include waving the foot, somersault on the perch or table, holding up wings, holding up objects with the foot, or tearing up a toy.

Providing an Appropriate Environment

The environment can be very critical to the bird's ability to be independent. Birds may perceive many things as dangerous that a large, predatory species such as a human would not. Location in the home should take this fact into account. Birds should be able to see approaching people and pets rather than having them appear from nowhere. Placing a cage on a wall right next to a door may be more stressful for a nervous bird. Parrots may even be sensitive to the emotional "energies" of those around them and can suffer from this increased stress.[21] Such things as marital difficulties, spousal abuse, child abuse, and loss of a loved one, even one the bird does not know, may indirectly affect some birds. These can be difficult subjects to approach with clients and must be handled delicately. People should be advised to seek professional counseling if such factors are involved.

Bonding

The whole point of having a pet is to bond with them in some fashion. While most birds' roles in a household are simple companions, occasionally birds are kept as surrogates for children, spouses, or parents. Sometimes birds, especially since they are long-lived, can serve as a last link to a loved one that has passed away.[22] When the behavior of a parrot causes this bond to be severed, the results can be devastating to the owner. Unfortunately, placement of these birds into these surrogate roles can lead to an unhealthy social environment. Ideally birds and owners interact as flock members, but not as mates. Social activities for birds within a flock may include foraging, playing, flying as a group, and other relatively dynamic activities. Allopreening and cuddling are done primarily with the mate. In companion birds, these interactions should be reserved for evenings and naptimes or when the bird is confronted with unfamiliar things.[19, 21] Many birds will beg for attention. Behaviors birds use to seek attention include shaking toys, sneezing, soft vocalization, displays, crouching and wing quivering, staring, and screaming.[14] Interactive dynamic attention given to a begging bird might teach more appropriate behavior.[19] Healthy social environments include social feeding (eating with the owners).[11] This can allow more socialization in a more casual atmosphere. It also gives an opportunity to demonstrate independent eating by eating in front of the bird and offering to share food.[19] Some species of psittacine birds are noted to spend all of their waking hours with their mates. "For such intensely social birds, life in an enclosure with no companionship must be the ultimate 'psychological torture.'"[6] Realistically, no one can provide 24-hour interaction with the bird. It is therefore best to avoid having the bird develop a pair bond with a person. In addition, birds that develop pair bonds with an owner will tend to be more aggressive. It is a myth that some species are "one-person birds." Interaction with only one person in captivity is contradictory to the psittacine social nature.[23] Birds should be encouraged to be accepting of multiple people. If reluctant, out-of-territory interactions such as step ups, rescues, or outings are recommended.[19] Rescues involve such things as a person who is not normally the favorite bringing the bird for a veterinary visit or grooming. Following the procedure and in this "hostile" environment, the person that the bird does not like starts to look very safe and comfortable to the bird. Outings are similar but simply involve taking the bird for a trip out of the home to an unfamiliar area. Again, the person becomes the most familiar thing to the bird. People disliked by a bird should practice step-up exercises in an area unfamiliar to the bird. This "home court advantage" will often result in a bird that behaves much better for a person it would normally bite.

Parrots' social behavior is both what makes them endearing to people and what often leads to undesirable or self-destructive behaviors. By attempting to understand the ways in which psittacine birds interact with one another, better methods of socializing these birds in home environments are possible. A balance between affection and independence is critical to psychologically healthy pet birds.

Motivation and Reinforcement

The concepts of motivation and reinforcement are explained to owners in the behavior class. The motivation for undesirable behavior must be removed. Desirable behaviors must be reinforced and undesirable ones must not be. Behaviors, both good and bad, exhibited by animals and people typically are initiated as a result of a particular motivation. For parrots motivations are typically simple things such as hunger, fear, play, social climbing, reproduction, or other things that would benefit the bird in the wild. In behavior modification, the motivation for a given behavior should be sought so that it can be removed or enhanced, depending on the desirability of the behavior. For example, the initial motivation for screaming may be hunger, pain, flock cohesion, or fear. These motivations can be easily removed by feeding the bird, treating the painful stimulus, calling to the bird, or removing the source of fear. Behaviors, both good and bad, generally continue to occur because they are being reinforced.[24] Inadvertent reinforcement of undesirable behavior is common among pet owners, especially with parrots and dogs. The reinforcement for screaming may come in the form of an excited verbal response, physical attention, being left alone, or even being given a treat of some kind. In addition to avoiding reinforcing bad behavior, it is important to reinforce good behavior. When a screaming bird is quiet, the owner should talk to or pet the bird.

Exercises

Step Up

One of the basic needs of a pet bird owner is the ability to transport the bird upon the hand. In order for this to occur the bird must learn to easily step onto the proffered hand. This is where the "step up" command comes into play. The handler states "step up" and moves the hand toward the bird. The hand must be very steady and positioned in a way that it is easy for the bird to step up on it. If the bird is not schooled in this exercise, it may require some coaxing to get it up on the hand. Sometimes one foot can be lifted and placed up on the hand, which is then gently lifted up. The bird must then bring the other foot up on the hand. As this process is repeated, the bird learns to step readily onto the hand. Some birds resist stepping up, not because they do not know what is requested but because they wish to exert control over the situation. In these cases, the handler should "follow through" with the hand, sweeping past the bird if it should hesitate. The motion is neither violent nor hesitant. It simply shows that the handler expects the bird to step up right away. This is one of the areas where these classes are very helpful. The instructor can monitor the motions and mannerisms of the handler and offer constructive criticism and demonstrate proper technique. It is remarkable how differently the same bird responds to different handling techniques.

STEP DOWN

Just as important to the bird owner is the ability to get the bird to step off of the hand. This is where the step down command comes in. The hand that the bird is perched upon is brought adjacent to the perch. The term "step down" is spoken. The bird is then encouraged to step onto the perch. The author prefers to have the bird step backward onto the perch. This makes the motion different from the "step up" motion, avoiding confusion. If the bird does not step onto the perch, the hand is lowered below the level of the perch. If the hand is in front of the perch the tail will then bump the perch and most birds will step back onto the perch. If not, one foot can be gently placed on the perch, and the other will follow as the hand is lowered.

STAY

This command is essential if parrots are to be allowed substantial time with the "flock" or family. The bird is simply placed upon the perch and the term "stay" is spoken. The handler then moves a short distance from the bird. Many birds will posture at this point, indicating the desire to move off of the perch. At this point the "stay" command is repeated. If the bird leaves the perch, it is replaced and the process is repeated. Increasing distances and times are then used to teach the bird to stay upon a given site.

Hooding

Hooding is a term taken from the time-honored falconry technique of placing a leather cap or hood over the head of the bird to reduce its reaction to visual stimuli. Rather than placing a leather hood, in this case a hand is simply capped over the head to guard the bird from perceived threats. Many birds will tolerate this immediately, while others will require desensitization. Owners are told to proceed slowly to prevent making the bird more fearful.

Carrier

Placing a bird into a carrying cage is a common maintenance procedure. In some cases, however, it can be a traumatic event. The method combines the preceding techniques to put the bird easily into a front-loading pet carrier. The bird is stepped up onto one hand, the other hand is cupped over the head, and then the bird is placed

backward into the carrier. A "step down" and a "stay" command are given. When the bird steps down, the carrier can be closed.

Towel

Desensitizing pet birds to towels makes other common maintenance procedures less stressful. Clients are instructed to slowly accustom the bird to being touched with and eventually wrapped up in a towel. Again it is important to move slowly to prevent making the bird more fearful of towels.

Owners are instructed to practice these exercises for 15–20 minutes daily. The amount of time in the classes is insufficient for the birds to become proficient. The class time is really for instruction of the owners. Their handling techniques should be honed so that the home training is more effective.

BENEFITS OF THE BEHAVIOR CLASSES

The performance level of the birds in the class has been highly variable. Each bird, however, has shown improvement throughout the class. The birds coming in with the poorest behavior often show the most improvement. The owners generally feel closer to the bird and have a better understanding of the bird's needs. Several have repeated the class or had another family member go through the class.

The bird behavior class has been very well received by the public. About four sessions are run per year, and there has been no difficulty in filling these slots. There have been between four and ten members in each class. This class has been a tremendous positive public-relations builder. The author has improved his own exam room demeanor by a greater understanding of parrot behavior. A project with such positive aspects also gives the instructor a lift in attitude. Clients bond with their birds better as a result of the obedience classes. Better behavior on the part of the bird and a better understanding of parrot's behavior on the part of the owner keep the frustration of both to a minimum. Several owners have decided to keep their birds instead of selling or placing them. Several people have started to handle their birds much more since taking the obedience class. They have been able to establish dominance and now they can handle the bird without chasing it around or being bitten. When owners have to administer treatments to their birds, those that have been to the class are able to comply with treatments better than before. One client that went through the class had a conure that was very cage territorial and, whenever he was brought in for boarding, his cage would be very dirty. After the owners had taken the class, they kept the cage much cleaner than before and the bird was easier to care for in the hospital. Most of the birds that have been through obedience classes are much easier to handle for clinical examinations. The birds have been to the hospital without having unpleasant procedures, so they are not stressed by their mere presence there. The other reason is that one of the exercises in the class is to play with the bird using a towel. These birds often allow the towel to be placed over them without a struggle. Obedience classes can also become a practice profit center. The material costs of running the class, including perches, photocopying, and the videotape, are minimal. The only other cost is the time of the person teaching the class. In the author's practice it is the veterinarian that teaches the class; however, a well-trained and experienced technician could fill the instructor's role. More important than the revenues from the class itself is the fact that clients who take this class bond with the practice. They can see that their veterinarian is not just interested in money or in the medical aspects of birds. They can see that the bird's well-being is considered important. This is something they tell their friends and family .

REFERENCES

1. Neville, P.F. 1997. "Preventing problems via social and environmental enrichment." Proceedings North American Veterinary Conference, pp. 31–32.
2. Anderson, R.K. 1990. Preventing needless deaths of pets: Putting dogs on their best behavior. *Veterinary Forum*, April, pp. 32–33.
3. Wilson, L. 1996. "Non-medical approach to the behavioral feather plucker." Proc Annu Conf Assoc Avian Vet, pp. 3–9.
4. Voith, V.L., and P.L. Borchelt. 1985. Fears and phobias in companion animals. *Compend Cont Educ Pract Vet* 7 (3):209–218.
5. Evans, J.M. 1985. *The Evans guide for counseling dog owners.* New York: Howell Book House.
6. Harrison, G.J. 1994. "Perspective on parrot behavior." In *Avian medicine: Principles and applications,* ed. B.W. Ritchie, G.J. Harrison, and L.R. Harrison, pp. 96–108. Lake Worth, FL: Wingers Publishing Inc.
7. Lafeber, T.J. 1983. *Let's celebrate pet birds.* Odell, IL: Lafeber Co.
8. Ramey, K., N. Moore, and J.R. Millam. 1994. "Affiliative behavior in captive breeding amazons parrots." Proc Annu Conf Assoc Avian Vet, p. 434.
9. Jochim, L., and J.R. Millam. 1994. "Behavior of orange-winged amazon parrots before and after nest box presentation." Proc Annu Conf Assoc Avian Vet, p. 435.
10. Millam, J.R. 1994. "Environmental enrichment stimulates egg laying in naive orange-winged amazon parrots." Proc Annu Conf Assoc Avian Vet, p. 436.
11. Athan, M.S. 1993. *Guide to a well-behaved parrot.* Hong Kong: Barron's.
12. Davis, C. 1997. "Behavior." In *Avian medicine and surgery,* ed. R.B. Altman, S.L. Clubb, G.M. Dorrestein, and K. Quesenberry, pp. 96–100. Philadelphia: W.B. Saunders Company.
13. Smith, I.L. 1999. "Basic behavioral principles for the avian veterinarian." Proc Annu Conf Assoc Avian Vet, pp. 47–55.
14. Rach, J.A. 1998. *Why does my bird do that: A guide to parrot behavior.* New York: Howell Book House.
15. Friedman, S.G., and B. Brinker. 2000. Early socialization: A biological need and the key to companionability. *Original Flying Machine* 2:7–8.
16. Horwitz, D. 1999. "Playtime: How to have fun with your pet." Proc North Am Vet Conf, p. 31.
17. Athan, M.S. 1997. *Guide to the quaker parrot.* Hong Kong: Barron's.
18. Linden, P.G. 1999. "Deliberate behavioral development: Stages, principles, and applications." Proc Annu Conf Assoc Avian Vet, pp. 269–271.
19. Athan, M.S., and D. Deter D. 2000. *The African grey parrot handbook.* Hong Kong: Barron's.
20. Blanchard, S. 2000. Teaching your parrot self-soothing techniques. *Pet Bird Report* 9 (6):52–53.
21. Clark, P. 2000. The optimal environment: Part IV, the social climate. *Pet Bird Report* 9 (6):26–31.
22. Harris, J.M. 1997. "The human-avian bond." In *Avian medicine and surgery,* ed. R.B. Altman, S.L. Clubb, G.M. Dorrestein, and K. Quesenberry, pp. 995–998. Philadelphia: W.B. Saunders Company.
23. Wilson, L. 2000. "The one person bird-prevention and rehabilitation." Proc Annu Conf Assoc Avian Vet, pp. 69–73.
24. Case, L.P. 1994. "Motivation and reinforcement: The keys to solving behavior problems in dogs." Proceedings Eastern Illinois Veterinary Medical Association Spring Clinic, pp. 1–6.

16
Clinical Evaluation of Psittacine Behavioral Disorders

Kenneth R. Welle and Liz Wilson

ESTABLISHING THE CONSULTANT/CLIENT RELATIONSHIP

The most important facet to establishing a consultant/client relationship is to first create an open and honest rapport with the parrot owner. Without this connection, it will be exceedingly difficult for the behavior consultant or avian veterinarian to accurately access the situation, and without this, it will be extremely difficult to assist in improving the situation. Judgmental language must be avoided at all costs, as this type of approach will often encourage owners to be dishonest with the interviewer in hopes of avoiding a negative response. This author (Wilson) finds that recounting her own mistakes with psittacine behavior can encourage owners to relax and talk openly.

IS THERE REALLY A PROBLEM?

Once a rapport has been established, the consultant must assess whether or not a problem actually exists. People often want to train their parrots to *not be parrots*, such as wanting to teach them to be quiet all the time, not to be destructive, and not to be so untidy. Parrots are inherently loud, destructive, and messy creatures, and trying to change them into something else is an exercise in futility. The end result is likely to be the bird losing its home.

Problems that require intervention with a consultation would include management problems such as an inappropriate environment (i.e., a parrot living in a bar), or an inappropriate social climate (such as clients having combative relationships with others in the environment). Additionally, there are the problem behaviors themselves, such as self-inflicted damage (i.e., feather destruction, self-mutilation), excessive fear, aggressive behaviors, and excessive vocalizations.

LEVEL OF COOPERATION FROM OTHERS IN THE ENVIRONMENT

The next step would be to evaluate the amount of assistance the consultant can expect from the owners. Do all the people in the environment want to resolve the problem with the parrot, or would they prefer the bird be gone? While some problems, such as biting, can be resolved on a one-on-one basis, problems such as excessive screaming require the cooperation of everyone in the environment. If even one person rewards unacceptable behaviors (such as the husband who would give his wife's African Grey Parrot [*Psittacus erithacus*] a piece of cheese to shut it up), then no improvement will be realized. Odds increase exponentially for a successful denouement if consultations include all family members whenever possible, especially with excessive noise.

Many behaviors in pet parrots may not initially seem problematic to owners, until further ramifications develop. A good example of this is the *one-person bird*. Many people are tremendously flattered by a bird's exclusive affection, and actually relish this situation, often (passively or otherwise) allowing the bird's aggression toward others in the household. These people usually do not seek assistance with this type of situation until the bird manifests further evidence of these problem behaviors, such as with feather destruction. Some owners will blatantly encourage aggression toward others, for example, finding it amusing to watch a little bird chase their spouse, and many behavior consultants believe that human laughter is a powerful reinforcement for the companion parrot.

An extremely common underlying factor with problem behaviors in companion parrots is that of inappropriate bond formation, as in overdependencies and/or the formation of a "pair bond" or "mate bond" with an inappropriate species like a person. Unfortunately, much of the lay literature still encourages this, and most owners see nothing wrong with "being their bird's mate." At least they see nothing wrong until the confused and extremely frustrated parrot begins manifesting unacceptable behaviors such as feather destruction, excessive screaming, severe aggression, and, in some cases, even self-mutilation.

It is an unfortunate reality that many people do not wish for their baby parrots to mature. The concept of neoteny is a powerfully appealing one, and many owners try to maintain their relationships on the level of cuddling instead of allowing the bird to mature and grow into the entity nature designed it to be. These people apparently hope to maintain themselves as a "bird mommy" forever, and frequently comment that they "want their sweet baby back" when their parrots start to mature. However, this approach is guaranteed to lead to a dysfunctional relationship.

Fear can be a problem with companion parrots, whether the bird fears the person or vice versa. Like all companion animals, parrots will form different relationships with different people in their lives, and some relationships are more combative than others. While biting is a common problem with companion psittacids, it is often not difficult to resolve, depending on the etiology. However, it is not easy for people who are afraid of parrots to control their charges. Parrots will not be comfortable with people who are not comfortable with them, and it is difficult to train parrots to be tolerant of people who are awkward and ill at ease around them. As prey animals, it is logical that they cannot relax when humans, for example, offer a hand to step up and then jerk the hand away when parrots reach with their beaks to stabilize the perch.

Occasionally, one encounters clients who, despite problem behaviors with their parrots, are averse to the idea of modifying what they perceive as "natural" behaviors. These people are often under the mistaken impression that all psittacine behaviors are instinctual, which is far from the case. Like most intelligent animals, parrots have a tremendous capacity for learning and adapting their behavior in response to environmental input.[1] In the wild, other flock members educate these birds. In captivity, unless educated by the humans with whom they live, psittacine birds have no idea how to behave. As a result, they often develop displacement behaviors that humans find distasteful, such as excessive screaming, feather destruction, and aggression.

A frustrating reality is the owner who has, consciously or otherwise, already decided to give up a parrot prior to seeking assistance in behavior modification. In this situation, working with a behavior consultant and/or avian veterinarian has the only function of assuaging the owner's guilt by allowing him or her to believe that he or she has "tried everything." Not surprisingly, a behavior consultation will not change the outcome in this situation, as the odds are against the owner being sufficiently motivated to make the necessary changes to accomplish anything positive with the bird.

TAKING THE BEHAVIORAL HISTORY

Unlike with medical problems, there is no testing that one can do to assist in evaluating behavioral disease. As a consequence, the behavioral history and observation are the only diagnostic tools available for evaluation of behavioral disorders.[2] However, problems arise when trying to evaluate psittacine behavior when the animal is in a veterinary clinic exam room, as the strange surroundings can substantially modify the animal's behavior. The same is true, to a lesser degree, of the behavior consultant doing an in-home visit, and this can somewhat limit the value of direct observation. However, within those limitations much can be learned if the consultant is astute.

As with any properly done physical exam, the examiner needs to work with consistency and a standardized form. A sample form is included in Appendix 16A. This enables the examiner to collect data in a somewhat organized manner and decreases the odds of forgetting to ask an important question. Some consultants prefer to send clients a form to fill out prior to the first appointment. This can save a tremendous amount of time, which is its greatest advantage. This can also weed out those who are not sufficiently dedicated to follow through, thereby saving time and frustration for the consultant. However, much can be learned with spontaneous answers, especially when dealing with more than one person in the environment, as contradictions can be confusing but also extremely revealing. As a consequence, other consultants prefer to ask the questions, watch and/or listen carefully to the way questions are answered, and then transcribe the information. This method is extremely time-consuming but can be quite valuable, as the client's tone of voice and body language, if present, can be quite telling.

EVALUATING THE ENVIRONMENT

For evaluating a parrot's environment, photographs can be useful, but nothing surpasses actually being there and walking through the space. Consultants can also request a somewhat-to-scale sketched floor plan of the room or rooms in which a parrot spends time (M.S. Athan, personal communication, 1998), which will aid in visualization. Clients are requested to label windows, walls, skylights, doors, and the bird's cage, plus important pieces of furniture like the television, the sofa, and the client's favorite chair. Clients are also asked to use a dotted line to indicate the traffic flow through the room(s). For in-hospital consults, video tours are valuable. Watching the video with blueprint in hand can give an adequate impression of the space in which a parrot lives. In addition, when it comes to truly evaluating a parrot's environment and its interactions with the humans around it, this author (Wilson) has found the use of videotapes to be priceless.

GETTING HONEST ANSWERS

It is critical that the examiner get as much information as possible about a situation, and this is not always easy. Taking a good behavioral history is quite an art form, requiring tact and a delicate touch. The interviewer must avoid judgmental behavior totally, as an accusatory approach can induce some clients to lie to avoid condemnation. As with any history taking, the interviewer must also avoid the use of leading questions, as these can encourage some clients to give the interviewer what they think he or she wishes to hear, rather than the truth.

It may be useful to start an interview with a reminder that the value of the consult is dependent on the clients being willing to provide complete and honest answers, and that it is not the interviewer's job to judge—only to get as much information as possible to increase the likelihood of being able to help improve the situation.

If the examiner is sympathetic and non-accusatory, the likelihood increases that honest answers will result. For instance, in a situation where physical abuse was likely but unstated, a consultant might talk about how awful it is to be around, for example, a screaming parrot. By commenting that the gut-wrenching noise makes it hard not lose one's temper and throw something at a screaming parrot, the consultant might succeed in prompting the owner to admitting to having done just that.

OBSERVATION OF BEHAVIOR

Observation of the patient's behavior can be the most challenging part of behavior work. The difficulty is that the method used to observe the behavior can add artifacts to the observations. Location and the very presence of the observer may influence the bird's behavior. Observation in the veterinary examination room can reveal how a bird responds to a frightening situation. Birds that calmly preen their feathers while in the examination room are generally birds that tolerate change well and are not afraid of strangers. Aggressive birds may be much more docile away from their home territory and will often allow handling by people they will ordinarily bite severely. Observation of a bird in its home environment during a house call is somewhat better. Here the bird is in familiar territory and will have fewer distractions. This method also allows the consultant a first-hand view of the environment. The consultant, however, will influence the behavior to some extent. Most birds alter their behavior somewhat in the presence of unfamiliar people.

Video recording the bird's behavior may be the most effective means. Not only can the consultant view the interaction between bird and owner, but also the camera can be set up to record the behavior of the bird when the owner leaves the area. This can be extremely useful information. Animals with separation anxiety often exhibit signs of distress in the initial minutes following the exit of the owner. This is frequently observed in videos of pet birds.

Experience dictates the necessity of limiting the amount of tape a client sends, and clients are asked to send no more than two hours of tape, with the explanation that otherwise, there won't be time to watch it all, so something important might be missed. The following is part of the information this author (Wilson) sends to prospective phone clients regarding what to film:

One of the primary purposes of the film is so I can watch a parrot's body language, so try to avoid things like filming your parrot against a sunny window during the day, etc. Telephotos are ideal, because then I can see the bird more clearly without your having to stick the camera in its face. If you can't film in ideal circumstances, then just do the best you can. Whatever you send will be better than nothing. Just remember that the better I can see the bird, the better I might be able to understand what is going on with it.

Also, film your parrot's body language as it interacts with you in a variety of circumstances (i.e., eating, playing, snuggling, etc.). Do the same with anyone else who routinely interacts with the bird. Film the bird's body language when it is hanging out in the cage (i.e., eating, playing, etc.), both when you are in the room and when you are not. This part will require a tripod so the camera can run without you. Film the bird's body language as you interact with other family members.

Lastly, please film the view that the bird can see from its cage, panning slowly around the room. Be sure to set up the camera two to three days prior to filming, so the bird will get accustomed to its presence. This is extremely important because otherwise the parrot won't relax and act normally.

The following case illustrates the value of evaluating videotapes. A client thought his three-year-old female African Grey was screaming when he left the room as a manifestation of a control issue, and from what the client described, the consultant (Wilson) agreed. As requested, the client filmed his interactions with the Grey and then left the camera running after he left the room. The client had watched the tape prior to sending it but did not see anything that changed his interpretation of the bird's behavior. However, this author (Wilson) saw something totally different when she reviewed the tape. Instead of showing irritation at the human ignoring its calls, the young Grey was panicking, chewing on her nails and flipping her wings, which this author feels can be evidence of stress in a Grey. So instead of a control issue, this bird was apparently suffering from a psittacine form of separation anxiety. If the author had based her recommendations solely on the client's interpretation of the situation, then she would have given incorrect information as to how to resolve the conflict.

OWNER'S BEHAVIOR

It is very important for the consultant to make observations of the owner's behavior as well. Very often, it is not the bird that is behaving poorly. Some owners simply do not know how to handle their bird properly. Simple adjustments in the manner used by the owner can immediately solve some problems. Owners that continually make excuses for the behavior of the bird or who make unreasonable concessions to avoid being attacked may be the cause of aggression in a bird. When the bird sees that biting effectively controls the owner, the biting is reinforced. It is often startling what owners think is reasonable. One of the authors (Welle) has had clients who admitted to taking all phone calls in the garage to avoid being bitten, or others who rolled on the floor to get a bird off of the shoulder.

EVALUATING THE DATA

Once the data has been collected, it should be carefully evaluated for information that may lead to a clinically relevant conclusion. Veterinary behavior as a clinical science is still in its infancy. This is particularly true with respect to pet birds. The etiologies of behavioral disorders, the minimum standards for the care of companion psittacine birds, and the reference values for the "normal" responses of parrots to various situations have not been established. These facts can make the interpretation of the behavior history difficult. Nonetheless, trends can sometimes be identified. Associations between anamnestic factors and certain behavioral traits sometimes can be made. This is the means by which clinical sciences develop. More importantly, evaluation of the history allows a customized plan of environmental and behavioral modification to be formulated for the patient at hand.

SIGNALMENT

Signalment is as important in behavior as in other medical fields. Species, age, and gender can give clues to the type of problem that may be present. Parrots that mature rapidly (e.g., Budgerigars, Cockatiels) are somewhat less likely to develop certain behavioral traits than those that mature very slowly (e.g., large cockatoos, macaws). These smaller, rapidly developing species must learn maintenance and social behaviors in a fairly short period of time and therefore lack the extreme flexibility of learning that slow-developing species possess. The slightly more rigid learning pattern prevents the development of some undesirable traits. Some species such as cockatoos tend to bond by means of physical touch, allopreening, and other contact, while others, such as amazon parrots, tend to use vocalization, visual display, and other means to bond. These tendencies will attract different types of owners and will often lead to different types of behavior. Many species are genetically identical to the wild counterparts while a few (Budgerigars, Cockatiels, Peach-faced Lovebirds) are truly domesticated. Some species appear to be more prone to develop aggression; others are more prone to anxiety or fear. Not all of these traits are genetically determined, and it is important not to automatically label a problem based solely on the species, but the species can give a clue to the likely source of a behavioral disorder.

The age of the bird is also important. Some behaviors may be normal phases of development in a young bird but are not normal later in life. Many parrots will go through a phase of regurgitation as the crop shrinks during weaning. Begging behaviors are normal in nestling and fledgling birds but should diminish as they mature. Many behavioral traits are blamed on reproductive hormones. Before making any such claim, it must be determined whether the patient has reached sexual puberty. For small psittacine birds, this will occur before they reach a year of age, while in medium to large parrots, reproductive hormones are not a significant factor until they reach two to four years or more in age. Likewise, behavior problems are not likely to be primarily of sex hormone origin if they begin many years after the bird has been sexually mature.

The gender of many psittacine patients is not known. While in some instances it may have little relevance, some behaviors will be very dependent on the sex of the bird. The sex of the bird should be determined when reproductive influence is suspected. During breeding season, wild male parrots will generally find and guard a nest site. For a pet bird this natural trait may lead to territorial aggression.

DEVELOPMENT

More important than signalment is the background of the bird. Parrots are altricial birds, completely helpless at hatching. Their behavior patterns are very open at this point and the period between hatching and independence is critical. Early development may affect a bird's confidence and sense of security. It can determine a parrot's intelligence, flexibility, and potential as a companion animal. During its time with parents, a wild baby parrot learns what to eat, what to fear, how to travel, and how to interact with other flock members. The same is true in domestic-bred companion parrots, except that in many cases the bird has human surrogate parents (see chapter 11).

Hand-rearing baby parrots has long been used both as a means of increasing production of chicks and as a means of raising psittacine birds with little fear of humans. While the techniques for hand-rearing physically healthy psittacids has been evolving for a long time, the process of socializing and educating these birds has often been ignored. It is evident that hand-rearing of parrots alone does not prevent fear of humans. Juvenile birds must be socialized rather than assembly-line fed. Psittacine birds that are raised with no clutchmates and receive minimal physical contact with the caretaker will not often develop into well-adjusted pets. These birds may not learn to socialize with other birds or with humans. Many will not learn to play or explore their environment. Any synapses that are not stimulated by early sensory experiences may be "pruned" by the brain and eliminated.[3] Many of these birds imprint on humans as both parents and potential mates, which can lead to many problems in older parrots. As stated by Harrison in *Avian Medicine: Principles and Applications,* "Birds raised by human foster parents will imprint as people, not birds. As they mature, their natural instincts to choose a mate may cause objectionable behaviors. . . . An imprinted bird will spend all of its time attempting to drive unwanted individuals, other pets or objects out of its territory, while trying to find one chosen person with whom to mate."[4] This species confusion is compounded when the human caretaker fails to continue the bird's education to include necessary skills for coping with the artificial environment. Psittacine birds that are hand-reared and that are not sufficiently socialized with other conspecifics may have difficulty in relating to other parrots in avicultural settings.[5]

In contrast, parent-raised psittacids that do not receive any human contact until after they leave the nest box are little different from a wild-caught fledgling in behavior. They have no previous experience with humans and will learn how to react by watching and emulating their parents. If the parent birds have remained tame pets, the offspring will often tame easily after fledging. Many breeding birds, however, are either untamed or have become aggressive or indifferent to humans during the breeding cycle, and their offspring will be much more difficult to tame. Perhaps an ideal situation is for baby birds to be raised by parents but handled regularly by humans prior to fledging. While this may seem like a simple solution, it may be difficult to accomplish. Some breeders may abandon the nest if they are disturbed excessively, some may injure or kill their offspring in their attempts to guard the nest box, and some may severely injure the person attempting to invade the nest. Some situations in a bird's history may predispose it to anxiety or insecurity. Psittacine birds that are weaned too early, forced to wean before they are ready, or sold unweaned to inexperienced handlers may have a difficult time trusting humans. Pet parrots are often sold at very young ages under the pretense of forming a "stronger bond" to the new owner. These birds have already been removed from the natural parents, and then before they even have a chance to finish growing, they are taken away from their new "parents." It does not take these birds long to figure out this pattern.

GROOMING

Veterinarians or other groomers of pet birds can cause substantial problems. Unfortunately, many feel that a wing trim, nail trim, or beak trim is an innocuous procedure and will perform it without instruction on technique or case selection.[6] Improperly performed these methods can lead to long-term problems. First, the trauma of a painful nail trim or beak trim can make even a hand-raised baby bird fearful of people. Secondly, a severe wing or nail trim can affect the balance and coordination of the bird. Likewise, single wing trims will unbalance a bird. Some birds fall frequently, leading to more fear and pain. When excessive numbers of feathers are cut, the new feathers that come in have no protection and therefore are prone to damage. A vicious cycle ensues, with terrified birds becoming fearful of any human contact because they are afraid of falling and injury. Finally, flight is a learned skill and can lead to a greater sense of confidence, and even intelligence.[7] Trimming the wings, especially very early, can deprive birds of this necessary development.

Routine flight feather and nail clipping are necessary for most companion parrots, but the overly aggressive handling and grooming of the past have been dramatically modified in the last few years, with more humane methods replacing these potentially destructive, outdated techniques.

The technique of swooping down from behind to capture a parrot in a towel is no longer required. This technique, aptly named the "Harpy Eagle Catch" by Blanchard, was developed when captive parrots were all wild-caught imports.[8] With hysterically terrified untamed birds, speed was at a premium and it was critical to get the parrots under control quickly, before they could injure themselves or their handlers. However, most parrots in the United States today are domestically raised and do not perceive humans as deadly predators. Hence, the Harpy Eagle Catch is not only unnecessary, it can be seriously damaging. Speer states that "The Harpy Eagle grab causes fear-induced behavioral disease".[9]

Thanks to Blanchard's work, one of the authors (Wilson) has developed what she calls the "Frontal Towel Approach." This approach does not use a predatory attack to get control of a parrot, so it is substantially less stressful for the bird. The eyes of prey animals like psittacine birds are located on the lateral aspect of the skull, so their peripheral vision warns them of a forthcoming predatory attack. Seeing the towel coming with the Harpy Eagle Catch appears to throw a bird into a full fight or flight response as it is captured.

Once this systemic response is initiated, the bird will frantically struggle to escape what it likely perceives as a deadly situation.

The Frontal Towel Approach does not initiate this terrified reaction. To place a tame parrot under restraint using this method, the handler does the following. Talking quietly to the bird (instead of the owner), the patient is stepped onto a hand, and the bird's feet are gently but firmly pinned by the handler's fingers (Figure 16.1). Continuing to talk softly and keeping the towel low, the handler catches one corner of the towel in the fingers of the hand on which the bird is sitting (Figure 16.2), then smoothly brings the towel up and around behind the bird (Figure 16.3), and lowers it over the bird's head (Figure 16.4). The animal is then gently put under restraint (Figure 16.5). If the handler moves smoothly from the pinning of the feet to the towel's approach, this author (Wilson) has found that parrots pay little or no mind to their feet being pinned, as the towel's approach consumes their attention.

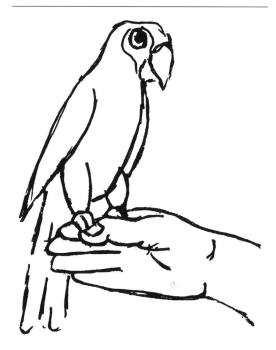

Figure 16.2. The parrot's foot is gently but firmly pinned with the thumb while the handler continues to talk softly and smile.

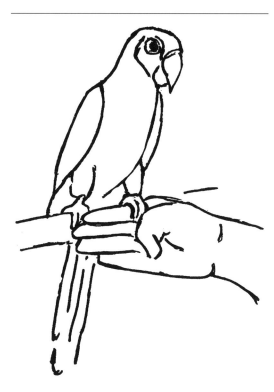

Figure 16.1. The parrot is stepped onto the hand and the handler greets the bird in a friendly manner.

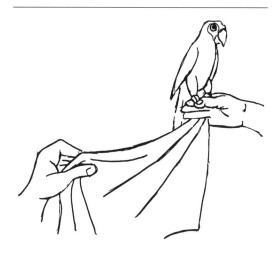

Figure 16.3. The handler catches one corner of the towel between the fingers of the hand on which the bird is sitting. Friendly talk and smiles continue.

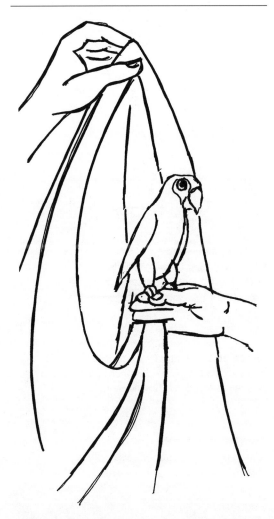

Figure 16.4. Continuing to talk calmly with a friendly facial expression, the handler then uses the other hand to slowly and smoothly bring the other end of the towel up . . .

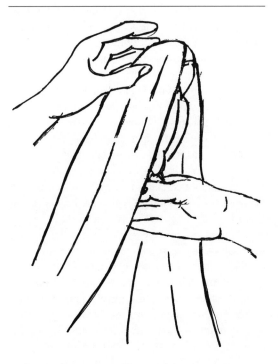

Figure 16.5. And the parrot's head is gently covered. Full restraint can now commence.

Even a parrot that is terrified of towels can generally be captured utilizing this technique. A frightened bird tends to flip backward from the hand as the towel approaches, but since the handler has the feet pinned, it cannot fall or escape. The towel is then wrapped around the upside-down bird, it is lowered to the table, and restraint is commenced as usual. While this approach is unquestionably more stressful than the previous one, the bird will still relax faster than it would with a predatory capture. Since avian veterinarians have been discussing the dangers of stress for decades, it seems reasonable to make every effort to avoid stressing the avian patient more than necessary.

Important note: There is danger of iatrogenic fractures when small birds like Budgerigars (*Melopsittacus undulatus*) and Cockatiels (*Nymphicus hollandicus*) flip backward. In situations such as those, this author (Wilson) immediately releases the feet so the bird escapes. Due to this potential, the toweling of small birds is often better accomplished via the old style grab from behind.

For that very reason, many educated bird owners have patterned their birds to be unafraid of being wrapped in towels. In the veterinary exam room, these owners will wish to towel their birds themselves, and then hand the towel-wrapped parrot to the veterinarian or veterinary technician. They will be justifiably disgruntled if a clinician chooses instead to undo this training with a predatory grab. If the veterinarian is not comfortable having the owner wrap the bird in this manner, then the veterinarian or technician can accomplish the towel wrap in the same friendly, non-aggressive manner.

It should be noted that, as with any restraint technique, practice is necessary for personnel to learn how to accomplish this maneuver confidently and smoothly. New handling techniques should *never* be attempted with compromised patients. Many hospitals have organized handling workshops for their personnel to develop confidence and proficiency with this capture method using their own pet birds prior to trying it with clients' birds.

As far as this author (Wilson) is concerned, it is absolutely unnecessary for tame birds to be grabbed from behind or by first darkening the room. This author has been using this frontal approach for over a decade and has yet to be bitten using it. More importantly, most parrots seem dramatically less stressed by restraint when captured in this manner.

PRIOR ENVIRONMENTS

Very often, birds that are presented for behavior problems are no longer with the family that originally purchased them. It is very common for a new person to adopt such a troubled bird assuming the problems must be due to abuse or neglect. While it is true that prior owners and environment may have caused or contributed to the current problem, it is not always due to a lack of trying. When the problem began before the current owner took possession of the bird, it is much more difficult to evaluate the root causes of the disorder. Sometimes the information regarding the previous home is available, but is often given in a somewhat slanderous fashion. The consultant should draw his or her own conclusions about the prior situation rather than taking the new owner's word that it was abusive. Parrots are social animals and need interaction with other birds or with humans. Often, due to fear, lack of time, or other factors, these needs are neglected. In rarer cases, teasing or even physical abuse may occur. These situations will very often have severe effects on the behavior of the patient, with manifestations often depending on the personality of the bird. Some may become aggressive, others fearful.

Just as common as neglect or abuse are situations where overbonding or pair bonding with the previous owner has occurred. This is particularly true with cockatoos, since people buy these birds because they love to cuddle. They therefore indulge in cuddling and petting at the expense of more active and independent play. The end result is a bird that pair bonds to a human, expecting constant and exclusive contact. When the person cannot meet these expectations, problems arise. When the new client adopts this bird, thinking the problem was due to a lack of attention, the cycle starts all over.

PHYSICAL ENVIRONMENT

An important part of the behavior consult is the evaluation of the physical environment of parrots. Factors that must be evaluated include size, construction, and cleanliness of the cage. Most birds spend the majority of their time caged and poor conditions can be extremely stressful. The location and surroundings of the cage can be critical as well. Some common household objects or sounds may be perceived as threatening to a bird. As prey species, parrots are naturally suspicious. Things that look completely innocuous to humans, such as clocks, portraits, or animal pictures, may cause anxiety in predisposed birds. Very loud noises are stressful to some birds, but total silence may encourage more severe reactions to normal household noises. Children and other pets can be very threatening to a bird. Erratic movements, staring, predatory tendencies, or just a lack of respect for personal space present not only a perception of threat but also potentially a real danger. Lack of any visual stimuli may lead to boredom and inflexibility. Cigarette smoke or other air quality issues can also result in stresses as well as causing health problems. Some areas may not allow a bird to "let down its guard." Cages that are placed in the center of a room force a bird to watch for danger in every direction. The same applies if the cage is placed against a large picture window or glass doors. If a doorway is on the same wall as the cage, surprise entry into the room can startle a nervous bird. These findings can add supportive evidence for anxiety-related behavior problems.

Birds that are isolated from all family activities will not develop normal social behaviors. If birds spend all of their time in one spot they tend to be easily stressed by changes. These birds may also be more likely to become territorial of their cage.[10] Conversely, if time is spent in various other locations, the bird may be more flexible. Perches or play gyms in an area of high activity can suggest that the bird has more casual socialization and sensory variation. Sleep cages in a separate room ensure sufficient dark and quiet for sleeping. Some birds commute regularly outside of the home. Traveling can also provide stimulation but can be stressful as well. The conditions under which the patient travels and the personality of the individual bird should be taken into account.

SCHEDULE

Most parrots are tropical or subtropical, where days are divided into 12 hours of light and another 12 hours of darkness. Birds getting less than eight to ten hours in a dark, quiet room are often stressed by sleep deprivation. Owners that simply cover the cage and yet continue to watch television in the room are deluding themselves into thinking that the bird is really sleeping.[11]

TOYS

There are several basic types of toys. Foot toys are those that are manipulated by the bird's feet; chewing toys are those that birds destroy or manipulate with the beak; climbing toys are those that the bird climbs, hangs, or swings upon; puzzle toys are those that require a bird to analyze, solve, and complete a task to receive a reward.[12] Some toys can serve as more than one toy type. Ideally, at least one of each type should be available to birds all of the time. When evaluating toys available to a patient, the type of toy, its size, construction materials, and suitability should be considered. Some toys intended as chew toys are too difficult for the bird to destroy, making it relatively uninteresting. The toys should match the size and preferences of the bird. Also important is the frequency with which the toys are changed. A playful bird will easily become bored with the same toys constantly available. Birds vary in their enthusiasm regarding toys. Birds that do not play with any toys may have never learned to play with toys. These birds are often more "dependent" on the owners.

SOCIAL ENVIRONMENT

Social interactions should be evaluated as well. Birds that have interactions primarily with one person will often become "one person" birds and are more likely to pair bond with this individual. Birds that interact with several people are less likely to do so. These birds are often much more independent. Nervous or anxious parrots and those pair bonded to owners often tolerate "alone time" poorly. This separation anxiety can lead to excessive vocalization or feather picking.

BEHAVIOR DESCRIPTION AND OBSERVATION

Finally, the owner's description of the behavior of the bird should be evaluated. These descriptions may be tainted by the owner's interpretation of the behavior, so it is important to emphasize to the owner that raw observations are what is desired. The overall behavior should be described in addition to any behavioral problems. The way in which the bird responds to various household members as well as to strangers, new situations, and other stimuli can give a great deal of information about the personality type of the bird and the possible motivation for various behaviors. Birds that are indifferent or frightened of people are unlikely to be using behaviors as a means of attracting attention. Likewise those that exhibit strong positive responses to all household members are unlikely to be trying to avoid attention. Birds with positive responses to some household members while they have negative responses to others may be overly dependent on one person. Birds that respond negatively to new people, places, or toys are often in a near-constant state of stress. The presence of certain sexual behaviors, such as regurgitation, masturbation, or nest building, can support a theory of a reproduction-associated problem.

A description of the problem behaviors and the circumstances in which they occur is very important since many behaviors occur only at certain times or in certain situations. From a description of the trigger, the behavior, and the consequences of the behavior, the consultant must determine what is actually occurring. This may be very simple in some cases, but can be very difficult in other situations. Owners often lack the ability to accurately describe a behavior. Occasionally a parrot will be presented to a veterinarian because of seizures when actually the "fits" are masturbation. Some types of behavior, such as regurgitation, can be normal in some circumstances but abnormal in others. It is important to get as many details about the behavior as possible. In addition, the frequency, the severity, and the timing should be recorded. Association with certain times or situations may give a clue as to cause, but it also helps to document these factors so that progress of treatment plans can be evaluated.

The owner's response to the behavior should be documented as well. In some cases the reactions may be reinforcing the behavior the owner wishes to eliminate. Reinforcement can come in many forms, some of which do not match the motivation the bird had for initiating the behavior. Food, drama, attention, or sometimes avoidance can be reinforcement in various situations.

More specific information to evaluate for specific behaviors can help narrow down the problem as well. For instance, with feather-destructive parrots, it is important to find out what parts of the body are affected, whether the bird picks when alone or when around people, whether other activities are interrupted while picking, and whether the picking seems to cause pain. This data can be critical when trying to diagnose the problem. A bird that only picks when alone may suffer from separation anxiety; a bird that interrupts other activities may have a true skin disorder that itches. These distinctions can help narrow down the hundreds of possible causes of a complicated problem.

DRAWING CONCLUSIONS

When all of the data has been evaluated, some conclusions must finally be drawn. Behavior is not an exact science and no two patients are exactly alike. Each diagnosis should be considered a theory. The validity of the theory can be tested by correcting the likely etiologic factors, applying behavior modification, and, in some cases, through the use of pharmaceutical therapy.

FOLLOW-UP

The evaluation does not end here. Follow-up to the problem is critical. Owners should be asked to start a journal of the bird's behavior. The frequency, severity, and timing of the episodes of undesirable behavior should be tracked. Any corresponding factors that are recognized should be tracked as well. This journal can have several benefits. The first is that the effectiveness of treatment can be documented. Most behavior prob-

lems that are successfully treated do not simply stop one day. They gradually attenuate in frequency and severity over time. If there is no record, owners may become discouraged and fail to comply with recommendations for sufficient time to resolve the behavior issues. The second benefit is that the additional data determined by the record keeping may add information that can help further define the problem.

REFERENCES

1. Welle, K.R. 2002. "Psittacine social structure: Applications to companion birds." Proc Annu Conf Assoc Avian Vet Specialty program.
2. Overall, K. 1997. *Clinical behavioral medicine for small animals.* Saint Louis: Mosby-Year Book, Inc., pp. 77–87.
3. Friedman, S.G., and B. Brinker. 2000. Early socialization: A biological need and the key to companionability. *Original Flying Machine* 2:7–8.
4. Harrison, G.J. 1994. "Perspective on parrot behavior." In *Avian medicine: Principles and application,* ed. B.W. Ritchie, G.J. Harrison, and L.R. Harrison, pp. 96–108.Lake Worth FL: Wingers Publishing Inc.
5. Styles, D.K. 2002. "Captive psittacine behavioral reproductive husbandry and management: Socialization, aggression control, and pairing techniques." Proc Annu Conf Assoc Avian Vet Specialty program.
6. Speer, B.L. 2001. "The clinical consequences of routine grooming procedures." Proc Annu Conf Assoc Avian Vet, Orlando, FL, August 22–24, pp. 109–115.
7. Linden, P.G. 1998. "Behavioral development of the companion psittacine bird." Proc Annu Conf Assoc Avian Vet, pp. 139–143.
8. Blanchard, S. 1994. Trust building towel handling techniques. *Pet Bird Report* 14:36–37.
9. Speer, B.L. 2001. "The clinical consequences of routine grooming procedures." Proc Annu Conf Assoc Avian Vet, Orlando, FL, August 22–24, pp. 109–115.
10. Blanchard, S. 1990. Phobic parrots. *Bird Talk Magazine* 90/8 (8):64–73
11. Athan, M.S. 1993. *Guide to a well behaved parrot.* Hong Kong: Barron's.
12. Wilson, L. 1996. "Non-medical approach to the behavioral feather plucker." Proc Annu Conf Assoc Avian Vet, pp. 3–11.

Appendix 16

Behavior History Form

Owner_____ Bird's name _____

Address_____ Species_____

Phone _____ Age_____

Work_____ Sex _____

FAX _____ Determined _____

E-mail_____ Color _____

Please check which of the options below that you would prefer.

☐ I would like to proceed with the behavior consultation and I agree to the fee of _____.

☐ I do not wish to proceed with the consultation but retain this for my bird's medical record.

☐ House call ☐ In-clinic visit ☐ Phone consult ☐ Video included

Medical and Grooming Information

My bird: *has / has not* been examined by my veterinarian in the past 6 months.

My bird: *has / has not* been examined by my veterinarian for this problem.

Have your veterinarian send a copy of your bird's medical record if he/she is not one of our patients.

My bird's wings are: ☐ *fully flighted* ☐ *clipped*

First wing trim was done: ☐ *before weaned* ☐ *after weaned* ☐ *when mature*

Wing trim style:

Wing trim is: ☐ *one side* ☐ *both sides*

Bird Source

I got my bird from: ☐ *a pet store* ☐ *a breeder* ☐ *a show* ☐ *shipped*

My bird was: ☐ *wild-caught* ☐ *domestic parent-raised* ☐ *hand-raised*

When I took my bird home, he/she was: ☐ *still being hand-fed* ☐ *just weaned*
☐ *weaned a while but sexually immature* ☐ *sexually mature*

If you hand-fed this bird, did you: ☐ *allow to wean on his/her own* ☐ *force weaning*
☐ *continue hand-feeding beyond six months of age*

Other than the breeder or pet store, my bird has had: ☐ *0* ☐ *1* ☐ *2* ☐ *several* previous owners

Prior to bringing my bird home I: ☐ *never* ☐ *occasionally* ☐ *frequently* visited him/her.

Environment

Describe the bird's cage. Give brand name, size, etc. _____

_____

_____

_____

_____

List all furnishings and contents of the cage. _____

_____

_____

_____

_____

How many hours per day does your bird spend in the cage?_____

_____

_____

_____

_____

Describe other areas where your bird spends time. _____

_____

_____

_____

_____

How much time is spent here? _____

_____

_____

_____

_____

List toys your bird has access to. _____

_____

_____

_____

_____

Draw a map of your house and put in the bird's cage and play area, as well as areas where family members spend time.

Sit or stand at bird height in the location of the cage. Describe everything you see and hear in all directions, including up and down. If you can photograph or video record this, much more information can be determined.

_____
_____
_____
_____

How many hours per day is your bird alone? _____

What sights, sounds, and other stimuli are available to your bird while you are gone? _____

_____
_____
_____
_____

When are the lights in the bird's area turned off at night?_____

_____
_____
_____
_____

When does light first come in the morning? _____

_____
_____
_____
_____
_____

Would you consider the light intensity: ☐ *bright*   ☐ *dim*   ☐ *moderate*

What types of lights are used in the area where the bird is kept? _____

_____
_____

Describe your bird's diet in detail. Give brands of pellets. Describe your bird's preferences._____

_____
_____
_____
_____

What is your bird's feeding schedule? _____

_____
_____
_____
_____

What are your bird's favorite treats? _____

_____
_____
_____
_____
_____

Are there any smokers in the household? _____

Do they smoke around the bird? _____

Are there any other sources of odors or fumes in the household?_____

_____

_____

_____

_____

How often and in what way is your bird bathed?_____

_____

_____

_____

_____

Do you dry the bird following a bath? How?_____

_____

_____

_____

_____

Your Bird's Flock

List all human members of the household. _____

_____

_____

_____

_____

List all of the animal members of the household. _____

_____

_____

_____

_____

List the ages of children within the household. _____

_____

_____

_____

_____

Who does the primary maintenance of the bird?_____

_____

_____

_____

_____

Who spends the most time with the bird? _____

_____

_____

_____

_____

Who does the bird appear to prefer? _____

_____

_____

_____

_____

Who does the bird appear to dislike?_____

_____

_____

_____

_____

Bird's Behavior

Would you say that your bird steps on your hand: ☐ *easily*   ☐ *hesitantly*   ☐ *rarely*

Is your bird allowed on your shoulder: ☐ *often*   ☐ *occasionally*   ☐ *rarely*   ☐ *never*

How does your bird greet you when you come home? _____

_____

_____

_____

_____

How does your bird greet other family members?_____

_____

_____

_____

_____

Describe your bird's play behavior. _____

_____

_____

_____

_____

Does your bird talk? ☐ *Yes*   ☐ *No*

Vocabulary: ☐ *<10 words*   ☐ *10–30 words*   ☐ *>30 words*

Does your bird use words appropriately? ☐ *Yes*   ☐ *No*

Does your bird like to be petted: ☐ *on the head*   ☐ *on the back*   ☐ *over the tail*

☐ *under wings*   ☐ *other* _____

When out of the cage, is your bird in physical contact with someone:

☐ *constantly*   ☐ *intermittently*   ☐ *rarely*   ☐ *never*

How well does your bird tolerate restraint?

☐ *doesn't mind at all*   ☐ *doesn't like it but tolerates it*   ☐ *gets very stressed*

How does your bird respond to the following situations:

Response	anxiety	fear	calm	happy	excited	aggressive	can't tell
Favorite approaching:							
Other approaching:							
Stranger approaching:							
Favorite opens cage:							
Other opens cage:							
Stranger opens cage:							
Favorite hand in cage:							
Other hand in cage:							
Stranger hand in cage:							
Favorite step up:							
Other step up:							
Stranger step up:							
Favorite petting/touching:							
Other petting/touching:							
Stranger petting/touching:							
Favorite hands food:							
Other hands food:							
Stranger hands food:							
Other approaching favorite:							
Favorite approaching other:							
Stranger approaching favorite:							
Favorite approaching stranger:							
Stranger approaching other:							
Other approaching stranger:							
Favorite to other transfer:							
Other to favorite transfer:							
Favorite to stranger transfer:							
Stranger to favorite transfer:							
Other animal approaches:							
Favorite out of vision:							
Other out of vision:							
Loud noises:							
New objects out of cage:							
New object in cage:							
Strange places:							

Does your bird exhibit any of the following sexual behaviors:

☐ *Regurgitation*   ☐ *Masturbation*   ☐ *Panting when petted*

☐ *Nesting*   ☐ *Egg laying*   ☐ *Aggression*

Specifically describe the situations in which these behaviors occur. _____

_____

_____

_____

_____

_____

Which behavior problems does your bird exhibit? Check all that apply.

☐ *Biting*   ☐ *Screaming*   ☐ *Feather plucking/ chewing*

☐ *Self-mutilation* ☐ *Irrational fears* ☐ *Other* _____

Describe these behaviors. _____

_____

_____

Specifically describe the situations in which these behaviors occur. _____

_____

_____

_____

Describe what you do when these behaviors occur. _____

_____

_____

_____

_____

For feather plucking, chewing, or self-mutilation, answer these questions.

What parts of the body are affected? _____

_____

_____

_____

_____

_____

DORSAL   VENTRAL

Draw where damage has occurred.

Are feathers pulled or damaged: (Check all that apply)

☐ *when they first appear?*   ☐ *when they start to open up?*

☐ *when they are mature?*   ☐ *when you're not home?*

☐ *when you're not paying attention?*   ☐ *when you're paying attention?*

Are the feathers: (Check all that apply)

☐ *pulled out at the root?*   ☐ *chewed in half?*

☐ *chewed/stripped lengthwise?*   ☐ *scratched with the feet?*

☐ *Have you seen bleeding?*   ☐ *Is the skin damaged?*

Does behavior interrupt:

☐ *playing?*   ☐ *eating?*   ☐ *other activities?*

This behavior can be interrupted by:

☐ *attention?*   ☐ *reprimand?*   ☐ *food?*

When this behavior occurs:

☐ *bird acts like it hurts?*   ☐ *bird acts like it itches?*   ☐ *bird acts like it doesn't bother him/her?*

Severity

☐ *Severe (most of bird devoid of feathers)*

☐ *Moderate (patchy distribution, may leave down alone)*

☐ *Mild (focal areas, most feathers intact)*

☐ *Questionable (unsure whether bird is really picking)*

Problem has occurred in: (Check all that apply) ☐ *winter*   ☐ *spring*   ☐ *summer*   ☐ *fall*

Problem appears worst in: ☐ *winter*   ☐ *spring*   ☐ *summer*   ☐ *fall*

17
Diagnostic Workup of Suspected Behavioral Problems

Susan E. Orosz

This chapter will focus on the diagnostic workup of two behavioral problems commonly encountered in avian practice, feather-damaging behavior and aggression.

FEATHER-DAMAGING BEHAVIOR

"Feather-damaging behavior" (FDB) is a term that describes those conditions where the companion bird plucks out, destroys, or barbers its own feathers (B. Speer, oral communication, Feb. 2003). It is often referred to as feather picking, but picking may be only a component to the entire process, so FDB is a more inclusive term. However, FDB represents a symptom and is not a diagnosis for a disease process even though it is often described in that manner. The term "FDB" should be used separately from the term "self-mutilation," as this condition represents self-destruction of at least the surface of the skin. Both conditions—FDB and self-mutilation—are often used as a diagnosis even though the true underlying cause and the diagnosis are obscure.

AGGRESSION

Aggression is often described in humans as a disturbed or psychological state, but in most animals it tends to be species-specific behavior that confers survival benefits to the individual or social group.[1] In a natural setting, the aggressive act is employed to protect valuable resources or as a self-defensive measure. Aggression would be involved in maintaining the integrity of a social group or acting to repel possible intruders. Aggression can be subdivided into a number of categories. According to Welle, in birds these cat-

egories would include fear aggression, possessive aggression, protective aggression, and territorial aggression.[2] Others have different classification schemes. For example, fear, pain, and stress-induced aggression can be considered defensive forms of aggression.[1] From the owner's perspective, the aggression takes the form of biting, as that is often why the owner brings the bird in for evaluation or considers sending the bird away to a sanctuary.

Fear aggression can be defined as aggression with signs of fear associated with withdrawal or passive and/or avoidance behaviors.[2] These are the birds that, when you approach, will bite when cornered and then retreat as quickly as possible. Protective aggression is aggression that is directed toward another person who approaches an object or, more commonly, a person the aggressor wishes to control.[2] In the natural setting this would be the male amazon that defends its mate when another male approaches. This scenario is commonly expressed by a client that tells you that the bird "always bites my husband when he approaches me, Doc." Protective aggression is consistently directed to a third party in the presence of a certain individual without an actual threat.[2] Territorial aggression is aggression that occurs in a defined area like a cage. It often intensifies as the recipient approaches and continues despite correction or attempt at interaction with the bird.[2] The most common example is when the bird is asked to step on the hand to get out of the cage, then the bird bites the hand—this is often described as cage aggression.

DIAGNOSIS OF FDB AND AGGRESSION

The diagnostic workup of FDB and aggression requires a thorough history and clinical examination. In human medicine, the history and physical examination represent approximately 80% of the information required to arrive at the diagnosis of the patient.[3]

The diagnostic tests ordered by the physician are used to rule in or out the working diagnosis or the differential diagnoses based on the findings derived from the history and the physical examination. In determining a behavioral diagnosis, the same criteria are required—a thorough history and examination. However, the examination is divided into two components, so it is more appropriate to describe it as a clinical examination. The clinical examination is divided into a physical examination and a behavioral examination.

The History

History taking is described in another chapter (chapter 16) but is mentioned here because of its importance in determining a list of differential diagnoses. The history must include a variety of questions not commonly asked in the traditional veterinary format.[2] This requires more time and a different approach to history taking than is usual. As suggested, the large number of questions that need to be addressed may require that the client(s) (and other people that play a role in the life of the patient) fill out at least some of the information before the veterinary visit. It may also require that the behavioral consultant's report (if available) be provided before the clinical appointment. This is important so that the avian clinician can review the material and develop a game plan before the patient arrives.[4]

Rearing History—Possible Factor in Development of FDB

In addition to the standard historical questions, the clinician—as well as the behavioral consultant—needs to ask the client questions to better understand the rearing of the patient, as this can have a major impact on the behaviors observed.[4] It has been suggested that some avian patients with FDB may have a similar condition to primates that exhibit self-injurious behavior (SIB). In a study on SIB in monkeys, maintenance of this behavior persisted or recurred despite attempts to change the environment, suggesting that this behavior has value to the individual.[5] Humans that self-wound expressed relief post-wounding of negative emotions that were apparently building up. This suggests that, in primates, the act of SIB is followed by an immediate sense of relief, which may occur in companion birds as well.[6, 7] Those studying primates with SIB noted that tension buildup was associated with an escalation of the animal's heart rate. This occurred within 30 seconds prior to the biting episode. It remained elevated during the biting episode and then would drop precipitously to baseline between 30 and 60 seconds after the episode was complete.[5] These data suggest that the self-injurious episode acts as a positive physiologic reinforcer of an abnormal behavior, making it difficult to quench or to provide relief with drugs. If this same scenario exists for some birds that exhibit FDB, then this may explain the lack of responsiveness to medical management.

Companion birds, like primates, are also very social animals. The rearing of their young chicks appears to involve a large number of interactions and learning experiences due to their altricial behavior as well as their complex social behaviors as psittacines. Bellanca and Crockett studied abnormal behavior in pigtail macaques (*Macaca nemestrina*), including SIB.[8] The amount of time spent in single housing regardless of rearing methods was linked to an increase in abnormal behavior. They looked at differences in rearing as it pertained to degrees of abnormal behaviors and SIB, and response to enrichment as a treatment. Their data is of particular interest to avian practitioners as the method of raising monkeys in an infant laboratory has some similarities to current avicultural practice of rearing chicks by hand, with only human interaction during the early stages and some interaction with chicks of similar ages. The monkeys were removed from their mothers while under five days of age and reared in single cages, although they could see and hear other infants.[8] At approximately 55 days of age, infants were allowed into a "playroom" with four to six other infants of the same species and approximate size and weight for 30-minute time periods at least five days a week. Not until they were weaned and at least six months of age were they group-housed. Anytime after that, they could be removed to individual housing for projects.

Results of the study showed that there were statistically relevant increases in locomotor stereotypies, self-abusive non-injurious behaviors that included hair plucking, self-stimulation, and other abnormal behaviors in the nursery-reared infants as compared to mother-reared infants.[8] Non-injurious self-abuse is considered as "potential SIB," and if it continues, in many cases it does lead to SIB. These behaviors appeared at nonspecific times later in life after placement in solitary caging. This occurred despite the fact that the monkeys were caged in rooms with other monkeys having visual, vocal, and auditory contact. For monkeys that had been mother-reared, then singly caged, abnormal behaviors that developed were much lower and were more effectively treated with enrichment, including social contact with a same-species monkey. Those that had been nursery-reared were more likely to be unresponsive to enrichment or even socialization. Many of these primates that were not mother-reared exhibited self-abusive behaviors or other abnormal behaviors that increased with time. In the observations of non-human primate self-abusive and hair-plucking behaviors, most worsen with time and many, depending on species, external stresses, and individual temperament, become SIB conditions in some of the more common primate species.[4]

What is different in the studies with primates, as compared with birds, is that no monkey was isolated in a room without some sort of contact (visual, vocal, auditory) with other monkeys of the same species, as institutions are not allowed to place a solitary animal in a room as primary housing. Such isolation is contrary to the Animal Welfare Act, Part D, Nonhuman Primates.[9] Many bird-owning households, on the other hand, have no other birds, let alone the same species, in visual, vocal, or auditory range of the newly purchased hand-raised bird. Often birds are weaned and placed into a household with no other birds. This would suggest that these situations may predispose the single companion bird to abnormal behaviors, as with primates.

It is important that the avian practitioner or the behavioral consultant ask about this scenario on the history form and take these concerns into account when developing a working diagnosis or determining the response to treatment. This does not mean that the clinician or the behavioral consultant should, when presented with a companion bird with FDB or any other behavioral problem, just throw up his or her hands and do nothing. It should instead provide *one* reason for the bird to have a problem and/or not respond to treatment. It also provides a backdrop to further understand this problem and a way of looking at research to improve a bird's outcome when living with humans. The primate data would also suggest that birds that were raised mostly by their parents and then separated from them at weaning have a better chance of responding to treatment. Orangewinged Amazons (*Amazona amazonica*) that met these criteria when singly housed and that developed FDB improved with environmental enrichment.[10]

The amount of time birds spent foraging in their natural environment may play an important role in understanding FDB, particularly with those birds that are separated at weaning. In Puerto Rican Amazon Parrots (*Amazona vittata*), for example, four to six hours are spent each day foraging for food and these birds often travel several miles between feeding sites.[11] In contrast, companion birds in our homes, like Orangewinged Amazon Parrots when provided a pelleted diet, spend approximately 30–72 minutes eating to meet their daily metabolic requirements without expending energy to travel to find food items or to manipulate them for consumption.[12]

These data suggest that companion bird species are highly motivated to forage for food over long periods of time, just like their wild counterparts,[10] and when foraging opportunities are not present, then abnormal behaviors such as FDB may develop. Chickens when not provided with foraging opportunities will also peck and do damage to feathers as a displacement for the lack of foraging.[13, 14] Therefore, the time spent foraging by the patient or interacting with toys would be important to obtain during the history.

From a clinical point of view, the study by Drs. Meehan, Millam, and Mench suggests that certain types of enrichments have the potential for greater use and hence success.[10] Orangewinged Amazon Parrots that were parent-raised until weaning developed FDB when placed into individual cages at weaning.[10] These parrots were divided into two groups after approximately 11 months post-weaning when the FDB began. One group received foraging enrichments while others were provided with physical enrichments. Foraging enrichments required that the parrots chew through barriers, manipulate objects through holes, and sort through inedible material and/or open containers to obtain food items while the normal ration was available. Physical enrichments included alternative perching sites, climbing or swinging opportunities, or providing moveable objects that could be manipulated with the feet or beak.

The study showed that the parrots used their enrichments within three days of introduction but that the use of the physical enrichments declined over time, while the use of the foraging ones remained stable.[10] Additionally, refeathering occurred within two weeks of introducing the items into the cages. Six of eight parrots demonstrated an improved feather score, which suggests that enrichment allows for foraging and reduces FDB but does not eliminate it. However, this study indicates that these types of foraging activities should be included as part of the clinical treatment regimen for FDB. This study also demonstrated that parrots in the enriched condition worked to access supplemental food items an average of 19–26% of their active time, even though their normal ration was available as a pellet. This would support the findings in chickens that in a barren environment and/or one without foraging opportunities, foraging attempts may be redirected toward their plumage as with FDB.[13–15] The quality and the availability of the foraging enrichments in particular contribute to the effectiveness of the response to the FDB.

Foraging may be important in the neural development of parrots, as in primates. A strong relationship was also found between the lack of behavioral opportunity for foraging and the development of stereotypic behaviors in parrots. There was evidence that there was an underlying neural compromise with stereotypies.[16] This suggests that neural dysfunction may result from a barren environment or the lack of enrichments that the parrots would be engaged in long term. It may also underlie abnormal, repetitive behaviors.[10]

The hypothesis would be that FDB can represent the avian counterpart to self-abusive non-injurious behavior and/or SIB in primates. If this were true, then feather damage could act as a coping strategy and should be physiologically reinforcing as with the change in heart rate (HR) in primates. No information is currently available to determine if there are HR changes in birds immediately prior to the feather-damaging event, but this needs to be investigated. The hypothesis would also include the effects of isolation and hand-rearing as an underlying factor in the development of the abnormal grooming behavior.[4]

This hypothesis suggests that new and important information be gathered during the history about hand-raising and weaning. This information is important for understanding the possible role of hand-raising practices and isolation of birds at weaning in the development of FDB. A form that takes these factors into account is provided in Table 17-1 as a guide in designing your history form. It is important that the clinical examination includes both a physical examination and a behavioral evaluation.[2]

Clinical Examination

There are two important aspects to the physical examination. The first is to document if there are physical changes that can be observed by the avian clinician. This would be most obvious with FDB. The second is to determine the extent of the changes observed. Documentation of these physical exam findings helps determine if there are any infectious or metabolic changes that produce a secondary behavioral condition. A feather-scoring system has been developed and presented in the literature for FBD and can be adapted for clinical use (see Table 17-2). It would be best to standardize a feather scoring system so that all professionals can then bring their data together to look at various parameters to further understand this problem and enhance treatment success.

From a clinical perspective, it is important to determine if there is damage to the feathers and where and how much damage has occurred. There may be situations where there is no visible damage to the feathers but the client reports that the bird is constantly chewing its feathers. Owners may be reporting normal behaviors that are thought to be abnormal. This most frequently happens when owners don't know how much time is spent in daily grooming. The other situation may occur when birds attempt to groom, but with little experience or learning from non-existent parents, they do not groom properly and spend much time doing a poor job. Owners may report feather loss when there is none. This most fre-

Table 17-1   Feather damaging/self-mutilation behavior form

Date of Clinical Examination_____
Owner's name_____
Patient's name_____ Species_____ Age_____ Sex_____

Owner's observations as told to clinician

Historical questions (Owner's report)	Yes	No	Unknown
Hen-reared			
Hand-reared			
Reared with siblings			
Reared with similar aged but different species			
Reared with non-similar aged birds			
At what age was the patient taken from the nest?	Description:		
Age when singly housed	Description:		
Age when placed as a single bird	Description:		
Describe social contact during hand rearing	Description:		
Describe weaning process and procedures	Description:		

Locomotor behaviors noted:	Yes	No	Unknown
Pacing back and forth on perch			
Somersaulting in the cage			
Bobbing head and body up and down			
Head flipping back and forth			
Running toes through beak			
Stretching			
Flapping of wings (i.e., flying in place)			
Flaring the crest when stresses			
Fluffing the feathers over the beak			

Self-stimulation behaviors noted:	Yes	No	Unknown
Head rubbing over uropygial gland and/or back			
Overgrooming			
Plucking over distal back and/or medial thighs			
Cuddling foot or extremity			
Vocalizations/screaming			
Tail and/or vent flaring			
Other:			

(continued)

Table 17-1 Feather damaging/self-mutilation behavior form (*continued*)

Clinical examination (observations in clinic)

Feather-damaging behaviors	Location:	Side preference:
Chewing feather shafts		
Chewing barbs		
Chewing remiges; primaries, secondaries		
Chewing rectrices		
Plucking and removing coverts		
Plucking and removing down		
Plucking and removing remiges		
Plucking and removing rectrices		
Self-mutilation and where		

Behavioral assessment   *(Record number of times for a 15-minute period)*

Observer's name:

Date:	Yes	Times/15 min	Not observed
Aggression			
Fear			
Pacing back and forth on perch			
Somersaulting in the cage			
Bobbing head and body up and down			
Head flipping back and forth			

Socomotor behaviors noted:	Yes	No	Unknown
Pacing back and forth on perch			
Somersaulting in the cage			
Bobbing head and body up and down			
Head flipping back and forth			
Running toes through beak			
Stretching			
Flapping of wings (i.e., flying in place)			
Flaring the crest when stresses			
Fluffing the feathers over the beak			

Self-stimulation behaviors noted:	Yes	No	Unknown
Head rubbing over uropygial gland and/or back			
Overgrooming			
Plucking over distal back and /or medial thighs			
Cuddling foot or extremity			
Vocalizations/screaming			
Tail and/or vent flaring			
Other:			

Table 17-2 Feather-scoring system (from C.L. Meehan, J.R. Millam, and J.A. Mench. 2003. *Appl Anim Behav Sci* 80:71–85)

Score	Description
(a)	Scoring system used for chest/flank, back, and legs
0	All or most feathers removed, down removed and skin exposed, evidence of skin or tissue injury
0.25	All or most feathers removed, down removed and skin exposed, no evidence of skin or tissue injury
0.5	All or most feathers removed, some down removed, patches of skin exposed
0.75	All or most feathers removed, down exposed and intact or feathers removed from more than half of the area, some down removed, patches of skin exposed
1.0	Feathers removed from less than half of the area, some down removed and skin exposed
1.25	Feathers removed from more than half of the area, down exposed and intact
1.5	Feathers removed from less than half of the area, down exposed and intact
1.75	Feathers intact with fraying or breakage
2.0	Feathers intact with little or no fraying or breakage
(b)	Scoring system used for wings
0	All or most primaries, secondaries, and coverts removed, down removed, skin exposed, evidence of skin or tissue injury
0.5	All or most primaries, secondaries, and coverts removed, down removed, skin exposed, no evidence of injury
1.0	More than half of coverts removed, down exposed and intact or more than half of primaries and secondaries removed, down exposed and intact
1.5	Fewer than half of coverts removed, down exposed and intact or fewer than half of primaries and secondaries removed, down exposed and intact or primaries and secondaries intact with significant breakage and fraying
2.0	Feathers intact with little or no fraying or breakage
(c)	Scoring system used for tail
0	All or most tail feathers removed or broken
1	Some tail feathers removed or broken or significant fraying of tail feathers
2	Feathers intact with little or no fraying or breakage

quently happens when the owner sees the apterylae spaces between feather tracts or pterylae when the bird is wet.[17]

As indicated on the form provided, it is important to determine more precisely the lesions as to their location, if there is a sidedness aspect to the picking, what part of the feather is being damaged, if the entire feather is being plucked out, and what type of feathers are being damaged. For example, the bird may only chew at the barbs of coverts on the ventral surface of the pectoral muscles. A bird with this condition would have a 1.75 score for the chest/flank back and legs portion of the scoring system but on the physical examination sheet the location and the extent of the lesion

should be indicated. With all feather conditions, drawings and/or photos help document the lesions and response to therapy and help with one's memory, particularly as most of these problems are long-term situations.

The physical examination is often described as consisting of two parts—observations followed by the actual hands-on palpation and auscultation. It is best to perform the observation and the behavioral examination at the front end of the visit after history taking. As indicated, often these abnormal behaviors are not observed in the office because the birds will not do them in a situation where they are not completely comfortable. Home visits help remove that variable but often just the presence of a "visitor" extinguishes the abnormal behavior. As suggested, proper video-taping helps skirt this issue. However, there are other times when the stress of this "new" environment brings out certain behaviors that the clinician can observe.

All abnormal behaviors of non-human primates are also evaluated in a systematic way, to classify them in categories such as affiliative, fearful, or agonistic.[4] The classification scheme allows for systematic and regular objective evaluation for effectiveness of treatment strategies. It also lends itself to accurate documentation of the behaviors and longitudinal assessments, unlike most evaluations of psittacine abnormal behaviors reported or observed by practitioners. Analysis also allows for species-specific normal behaviors, such as regular grooming or lip smacking in primates, to be recorded as percentage of time of the day, which may point to other learned behaviors (i.e., the animal never learned proper behaviors from older individuals). By classifying these behaviors, the veterinarian or behaviorist can work on training to manage specific problems, to overcome fears, train out some aggressive tendencies, or encourage affiliate behaviors.[4]

As indicated on the form provided in Table 17-1, locomotion-based behaviors are distinguished by self-stimulating behaviors under FDB but should be addressed for all abnormal behaviors as well. The behavioral assessment should record those behaviors within a defined period of time (defined here, e.g., as 15-minute blocks). This is important so that true changes can be noted over time and with treatments. We tend not to approach behavioral examinations from this perspective, but it is required when documenting abnormal behaviors in primates. Without this rigor, it is very difficult to assess changes scientifically.[4] However, primates are often videotaped in their normal caged environment and the behaviors counted. For the avian patient, videotaping them at home and having the professional review the tape is best.

From the perspective of aggression, it may be very difficult to assess territorial aggression in the exam room, as usually the companion bird is aggressive with its home cage. However, the tail fanning and flashing eyes of male amazons often indicate aggression. But often those signals are missed by the client or others. If these are not understood, when the client asks the bird to step up, he or she is asking to get bitten.[18] This would be a normal behavior that is misinterpreted as abnormal, but the understanding of why the owner gets bitten needs to be addressed. A better understanding of the normal reproductive physiology would help the owner understand the common mistakes or miscues that are made in the home.[18]

Observations concerning physical changes should be noted on the examination form. The bird's mentation, along with posture and stance, are important indicators of behavioral problems or disease. For example, one amazon patient was observed in my practice that bore its weight on mostly the left side of the body while the right side of the bird was mostly plucked over the back, hip, chest, and medial and lateral thigh. This patient had severe arthritis of the right hip. Other symptoms of disease need to be noted during the observation phase. Pectoral muscle mass, feather quality, and how the contour feathers lay are important to notice. They may indicate a tumor or fat deposition suggesting a lipoma. The number and quality of the droppings need to be inspected because increased urates suggest problems with the kidneys, for example. The nares, beak, and eyes should be given scrutiny to look for abnormalities. Although the form provided (Table 17-2) concentrates on the feathers and their quality, the coloration, iridescence, and the lay of the feathers against the body wall are also important and need to be noted. It is important to perform both portions of the examination in a step-wise fashion and in the same order for each patient.

The second part of the physical examination is the hands-on palpation and auscultation of the patient. As suggested in other chapters, it is important to make the toweling and physical part as stress free as possible. If often helps to tell the bird what you are doing prior to the event and to use a slow and methodical wrapping of the patient as described previously (E. Wilson, personal communication, August 1999).[19] The handling portion should be done in the same manner with each patient so that no part is forgotten. However, the problem(s) of the patient dictates where the clinician will concentrate his or her physical investigation. With skin and/or feather problems, a head loop helps to magnify and examine the components of the integumentary system. Several blood feathers in the affected area can be plucked and the pulp of the shaft used for a culture and/or a cytology. This should be done at the end of the handling phase.

In terms of diagnostics, it is best to let the avian patient calm down after its travel to the veterinary hospital, then perform the history, the observation phase of the physical examination, and the behavioral phase if there will be limited handling. If a CBC or plasma for a biochemical analysis needs to be part of the workup for the particular patient, it is best to obtain the blood sample prior to a significant amount of time spent handling and time spent in the towel. This is important when interpreting laboratory results as the stress of handling and traveling can alter the CBC results, with the lymphocycte count tending to decrease and the heterophil count and the WBC increasing over normal blood counts.[20] Elevation of several enzymes including AST and LDH can occur with toweling.[21] After the blood has been collected, the remainder of the physical examination can be completed. It is often best to start at the head, examine the oropharynx and take a choanal swab for a gram stain if one is performing a general health check, and proceed caudally down the remainder of the body with special emphasis at examining the structures of the integumentary system. There may be a reason to perform a skin scraping or take feathers for examination of parasites as well. The examination can then be completed with the remainder of the behavioral portion, if necessary. It is always best to make observations relating to behavior prior to toweling. However, the clinician should observe the patient immediately after handling. It is important to check the respiratory recovery time and watch for any abnormal behaviors, as stress may induce them.

DIFFERENTIAL DIAGNOSES FOR FDB

After the physical examination, one can narrow the differential list into one of two possible but unfortunately overlapping general categories for diseases that affect the integumentary system.[22, 23] These would be inflammatory skin and feather diseases and non-inflammatory skin and feather diseases that are often assumed to be non-infectious. Feather-damaging behavioral conditions would be a subset of the latter category. Inflammatory skin diseases include viral, fungal, bacterial, and parasitic infections that may cause disease symptoms.[22] Trauma results in other in-flammatory disease conditions. Common viral diseases that affect the integumentary system of psittacine birds include papillomavirus, poly-omavirus, avipoxvirus, and psittacine beak and feather disease (PBFD) virus or avian circovirus. Trauma includes several types of conditions including tail trauma, split sternum (often in African Grey Parrots), other traumatic conditions to the skin, and damage to blood feathers.[22, 24]

Papillomavirus is thought to result in wart-like dermal papillomas on unfeathered areas of the integument. These lesions have been observed as multiple cutaneous papillomas of the face on a Timneh African Grey Parrot, the legs of European Chaffinches and Braming's Finches, and the commissures of the bills of Canaries.[22, 24, 25] Cutaneous herpesvirus lesions can be confused with dermal papillomas. Herpes lesions present as wart-like lesions or thickenings of the skin and are often found on the feet or legs, particularly of cockatoos and macaws. In these types of birds they may show up as a flat, raised plaque or a roughening of the skin with depigmentation. The gross appearance is characteristic and diagnostic.[22, 24, 25] Biopsy with histopathology and surgical incision can be performed but is not recommended normally.

Polyomavirus often results in abnormal feathering of Budgerigars, particularly in chicks. Chicks affected between 7 and 15 days of age often have ascites and have changes of the primary and secondary flight and tail feathers or these feathers may be absent. Feathers demonstrate thickened shafts with hemorrhage. Feather abnormalities are uncommon in larger psittacines but may be found in those recovering from infection. These larger species often present with subcutaneous hemorrhages, hemorrhages in the feather shaft, and reduction in the numbers and changes in the morphology of down and contour feathers. Diagnosis is by biopsy with histopathological examination for characteristic lesions. A PCR probe is also available for diagnosis.[22, 24]

Avipoxvirus affects most of the families or groups of birds with some cross-infection depending on the group.[25] Infections from avipoxvirus produce symptoms that typically present as either a wet or dry form. Canaries and other related species can also present with a septicemic form. The dry or cutaneous form demonstrates raised papules, pustules, and/or nodules that can rupture to form crusts or scabs on non-feathered areas. Wild-caught Blue-fronted Amazons and young *Pionus* parrots are considered the most susceptible for this disease. Diagnosis is based on the gross appearance of the lesions and the presence of large Bollinger bodies, which are eosinophilic cytoplasmic inclusions observed histopathologically.[22, 24, 25]

PBFD affects a large number of species; however, those most commonly affected include birds from Africa, Asia, and Australia. The chronic form of the disease is associated with abnormal feathering, including dystrophic feathering with retained feather sheaths, blood in the umbilicus of the feather shaft, clubbing of the feathers and other abnormal feather shapes, multiple stress bars on the feather vane, and annular constrictions of the base of the feathers. Some birds may only exhibit feather changes while others show only beak abnormalities. Lesions of the beak include ulceration and an unkempt appearance with elongation, beaks that are weak and fracture easily, and palatine necrosis.[22, 24, 25] Beak lesions are observed more commonly in Sulfur-crested Cockatoos (*Cacatua* sp.), Umbrella Cockatoos (*Cacatua alba*), and Moluccan Cockatoos (*Cacatua moluccensis*).[22] Lories and lorikeets appear to be infected with a variant of PBFD. These birds exhibit less obvious feather lesions and their feathers may only appear dull. Lovebirds may also present with dull feathering with broken feathers.[24] Diagnosis is made through histopathology of an affected feather in combination with a PCR probe to help confirm the disease. Blood can also be drawn to determine if there are circulating viral particles that can be detected with the PCR probe. The PCR technology differs between lories and non-lories as the test has to be altered to include these species. In some of the species not confirmed using PCR technology, diagnosis is made by examination with the electron microscope of the biopsy sample.[26]

Fungal diseases affecting the integumentary system are not common in companion birds. It is difficult to distinguish fungal isolates from the skin causing disease from those that are part of the normal flora. Fungal organisms associated with integumentary disease include the common dermatophytes *Trichophyton* sp. and *Microsporum gypseum,* along with other mycotic organisms *Malassezia, Penicillium* sp, *Cryptococcus neoformans, Aspergillus* sp, *Candida* sp., *Mucor* sp., and *Rhizopus sp.* Some of these organisms produce scaly skin encrustations, possible hyperkeratosis, and patchy feather loss often affecting the head, neck, and breast. Cryptococcosis presents more commonly with respiratory and/or neurological signs. When it affects the integumentary system it is associated with granulomatous lesions of the face or beak. Candidal lesions often involve the rictus or commissures of the bill, the epidermal area around the nares, and the feather follicles on various locations around the body. *Penicillium* and *Aspergillus* sp. are often isolated from non-symmetrical erosive lesions of the beak. These lesions may also be associated with neoplasia such as squamous cell carcinoma, nutritional deficiencies, or poor husbandry practices.

Diagnosis of fungal organisms on the surface of the skin may be through cytology, histopathology, and/or culture. Histologic examination for dermatophytes is important, as a positive culture result may be from a contaminant. A diagnosis of *Malassezia* may be based on exfoliative cytology of the characteristic footprint-shaped yeast cells with confirmation by histopathology of the skin and/or feathers. Cryptococcosis can be confirmed by finding the characteristic yeast with its thickened capsule on histopathological or cytological examination. *Candida* histologically presents as a basophilic yeast with a thin capsule on gram stains while *Aspergillus* and *Penicillium* sp. have basophilic hyphae, which are much larger than gram-positive rods, with conidia.[22]

Bacterial infections may be primary or secondary and may be focal or generalized. The most common isolate from folliculitis is *Staphylococcus* sp., and it is associated with swelling and reddening of the area.[22] Generalized bacterial dermatitis is associated with soft tissue swelling and with flaking, reddening, or other discolorations and crusting of the skin. These types of lesions are often pruritic, resulting in self-trauma. Diagnosis is based on gross appearance, histopathology, and/or culture results. Secondary bacterial infections can often result post-trauma, including FDBs that are psychologic in nature. Grossly there may be swelling, necrosis, and/or cellulitis. It is more difficult with these secondary infections to identify the causative organisms as results are based on histopathology and findings from cultures.[22,24]

Mycobacterial infections can appear as wart-like growths, flaking swellings, or granulomas often on the head or in the oropharynx. These tend to not be pruritic and require biopsy with histopathological observations using acid fast staining for diagnosis.[22]

There are a number of parasitic diseases that affect the integumentary system in birds. They are often species or at least genus dependent. Mites are a common problem in chickens, with them harboring *Knemidokoptes mutans,* while Budgerigars and Canaries are infected with *Knemidokoptes pilae*. Other species affected with *Knemidokoptes* have included Gouldian Finches, Cockatiels, amazon parrots, Ring-necked Parakeets, Scarlet-chested Parrots, Princess Parrots, and Yellow-fronted Kakariki.[22] Mites are transmitted from bird to bird or by transmission in the nest to unfeathered chicks. Mites can often be diagnosed with a skin scraping. *Knemidokoptes* mites are often numerous and more easily observed compared with eternal mites that may not remain on the patient long enough to find them.[22]

The red mites of various species of birds (*Dermanyssus* and *Macronyssus* sp.) can be observed on the external surface of the feathers of fowl and wild birds but may not cause feather damage. They have been reported in Canaries and occasionally in Budgies. These mites are noted as nocturnal feeders and are not observed on the bird during the day. They can be found by placing a white cloth on the bottom of the cage for subsequent examination. They take a blood meal at night, so the patient may show only signs of anemia without the presence of the mites on the feathers.[22]

Myialges or the mite *Metamichrolichtus nudus* feeds on the skin, burrowing into its surface to form pits. Birds with these mites are pruritic, with feather loss around the head. They are often hyperkeratotic, and erythematous as well. Grey-cheeked Parakeets (*Brotogeris pyrrhopterus*) are more commonly affected. A louse or hippoboscid fly is required as a transport host to other birds for infection to be spread. Quill mites are more commonly associated with passerines. The *Metamichrolichtus* mites may be observed on a skin scrape while the quill mites may be observed in the powdery quill material or the broken feathers when examined microscopically.[22]

Biting lice often produce pruritis, mild to moderate feather damage, and hyperkeratosis depending on the degree of infestation. They are more commonly associated with gallinaceous birds, pigeons, and wild birds but have been reported occasionally in psittacine birds. Lice are host specific and do not survive long in the environment. Lice eggs can be found on the primary and secondary flight feathers or on feathers around the vent.[22]

Non-infectious causes are often considered non-inflammatory but this may not be the case. Perivascular dermatitis is considered a non-infectious disease process that is diagnosed by biopsy of skin for an infected area and a non-affected area. It is similar to lesions observed with hypersensitivity dermatitis in mammals with perivascular infiltrates of lymphocytes, plasma cells, eosinophils, and other inflammatory cells.[23] Histopathologic findings include the presence of edema, vascular hypertrophy, hyperplasia of the epidermis, and hyperkeratosis, depending on the length and severity of the lesions. These findings are consistent with other conditions associated with pruritis, suggesting that some birds with FDB are pruritic and may express some type of hypersensitivity reaction. Preliminary data suggest that there is a greater incidence in Blue-and-Gold Macaws with a lesser predisposition in amazon parrots and Eclectus Parrots.[23] It was found to be uncommon in African Grey Parrots.

Another non-infectious cause of FDB is from aberrant behaviors developed as a consequence of hand-rearing. There may be other causes as well that result in the symptom of feather damage and this condition has often been described as psychogenic feather picking.[23] Affected birds appear clinically with symptoms similar to those that present with perivascular dermatitis.[23] It is particularly important that biopsies are taken from both affected skin and unaffected sites. Inflammation can be observed histologically from the affected sites because of the trauma involved in this psychogenic form. But in these birds, inflammatory indicators are not observed in the "non-affected" biopsy samples, unlike those birds that exhibit perivascular dermatitis. Preliminary data suggests that African Grey Parrots, cockatoos, and Cockatiels are more likely to present with the psychogenic form of FDB in review of biopsy samples submitted.[23]

Feather dysplasia is another form of FDB and

can result from a variety of etiologies, some of which are undetermined. This condition describes abnormal growth patterns of the developing feathers and has been likened to the follicular dysplasia of the hair follicles of dogs.[23, 24] However, abnormal growth can result from a variety of diseases and may be of an infectious as well as a non-infectious one. Birds may develop feather dysplasia as a consequence of a congenital condition, an inherited problem, hormonal or metabolic conditions, nutritional problems, spontaneous situations, infectious agents such as PBFD virus, and other suspected but not confirmed viral etiologies. For example, polyfolliculitis syndrome is more commonly associated with lovebirds, Budgerigars, parrotlets, and Cockatiels. It appears as multiple quills projecting from a single feather follicle.[22] Its etiology has not been determined, but it is suspected to be viral in lovebirds.[22, 24]

DIFFERENTIAL DIAGNOSIS FOR AGGRESSION

Aggression is often diagnosed through the clinical examination and the history provided by the owner. Commonly owners report that the bird is biting someone in the family, often the spouse. Most of the time the bird has "chosen" the other spouse as its mate and is just defending their relationship. It is important to understand the cues that the human(s) and bird are providing each other in this scenario to understand if the aggression is from a bonding/mate problem.[18] The reason for the aggression may be purely behavioral with no underlying physical problem, or it may have a physical component. Often male amazons become aggressive around the time of the breeding season, which would be normal behaviorally but very difficult for a pet-oriented owner to handle. Even though one might be able to determine the aggression is territorial or protective and might be from breeding activity, it would be best to perform some diagnostics to confirm or refute the working diagnosis. In this scenario, it would be important to establish the sex of the bird and to run a hormone panel to determine if the bird is in the culmination phase of the breeding cycle. The hormone panel most commonly used in birds is the ferret panel at the University of Tennessee, as it provides the male and female sex hormones along with some of the metabo-

lites.[27] The sex steroid hormones are not species dependent and can be measured in a variety of species using the same type of testing protocol, while the protein hormones cannot.

Another way to determine if the bird has increased sex hormone levels is to observe the size and quality of the gonads by endoscopy, inferring that the hormone levels are elevated. Training owners to understand when birds are aggressive is the first step in avoiding the problem of biting. The next step is to teach the bird and the owner basic commands and ways to discipline the bird.[28] Positive reinforcement and rewards for good behavior help shape a positive attitude for the companion bird with its owner. These may be taught by the clinician or the behavioral consultant with recheck appointments tailored for the individual situation.

Other diagnostic tests for birds exhibiting aggression could be those that check the function of the liver and brain. Plasma biochemical analyses should include an AST, CPK, albumin, total protein, glucose, cholesterol, and bile acid levels to help determine normal liver function. Most commonly, aggression from altered brain function would require a neurologic examination and other diagnostic tests such as a CT scan and/or electrodiagnostics. Pain may also make birds appear aggressive to the less knowledgeable, as they often bite when in pain. Therefore, the astute clinician needs to observe the bird carefully and monitor the bird's behavior in the exam room to determine the diagnostic tests that need to be run.

DIAGNOSTIC TESTS FOR FEATHER-DAMAGING BEHAVIOR

Diagnostic tests should be tailored to the individual bird and the findings from the history and clinical examination. They should be based on the working diagnosis or the list of differential diagnoses. In the case of FDB, the diagnostic workup plan should center on diagnostics involving the integumentary system. Although the inflammatory diseases of the integument overlap with those in the non-inflammatory category, that does not mean that the shotgun approach of diagnostic testing is indicated. Most clients are exasperated that they spent a large amount of money with no results. It is important to tailor the tests to the individual bird and to explain to the owner what the tests may or may not show in helping to arrive at a diagnosis. Education is extremely important for these owners. As clinicians, one should stress to the owner that they should not expect the bird will go home after one visit and grow back its feathers and look perfectly normal. Owners need to understand that many birds will stay the same, while others will improve but not return to "normal" depending on the diagnosis and the degree of trauma to the skin and feather follicles. This is particularly true at this point with our understanding of FDBs. Psychological FDB birds may improve for a while and then relapse. With attention from clinicians and behavioral consultants, they may improve again. It is important to look at the triggers for FDB to find the underlying cause(s) for possible resolution. The bottom line is that once the companion bird starts damaging its feathers, it is not going to be a "quick fix." It will require diligence on the part of the owner and will be costly. It is important that the owner understands that on the front end.

Clinically speaking, a minimum database is often referred to when describing a workup for a particular disease condition. However, the minimum database for birds exhibiting FDB or other integumentary problems is not set in stone. With most disease processes, the minimum database is a CBC and plasma biochemical analyses with the possible inclusion of a plasma electrophoresis (EPH).[29] The CBC is a general indicator of overall health and will not provide any clues about a specific disease. Most birds with FDB will not have any changes in the components of their CBC. However, those that mutilate or cause damage to their skin may have an increased white blood cell count (WBC) with a heterophilia and those that have lost a significant amount of blood may demonstrate anemia. In chronically ill birds, there may an increased WBC with a monocytosis. The CBC can also be used to monitor the response to treatment, particularly for those birds with an infectious dermatitis.[29]

The plasma biochemical analysis is an indicator of general organ function. Those birds that have been picking will often have an increased aspartate aminotransferase (AST) level because this enzyme is released with liver damage and that of muscle cells that can occur with picking. Additionally, picking birds can have an elevated creatinine phosphokinase (CPK), an enzyme that elevates only with muscle damage. Most commonly

in birds with FDB, both enzymes will be elevated. If only the AST level is elevated, then there is concern that there may be liver damage. Liver damage, in mammals, is known to result in pruritis and may be involved in the underlying cause of the problem.[29] Elevation of the AST value is also observed in birds that have increased gonadal hormones. Uric acid levels are associated with renal disease and may help explain some birds that pick only over their synsacrum. Other birds that are in the culmination phase of the breeding cycle often pick in this area, along with the lateral thighs and flanks. Lower than normal levels of plasma proteins may be associated with liver disease (where some are manufactured), problems with filtration in the kidneys, and problems with ingestion from the GI tract (observed in proventricular dilatation disease, PDD).[29]

Plasma electrophoresis provides general information about the health of the avian patient but does not provide a specific diagnosis. The EPH should be used in conjunction with the CBC and plasma biochemical analysis. Many birds with FDB will have normal values, suggesting that often there is no specific infectious disease entity that causes the underlying problem. However, those patients with an increased beta fraction are associated with an acute infectious disease while an increased gamma fraction is associated with a chronic infection. This gamma fraction may often be elevated with chronic pickers, especially those with damage to the skin.[29]

Sex Determination

It is important to know the sex of the bird as a guide to understanding the relationship to the disease process. Sex determination can be performed by rigid endoscopy or by PCR or other recent technologies using the feather or blood.

Fecal Examination

Fecal examination can provide information about the general health of the bird but does not indicate a diagnosis for most feather pickers except for those with *Giardia*. Trophozoites can be observed on a slide of fresh droppings at 20–40X while the cysts are best seen with an iodine stain. *Giardia* ELISA tests designed for dogs may not be appropriate for birds as the testing has not been confirmed to cross-react between birds and dogs. Nematodes have been associated with "poor doing" and pruritis, but most companion birds are not exposed to the conditions for them to be a problem.[24, 29]

Skin Scraping for Parasites

Skin scrapings for cytological examination for parasites is a common procedure in mammals that are pruritic but uncommon in birds. *Knemidokoptes* sp. mites and *Metamichrolichus nudus* are two of the most common types of mites in avian species. The former species of mites do not typically result in pruritis, while the second type, most common in Grey-cheeked Parakeets, is highly pruritic.[22, 29] The same technique can be used as in mammals to obtain the sample. However, care must be taken to not tear the skin as it is thinner than that of mammals.[17]

Heavy Metal Assays

There is anecdotal information that suggests that heavy metal toxicosis, namely lead and/or zinc, may cause FDB. However, data on zinc toxicosis suggest that birds develop pancreatitis and do not become pruritic. Pruritis and feather damage do not seem to be a manifestation of lead toxicosis.[30, 31]

BACTERIAL AND FUNGAL CULTURES

Bacterial and fungal cultures should be reserved to areas of the integument that are abnormal. Choanal and fecal cultures only reflect the microorganisms from these regions and would imply overall health but not specific problems that cause the bird to have FDB.[29]

In abnormal areas, samples for cultures can be paired with Gram stains to make a diagnosis. A deep culture is recommended over a superficial one. Often therapy can be initiated based on the Gram stain while waiting for culture results, particularly with fungal cultures. Histopathology can also help in arriving at a diagnosis, and biopsy samples are recommended when a culture is taken.[22, 24]

Feather pulp cultures and Gram stains may be useful in some patients with FDB, as the picking may cause damage that produces a secondary infection. The history and clinical examination may help determine if the infection is secondary or primary.[22] Often Gram stains of the pulp cavity may be misdiagnosed as a fungal infection, as the nucleus of ruptured red blood cells can appear as

yeast-like organisms (S.E. Orosz, personal observation, 2003).

Histopathology of the Skin or Feathers

A skin biopsy including a feather follicle, particularly an immature one, is important for diagnosing an infectious or inflammatory condition.[22, 23] It is important to take a biopsy of the skin from an affected area and one from a noninfected one. Samples should also be clearly marked in order for the pathologist to make an appropriate interpretation. Results from the histopathological examination can help rule in as well as rule out a number of infectious causes of FDB such as viral, bacterial, parasitic, and fungal diseases. It is also important for determining if there is evidence of perivascular dermatitis. When there is evidence of disease while the culture results are negative there can be a number of explanations for the cause. Negative aerobic cultures occur when an anaerobic organism is present, when the patient is on antibiotics, and when the cultures are not handled properly. When the histopathologic results suggest the skin is normal, then the diagnosis of FDB is more likely to be psychological in origin.[22]

Intradermal Skin Testing

Early results developing the use of intradermal skin testing for birds have not been promising. It is assumed that if these tests were developed to the level as for mammals, then desensitization might also reduce the prevalence of FDB. Unfortunately, these tests have not indicated that allergens play a major role in FDB.[29]

Testing for Aspergillosis

Aspergillosis is not a common diagnosis for FDB and the *Aspergillus* organisms may affect the beak more often than the feathers. Measuring the titers or antibodies of *Aspergillus* sp. from blood samples does not help determine if this may be the cause for integumentary problems. Fungal cultures, exfoliative cytology, and histopathology of biopsy samples are more appropriate to make a diagnosis.[22, 24]

Viral PCR and Other Test Procedures

Psittacine birds with FDB are often tested using viral PCR probes for avian polyomavirus and PBFD, as these two viruses can affect the feathering of psittacine birds.[22, 24, 25, 29] Polyoma-virus may cause feathering abnormalities of the smaller species including Budgerigars and finches, but the test performs poorly with these smaller species. The PCR test for PBFD may be considered in the old world species as these birds are affected more commonly compared with the new world species. The virus in the chronic form of the disease can produce feather and/or beak dystrophy, which may be mistaken for mutilation of the feathers. In smaller species and less common ones, histopathology of a feather biopsy with its surrounding skin may be required, along with electron microscopy of the sample.[26]

Whole Body Radiology and Ultrasound Evaluation

Whole body radiographs may be useful when a patient picks or mutilates over a particular area or to diagnose those with PDD. Some birds with PDD may also be pruritic and have FDB.[29] Dilation of the proventriculus can be observed radiographically as an organ shadow that passes from rostral to caudal and extends beyond the liver margin on the left side on a VD view. It may be diagnosed using barium to coat the proventriculus to delineate it if it extends beyond the liver margin. Additionally, birds with PDD have altered motility of their proventriculus and gizzard (ventriculus), and those changes can best be observed using fluoroscopy.

Some birds with organ dysfunction may be pruritic, as is the case with liver disease, or may pick over a localized area where the organ is situated, as with the kidneys. When there is suspected organ dysfunction, ultrasound evaluation of the organ can be performed with a possible fine needle aspirate as a biopsy.[29]

REFERENCES

1. Dodman, N.H. 1998. "Pharmacologic treatment of aggression on veterinary patients." In *Psychopharmacology of animal behavior disorders,* ed. N.H. Dodman and L. Schuster, pp. 41–63. Malden, MA: Blackwell Science.
2. Welle, K. 2003. "Evaluation, diagnosis, and modification of behavioral disorders." Proc MASAAV Avian Med Surg Conf, pp. 176–191.
3. Sackett, D.L., S.E. Straus, W.S. Richardson, W. Rosenberg, and R.B. Haynes. 2000. *Evidence-based medicine: How to practice and teach EBM,* 2nd ed. London, England: Churchill Livingstone.
4. Orosz, S.E., and C.J. Delaney. 2003. "Self-injurious behavior (SIB) of primates as a model for feather damaging behavior (FDB) in companion psittacine birds." Proc Annu Conf Assoc Avian Vet: Avian Specialty Advanced Program—Another Feather Picker: That Sinking Feeling, pp. 39–50.
5. Novak, M.A. 2003. Self-injurious behavior in rhesus monkeys: New insights into its etiology, physiology, and treatment. *Am J Primatology* 59:3–19.
6. Jones, I.H., and B.M. Barraclough. 1978. Automutilation in animals and its relevance to self-injury in man. *Acta Psychiatr Scand* 58:40–47.
7. Haines, J., C.L. Williams, K.L. Brain, and G.V. Wilson. 1995. The psychophysiology of self-mutilation. *J Abnorm Psychol* 104 (3):471–489.
8. Bellanca, R.U., and C.M. Crockett. 2002. Factors predicting increased incidence of abnormal behavior in male pigtailed macaques. *Am J Primatol* 58 (2):57–69.
9. USDA. 1985 and amendments. Animal Welfare Act, Subchapter A, Animal Welfare, Subpart D—Specifications for the Humane Handling, Care, Treatment, and Transportation of Nonhuman Primates; Paragraph 3.81, Environment enhancement to promote psychological well-being; Animal Plant Health Inspection Service, USDA.
10. Meehan, C.L., J.R. Millam, and J.A. Mench. 2003. Foraging opportunity and increased physical complexity both prevent and reduce psychogenic feather picking by young Amazon parrots. *Applied Anim Behav Sci* 80:71–85.
11. Snyder, N.F.R., J.W. Wiley, and C.B. Kepler. 1987. *The parrots of Luquillo: Natural history and conservation of the Puerto Rican parrot.* Los Angeles: Western Foundation of Vertebrate Zoology.
12. Oviatt, L.A., and J.R. Millam. 1997. Breeding behavior of captive orange-winged amazon parrots. *Exotic Bird Rep* 9:6–7.
13. Huber-Eicher, B., and B. Wechsler. 1997. Feather pecking in domestic chicks: Its relation to dust-bathing and foraging. *Anim Behav* 54:757–768.
14. Huber-Eicher, B., and B. Wechsler. 1998. The effect of quality and availability of foraging materials on feather pecking in laying hen chicks. *Anim Behav* 55:861–863.
15. El-lethey, H., T.W. Jungi, and B. Huber-Eicher. 2001. Effects of feeding corticosterone and housing conditions on feather pecking in laying hens (*Gallus gallus domesticus*). *Physiol Behav* 73: 243–251.
16. Garner, J.P., C.L. Meehan, and J.A. Mench. Cage-induced stereotypy in parrots and brain dysfunction: Parallels to schizophrenia and autism. Submitted.
17. Orosz, S.E. 2003. "Anatomy and physiology of the integumentary system." Proc Annu Conf Assoc

Avian Vet: Avian Specialty Advanced Program—
Another Feather Picker: That Sinking Feeling, pp.
3–12.

18. Speer, B.L. 2003. "Sex and the single bird." Proc
Annu Conf Assoc Avian Vet, pp. 331–343.

19. Hooimeijer, J. 2003. "A practical behavior protocol
for dealing with parrots." Proc Annu Conf Assoc
Avian Vet, pp. 177–181.

20. Speer, B.L., and P.H. Kass. 1995. "The influence
of travel on hematologic parameters in hyacinth
macaws." Proc Annu Conf Assoc Avian Vet, pp. 43.

21. Orosz, S.E., J.M. Grizzle, J.W. Bartges, N.K.
Zagaya, A.K. McGee, J. McGinn, and C. Cray.
2000. "A critical care diet for use in parrots." Proc
Annu Conf Assoc Avian Vet, pp. 7–9.

22. Reavill, D. 2003. "Inflammatory skin diseases."
Proc Annu Conf Assoc Avian Vet, pp. 13–24.

23. Garner, M.M. 2003. "Avian noninfectious skin disorders." Proc Annu Conf Assoc Avian Vet, pp.
21–24.

24. Koski, M.A. 2002. Dermatologic diseases in
psittacine birds: An investigational approach.
Semin Avian Exotic Anim Med 11 (3):105–124.

25. Gerlach, H. 1994. "Avipoxvirus affects most of the
families or groups of birds with some cross infection depending on the group. Viruses." In *Avian
medicine: Principles and application,* ed. B.W.
Ritchie, G.J. Harrison, and L.R. Harrison LR, pp.
862–948.. Lake Worth, FL: Wingers.

26. Woods, L.W., and K.S. Latimer. 2003. Circovirus
infection of nonpsittacine birds. *J Avian Med Surg*
14 (3):154–163.

27. Pollock, C.G., and S.E. Orosz. 2002. Avian reproductive anatomy, physiology, and endrocrinology.
Vet Clin North Am Exot Anim Pract 5 (3):441–474.

28. Speer, B.L. 2003. Avian medicine today: Setting
the standard. *Proc Bayer Exotics Symp* 25 (3A):
21–31.

29. Rosenthal, K.L. 2003. "Diagnostics: Please let
there be an answer." Proc Annu Conf Assoc Avian
Vet: Avian Specialty Advanced Program—Another
Feather Picker: That Sinking Feeling, pp. 25–30.

30. Speer, B.L. 2003. "Zinc toxicosis: Separating fact
from fiction." Proc 24th Annu Conf Avian Med
Surg: MASAAV, pp. 156–159.

31. Levengood, J.M., G.C. Sanderson, W.L. Anderson,
G.L. Foley, P.W. Brown, and J.W. Seets. 2000.
Influence of diet on the hematology and serum
biochemistry of zinc-intoxicated mallards. *J Wildl
Dis* 36 (1):111–123.

18
Aggressive Behavior in Pet Birds

Kenneth R. Welle and Andrew U. Luescher

Biting is one of the most common and definitely the most serious behavior problem in any pet. Parrots are no exception. Psittacine aggression is one of the more serious of behavioral problems for pet bird owners. The strong jaws and hooked bill of parrots can inflict serious pain and do substantial damage to the owners. Aggression in parrots takes the form of biting or lunging at a person or another bird. Parrots will use biting as a last resort for protection and to guard resources. They also are very intelligent. Their experience will determine what behaviors are most effective to accomplish the goals they are looking to achieve. Some birds will learn that aggressive behavior is very effective, while others may find another strategy works best for them.

While the aggression of an individual bird can have overlapping and interacting etiologies, it is helpful to categorize the problem in order to treat it. As in any other species, aggressive behavior has several etiologies.[1] Aggressive behavior etiologies in pet birds include fear, conditioning, territoriality, and attachment to a mate. Diagnosis of any behavioral disorder is based upon the behavioral history, testing the bird's response to various situations, and direct observation of the bird. Specifically, the signalment, a description of the environment and social interactions, and a description of the aggression, the circumstances in which it occurs, and the owner's reaction to the behavior are critical to the assessment of a biting bird.[2] It is particularly important to see the bird's interaction with owners and other people. Aggressive birds will often behave much better in the veterinary hospital or other unfamiliar place than in their home environment. If all of the observations are made away from the home territory, the true behavior of the bird may not be noted. A house call, or better yet, videotapes of the bird and owner at home are a much preferable means of assessing the behavior.

FEAR BITING

With parrots being a prey species, fear is one of the most common motivators for biting. A bird that is frightened by people is simply trying to defend itself. There does not appear to be any age or sex predilection. This is technically not a behavior problem. Biting is a perfectly reasonable reaction to something thought to be a threat. The real problem is the fact that the bird perceives someone as a threat. The reasons that this occurs vary. Wild birds naturally fear humans. The process of capture, shipping, and sale does little to reduce these fears. These wild-caught birds, however, are less common than in years past. Most of those remaining have had years to either reduce or confirm their fears of humans. The vast majority of pet birds are captive bred and have lived their entire lives around humans. While most Budgerigars and many other small psittacine birds are parent-reared, most larger parrots are raised by humans. Their fears of humans are much more difficult to explain. While overt abuse would readily explain a bird's fear of humans, there is little evidence of such abuse in most cases. Certain species are more likely to develop fear of people despite the fact that they have been raised around them. African Grey Parrots are well known for this problem. The factors involved vary. Sometimes these birds are not socialized adequately when young. Some may have had excessively severe wing trims, causing them to be somewhat clumsy. These birds will then have frequent falls, feather and beak breakage, and other painful events that make them fear coming out of their "safe haven" within their cage. The complexity of the early environment has an effect on emotional stability, too (see chapter 11), and many hand-raised birds are kept in a severely restricted environment until fledging.

There are certain features to this type of biting that are relatively easy to recognize. Usually, these birds only bite when cornered or caught. They will not often attack or chase someone. They may learn to attack rather than retreat when the cage door is opened, but they will generally try to get past the handler rather than defend the cage. Fearful vocalizations such as growling or screaming will often precede or accompany the biting. Many will be "cage bound," very reluctant to leave the cage even on their own. When they are presented to the veterinary hospital, they will be extremely stressed, often vocalizing almost constantly. They may begin to cower, pant, or thrash about when the cage is approached. A stress leukogram is very common with these birds. Most affected birds will not allow handling by anyone, although occasionally birds will be fearful of a particular person, gender, behavior, or a physical characteristic of a person. One behavior, which is very likely to initiate biting, is when people offer a hand and then jerk it back when the bird reaches out with the beak. Many fear biters are somewhat clumsy and they may have fallen when people have pulled the hand away from the beak.

Treatment of this problem requires a lot of patience. Affected birds should be gradually desensitized to the presence of people. Depending on the severity, initial contact may have to be limited to basic care of the bird. If the bird accepts anyone, that person should do all of the basic maintenance until the bird learns to accept others. As the bird begins to remain calm in the presence of the feared person, then eye contact and vocal interaction can be tried. In extreme cases, anxiolytic drugs can be used to facilitate the early stages of treatment. When basic non-contact communication has progressed to a point where the bird is calm, then handling can be tried. Since the bird is already fearful, coaxing and reward should be used here. A favorite food item should be reserved for this purpose. It may be necessary to restrict food slightly to encourage the bird to take a treat. Initially a treat should be placed on the floor, in the food dish, or on the roost, and the hand withdrawn less and less far, so the bird gets rewarded for approaching the hand. Then basic operant conditioning can be used to pattern the bird to step out of the cage, and finally onto the hand. Clicker training would be an excellent method to deal with fearful birds (see chapter 20). The voice should remain calm and coaxing at all times. If the biting is severe, it may be necessary to use a handheld perch or even a protective glove for initial handling. Despite warnings about gloves causing greater fear, used properly, they can be useful tools. Falconers have used gloves for a thousand years, and they have never made their charges more fearful of humans. When using handheld perches or gloves, it is important that the bird is desensitized to them before sticking them up to the bird's chest. This can be achieved simply by laying them a little closer to the cage every day, and eventually moving them gently at decreasing distances to the cage while the bird eats its favorite treat. The glove should only be used as a perch for the bird, never to grab or restrain it. The advantage of the glove or perch is that it can give the handler more confidence to hold the bird steady than a bare hand. A stable dowel or glove is much better than a hand that is pulled away. If there is any indication that gloves have been used for restraint in the past, they should not be used with that particular bird. Punishing a fear biter is contraindicated. The biting behavior in this situation is a normal response. The situation is abnormal and this is what should be addressed.

The prognosis for fear biting is fair. Success depends on the patience and commitment of the owner. The speed of progress will depend on the severity of the fear. Birds that have very generalized fear of humans will require a greater length of time than those that simply fear hands. The ability of the owner to offer a steady hand to the bird is critical as well. If a stable perching surface cannot be offered to the bird, then stepping up will rarely occur.

CONDITIONED AGGRESSION

This type of aggression is often called dominance aggression. Dominance aggression is a controversial classification. The term implies a social order maintained by subtle, species-typical cues that serve to minimize aggression. This communication is not possible between birds and people. However, birds can easily be conditioned to be aggressive by a person backing off or in other ways rewarding the aggression (see chapter 20). Fear aggression, mate-related aggression, and territorial aggression are very easily conditioned that way. Also, if the bird was able to control the owner's behavior for some time, and then the owner does not comply with the parrot's expectations, there is what is called a "frustration effect" that easily results in an outburst of aggression. If then the owner does act according to the parrot's expectations, this aggression is reinforced. If the aggression is consistently successful, the bird becomes very confident in using aggression, so a fear aggression may change into confident, or offensive, aggression.

This type of aggression may occur in any species but is particularly common in amazons and macaws. It occurs more often in mature than in juvenile birds. It has been suggested that male birds are affected more commonly, but the gender of many birds is undetermined. In dogs, the analogous problem is most commonly seen with owners with anthropomorphic, and thus inconsistent, involvement with their pet, and in first-time dog owners.[3] In parrots it seems to occur more commonly with birds belonging to people with little experience with birds. It also occurs more frequently in larger species of birds. This is more likely due to the fact that more people will be intimidated by larger species than the fact that these birds are particularly aggressive. Affected birds have often learned to manipulate the owner to their wishes. The owners' behavior may be as useful for a diagnosis as is the bird's behavior. They often will make excuses for the bird's behavior, take extraordinary measures to prevent upsetting the bird, or otherwise defer to the tantrums of the bird.

These birds will show a particular pattern of aggression. The bird may bite certain family members but not others. When the interactions are observed the ones bitten are less confident and assertive with the bird than those that are not bitten. The biting does not appear to be influenced by the bond between bird and owner; the person bitten may be the bird's favorite person. Biting may occur when the owner tries to get the bird off the shoulder, put the bird in a cage, or remove the bird from the perch. These birds may occasionally bite when the owner stops petting them. The owners often blame themselves for the bite and will comply.

For most animals, loss of control over the environment, alongside loss of the ability to predict what is going to happen, is very stressful. This is most certainly true for intelligent animals such as parrots. They therefore strive to have control over the environment. If the owners do not establish the contingencies between the bird's behavior and the effects it has, the birds will. This is not an abnormal behavior, but simply necessary for the bird's well-being. Consistency in interaction with the bird and training will give the bird control and make the environment predictable in a manner that is also acceptable to the owners. The bird simply has to do the right behavior to get what it wants, and the bird also learns when such behavior is going to pay off and when not. Aggressive birds have been patterned to use aggressive behavior to control the behavior of their owners, who have been patterned to comply. Both owner and bird may be resistant to changing the situation. After years of being bitten, the owner will be hesitant to be assertive with the biting bird. The bird will initially be a bit confused and will try to re-establish control. Aggression may get worse before it gets better. In some cases, the bird will benefit from placement in a home with a more confident and consistent handler.

The wings should be trimmed to give the bird one less means of controlling situations. All handling should take place in neutral territory. If there are any household members that can safely handle the bird, they should bring the bird to the neutral area. If no one can safely handle the bird, the owners should be schooled on safe towel capture and restraint of the bird. Once in a neutral site, out of the sight of the cage, step-up exercises should be practiced. The owners should be coached on confident and consistent handling techniques. If the owner cannot keep the hand in front of the bird without withdrawing from the beak, then a perch or gloved hand should be used. All of the precautions regarding the use of perches and gloves discussed previously should be followed here as well.

The shoulders should be considered off-limits. This can be challenging in its own right if the bird is accustomed to riding on the owner's shoulders. Hand position should be higher than the elbow so the bird does not just climb up onto the shoulder. Birds are reluctant to slide down the arm to the elbow and then up the upper arm to the shoulder.

To prevent the bird from jumping to the shoulder, the feet may have to be restrained. Placing a towel or other object on the shoulder may discourage the bird from jumping on the shoulder. If the bird jumps onto the shoulder with the towel on it, the towel and bird are quickly removed.

The owners should be taught to recognize threat behavior. When the bird displays threat behavior, or a bite occurs, the bird should be given a command and rewarded for the appropriate behavior. In this way the owner does not have to use a punishment but rather teaches the bird appropriate behavior. The beak should not be "grabbed" or "thumped," as this can escalate the aggression. Birds should never be hit. Yelling or other types of drama can actually be entertaining for some birds, so the victim should always remain calm. The very effectiveness of the bite is what reinforces the behavior. Unless there is a significant anxiety component to the aggression, drug therapy is not indicated for this problem.

Prognosis is fair for the bird but guarded for the relationship between the owner and bird. The longer the duration of the problem, the more difficult it is to reverse the problem. One client of one of the authors (Welle) had a Scarlet Macaw that for eight years had controlled her by biting. Although the author established that this would not work with him within one session, the macaw still viciously attacked the owner whenever she did not comply with the bird's wishes. It is difficult for a bird with eight years of experience showing it can manipulate a person by biting to unlearn this behavior. However, the birds quickly learn that a new person cannot be controlled, and so they will no longer try as hard.

TERRITORIAL AGGRESSION

Territorial aggression is particularly common in certain species. Quaker Parakeets are well known for this trait. Conures, miniature macaws, African Grey Parrots, and amazon parrots are also prone to develop this problem. Breeding birds of all species tend to be territorial about their nest area and cage (Figure 18.1). In these birds, this behavior is considered desirable. Guarding of the nest territory is an important breeding cue. While the sex of many avian patients is unknown, it appears that territorial aggression is somewhat more common in males than in females.

Diagnostic criteria for territorial aggression are

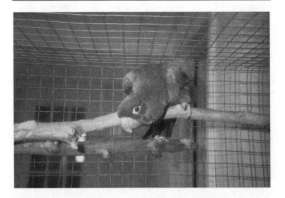

Figure 18.1.   Territorial behavior is normal in breeder birds such as this Mitred Conure (*Aratinga mitrata*).

very simple. Territorial aggression occurs when the bird is in or on its cage, playpen, or other living area. If this is not the case, the aggression cannot be territorial aggression. Aggressive behavior must be limited to these areas. It is possible, however, for a bird to exhibit both territorial aggression and other forms of aggression. Some fearful birds will appear to have territorial aggression because they attack when a hand comes into their cage. These birds have learned that there is no retreat within the cage and therefore will attack a hand as it enters the cage. The way to distinguish between the two is by observing the other behaviors. If fearful vocalizations occur, if the aggression occurs at locations other than the primary living space and the bird is intolerant of handling under various situations, the problem is more likely to be fear biting. However, fearful birds can attack in a confident way, without showing fear, if they have learned that the aggression works in getting the owner to withdraw. If the bird attacks without vocalizing or when the cage is not opened, but when away from the cage exhibits no fear or aggression, the problem is more likely territorial aggression.

Behavior modification for territorial aggression is multifaceted. In order to achieve the specific goals, general obedience training is essential. The step-up command should be automatic for the bird. This command is an important training tool. To avoid injury to the owner, the bird should be removed while servicing the cage. Owners should be schooled on atraumatic but secure towel restraint of the bird if necessary. Birds that will not leave the cage without biting should be caught and carried to a separate area. Some birds can be safely handled following voluntary exit from the cage. This will facilitate the other training measures.

An attempt should be made to make the bird less dependent on the cage. This helps both in the prevention and treatment of territorial aggression. Birds that spend most or all of their time in one cage can become viciously aggressive about defending it.[4] In the wild, birds roost in the same area each night. During the day, they travel to other locations to forage, usually with their flock. A two-cage housing system helps provide a more natural system (see chapter 26). A large, well-furnished cage or playpen should be used during the daytime to encourage activity. The cage should be rearranged frequently to promote adaptability in the bird. During the night, a smaller roosting cage with rather spartan accommodations should be used. Each morning the bird can be transported to the larger cage and each evening to the roosting cage. If further measures are needed, the bird can be meal fed twice daily in another location.

The bird should be integrated into the family social unit. Portable perching stations allow the bird to sit close to the activity of the family. This, combined with consistent handling and training, provides the bird with the social skills needed to be well-adjusted pets. The two-cage housing system described previously forces owners to handle birds at least twice daily to transport them.

Regularly scheduled handling and training sessions are important for maintaining socialization and control. The step up, rewarded with food treats, is especially important. A narrow T-stand should be used initially to train the bird. The T-stand is like a leash on a dog: it prevents the bird from moving too far. The T-stand is initially placed in a location away from the cage (different room). As training progresses, the T-stand can be moved closer and closer to the cage. Eventually, the step up can be practiced in the cage. This necessitates a widely opening cage door. The training should first be done by the person having the least problems, and then by other people. Every new person has to start over from the beginning, with the T-stand far away from the cage.

Psychotropic drugs are not generally indicated in the treatment of territorial aggression in birds.

The chemical basis of aggression is unknown in birds. Additionally, the prognosis for treatment of territorial aggression with behavioral modification alone is favorable.

MATE-RELATED AGGRESSION

Parrots are prone to developing unhealthy pair bonds with one of their owners. While a bird may bond to more than one person, only one is chosen for a mate. However, if the chosen mate is the only one who ever handles the bird, the aggressive tendencies will be much worse. Mate-related aggression occurs most commonly in hand-raised birds of larger parrot species. Amazon parrots, macaws, cockatoos, and Quaker Parrots are all commonly affected. Male birds are most often affected. The behavior often begins or becomes more serious at sexual maturity or during breeding season.

The aggression will most often occur in situations where the bird's favorite person is approached by someone else, such as another family member. The aggression may be directed toward the rival or paradoxically redirected toward the favorite person. Occasionally, an inanimate object such as a telephone, or a cavity such as an open drawer, may trigger the aggression. Unlike most other types of aggression, these birds will often attack or chase their victims. They are often exceptionally cuddly at other times, at least toward the favorite person.

To help minimize mate-related aggression, the bird should be socialized appropriately. The person to whom the bird has pair bonded should work to develop a more platonic bond. Interactions should be more active and dynamic, avoiding cuddling and petting. The bird should not be allowed on the shoulder. This position in close proximity to the face encourages pair bonding. Additionally, the damage done with a bite can be much greater. All members of the household should take the bird to novel, unfamiliar places so they can be seen as the familiar, comforting figure. In these locations, basic commands such as "step up" and "step down" should be practiced by all family members. The favored person should do all of the unpleasant tasks such as grooming, and otherwise largely ignore the bird until the problem is resolved. Only non-favored people should give favorite treats.

The attacking bird should be gently captured in

a towel and placed in the cage or other controlled area. Owners should be taught how to safely and effectively towel restrain these birds. If the owner can predict the aggression, the preferred person could leave swiftly and therewith remove the cause of the aggression.

In some cases, the aggressive behavior can be reduced with hormonal therapy. Leuprolide acetate can reduce the sexual hormones and thereby reduce the intensity of the aggressive behavior during the initial phases of behavior modification. Orchiectomy can reduce aggressiveness in some cases.[5]

REDIRECTED AGGRESSION

Occasionally, the person who provided the stimulus for the bite is not the one bitten. If a bird cannot reach the person it intends to bite, it will sometimes bite whomever happens to be close. Redirected aggression is not a diagnosis but refers to a mechanism that modifies other types of aggression. Frequently, it is mate-related aggression that gets redirected, in this case usually to the bonded person because he or she is usually close by. To treat the problem of redirected aggression, the aggression that is redirected needs to be addressed.

INTRASPECIFIC AGGRESSION

Aggression toward other birds represents another common problem in companion and avicultural birds. Many bird owners have more than one bird and injuries of one by another are relatively common. In aviculture, pairs must be kept together in the breeding season in order to produce offspring, so safe congregation is crucial. In many cases the causes for aggression between birds are the same as aggression toward humans. Fear, territorial defense, and mate-related aggression can all play a role. Often, however, the problem is a result of a lack of adequate flock social skills in the birds involved.[6] Many pet and breeding birds today have had little or no experience with other birds. They have not learned from parents or other flock members how to behave in a socially acceptable manner. The result may be aggression exhibited by or toward the poorly socialized bird. While some authors advise that parrots should be socialized specifically as replacement breeders, others advise keeping parrots as pets for only the first several years and then placing them into breeding collections.[7]

In pet birds, simply housing birds individually and supervising them when they are not confined can often avoid the problem. If cages are placed in proximity, the birds may become increasingly tolerant of the other bird. Care must be taken, especially when one bird is loose and the other is confined. It is very common for foot injuries to occur when a bird climbs on the cage of another bird, resulting in a bite to the foot from the confined bird. Occasionally conflicts arise because of limited access to resources. Mild aggression can sometimes be alleviated by providing extra resources, such as perching space, food and water dishes, and toys. Overcrowding can easily lead to aggression and is a major stressor for any captive animal.

Aggression toward mates is a very common problem, especially in cockatoos (see chapter 22). Male breeding parrots defend their territory vigorously. If the proximity of another pair stimulates aggressive behavior, this can be redirected toward the female. Visual barriers, at least in the area of the nest site, can help avoid this problem. It is also possible that the pair bond is dissolving.[8] While the pair bond is usually permanent, occasionally parrots will leave a former mate for another. By allowing flocking in the non-breeding season, the birds can either re-establish the pair bond or form a new pair prior to the next season.[6]

CONCLUSION

Like any behavioral disorder, improvement will usually occur slowly and gradually. Owners should be advised to keep a journal of their bird's behavior. The frequency, severity, and nature of any occurrence of aggression should be logged. A reduction in the frequency or severity of aggression indicates that the treatment plan is working. The patient should be re-evaluated every six to eight weeks and the client should be interviewed to determine if the treatment plan is being followed correctly. Alterations can be made if adequate progress has not been made. In cases where the problem has not improved, the diagnosis should be reassessed. Depending upon the severity of the problem and the personality of the owner, placement of the bird into a new home can be considered. If this situation occurs, the veterinarian should coach the new owner so that the same cycle does not begin again.

REFERENCES

1. Welle, K.R. 1998. "Psittacine behavior." Proc Annual Conf Assoc Avian Vet, pp. 371–377
2. Welle, K.R. 1999. *Psittacine behavior handbook.* Bedford, TX: Assoc Avian Vet Publication Office.
3. O'Farrell, V. 1995. "Effects of owner personality and attitudes on dog behaviour." In *The domestic dog,* ed. J. Serpell, pp. 153–158. Cambridge: Cambridge University Press.
4. Athan, M.S. 1993. *Guide to a well-behaved parrot.* Hong Kong: Barron's, pp. 36–54.
5. Bennet, R.A. 2002. "Reproductive surgery in birds." Proc Atlantic Coast Veterinary Conference.
6. Styles, D.K. 2002. "Captive psittacine behavioral reproductive husbandry and management: Socialization, aggression control, and pairing techniques." Proc Annu Conf Assoc Avian Vet Specialty Program.
7. Clubb, S.L. 1998. Captive management of birds for a lifetime. *JAVMA* 212:1243–1245.
8. Clubb, K.J., S.L. Clubb, S. Phillips, and S. Wolf. 1992. "Intraspecific aggression in cockatoos." In *Psittacine aviculture: Perspectives, techniques and research,* ed. R.M. Schubot, K.J. Clubb, and S.L. Clubb, chapter 8. Loxahatchee, FL: Avicultural Breeding and Research Center.

19
Parrot Vocalization

Laurie Bergman and Ulrike S. Reinisch

The ability to vocalize is arguably both one of the most and least endearing traits in a pet parrot. The popularity of some species of parrots as pets, such as African Greys, derives from their ability to speak, to mimic human speech and other noises. However, parrots' ability to vocalize and normal patterns of vocalization often become problematic for pet bird owners.

Naturalists have noted several features about psittacine vocalizations in the wild that have relevance for the captive management of these birds. First is the daily pattern of vocalization. In most species of parrots, especially those commonly kept as pets, such as amazons, macaws, and cockatoos, the flock will be quiet from sunset until the next dawn (Snyder 1987; Rowley 1990). At daybreak, the flock will vocalize and fly around the roosting area before setting out to forage for the day in a different location. Again, as dusk approaches, after the birds have returned to the roosting area, there is a period of vocalization.

In a household setting this pattern can lead to problems, especially when birds vocalize at sunrise and owners or their neighbors are not ready to wake up. Owners may also complain of birds "screaming" when they come home from work. Vocalizations at this time of day may be due to a combination of factors—greeting the returning "flock member" and normal, pre-sunset, vocalizations. The first step in treating these problems is owner education. Pet parrot owners must be aware that their birds, no matter how bonded they are to people and even if bred in captivity and hand-raised, are still wild animals. With the possible exceptions of Cockatiels and Budgies, pet parrots do not meet the basic definition of domesticated animals in that pet parrots are not genetically different from wild parrots as a result of se-

lective breeding (Hurnik 1995). As a starting point in treating any pet bird behavior problem, owners must understand that they may be able to modify the expression of their birds' normal behaviors but won't be able to completely eradicate these behaviors. In the case of morning and evening vocalizations, once owners understand that their birds will still vocalize twice daily, then they are ready to start to shape those periods of vocalization into more acceptable ones. Most species of parrots that are kept as pets are tropical or semi-tropical (Forshaw 1989). To replicate natural conditions they should be receiving close to 12 hours of light and 12 hours of dark each day. One easy way to control vocalizations is to control the bird's dark/light cycle. Covering cages or having birds sleep in a dark room allows owners to set when "sunrise" occurs. Most parrots will not vocalize in the morning until after daybreak. Likewise, owners may be able to shift evening vocalizations by controlling when "sunset" occurs. Owners can also redirect these natural periods of vocalization into more acceptable behaviors by giving the bird another activity to perform at these times. For example, in the evenings the owner can take advantage of the bird's natural proclivity to vocalize by using this time to teach the bird new phrases or sounds to say. Alternately, owners can pre-empt and reduce some of the vocalizations by giving the bird a new toy or special food at the times that it is likely to vocalize. It is important that the toy or treat be given before the bird starts to vocalize. If this is not the case then the bird may learn that by yelling it earns a reward.

Naturalists have also noted several different types of vocalizations from wild parrots. These include alarm calls, contact calls, food begging calls, and interspecific agonistic calls. Many of these vocalizations are learned by parrot chicks from their parents and flock mates. Naturally cross-fostered Galahs (*Cacatua roseicapilla*) that were reared by Pink Cockatoos (*Cacatua leadbeateri*) have contact calls like their foster parents, not like their own species. Budgerigars (*Melopsittacus undulates*) that are reared in isolation not only exhibit abnormal vocalizations but also abnormal behaviors. Among these abnormal behaviors is evidence of social bonding to inanimate objects exhibited by warbling as though courting selected objects (Farabaugh & Dooling 1996). A hand-reared pet parrot will not have the exact same vocalizations as its wild relatives, but it will show similar patterns of vocalizations and uses of vocalizations.

Because almost all species of psittacines are highly social, as flock dwellers parrots have developed a variety of vocalizations that serve exclusively or primarily as contact calls. These are calls that serve to identify where other members of the flock are and help promote flock cohesion. Unfortunately, most pet parrots are not maintained in flocks. Even if there are other birds in the household parrots often form inappropriate pair bonds with their owners. When separated from the owner these birds will vocalize. Initially they may give contact calls, which may progress to more distressed and anxious vocalizations if they receive no response to the calmer contact calls. In some birds this vocalization may only take place when the owner leaves the house. Other birds may give contact calls every time their owners leave their sight. One way to address this problem is by having the owner maintain auditory contact with the bird when in another part of the house. For some birds this can be as simple as hearing the owner whistling or talking while in another room. The owner's vocalizations need not be in response to the bird's contact calls but can begin when he or she leaves the room before the bird begins to vocalize.

In more severe cases the bird should be treated for separation anxiety. This treatment begins by reducing the bird's dependence upon the owner while the owner is at home. This is accomplished by limiting interactions with the bird, by making the interactions more structured through positive reinforcement-based training, and by providing the parrot with alternatives to interacting with the owner. These alternates can be toys, especially food-dispensing toys or toys that can be chewed up or shredded, or special food treats, especially challenging foods like nuts that must be cracked or whole fruits. Other visual and auditory stimuli, like television or radio, can help give the parrot another focus for its attention. The other part to a separation anxiety treatment plan is using a series of very short departures to desensitize the bird to being left alone. These departures must be brief enough that the bird does not experience any anxiety whatsoever. During these practice departures the parrot is provided with special food treats and toys to give it opportunities for other more rewarding behaviors than calling out to its owner.

Vocalizations that serve as alarm calls have also been identified in a number of parrot species. In some species, such as Cockatiels (*Nymphicus hollandicus*) and the Red-rumped Parrot (*Psephotus haematonotus*), several different types of alarm calls that indicate varying levels of distress have been identified (Pidgeon 1981). In a pet situation owners may hear these calls in response to actual or perceived threats to the birds. Many owners are able to identify the function of these particular vocalizations and realize that their birds are distressed and not "just screaming." This knowledge may allow the owner to respond to the screaming by removing the stimulus that is causing the alarm. For example, one of the author's (Bergman) Indian Ringneck Parakeets would only give an alarm call if a dog was near his cage. The owner learned to call the dog whenever she heard the bird's alarm call. Once the dog moved away from the bird's cage the bird would stop calling and relax.

Alarm calls can become problematic. By nature these calls tend to be loud and of a frequency that carries well in order to warn the entire flock and possibly drive away threats (Fernandez-Juricic et al. 1998). A pet parrot that alarm calls frequently can be quite disturbing to the people who must live with or near the bird. Furthermore, a pet parrot that is alarm calling frequently is a welfare issue. These vocalizations are given when the bird is in distress. The presence of frequent alarm calls can indicate a poor husbandry situation in which a bird is being kept in a distressing environment.

The first and most important step in treating a parrot with excessive alarm calls is to identify and remove the stimuli that are provoking the vocalizations. These stimuli may be inanimate objects in the bird's immediate environment (e.g., toys, cage furniture) or anywhere within the bird's line of sight. Other possible stimuli are people or other animals. Remembering that pet parrots are wild animals that are a prey species in the wild can help to identify the source of the bird's alarm. Alarm calls may be elicited by seeing potential predators, dogs, cats, birds of prey, snakes, and so forth in the house, through a window, or in pictures or on television.

Often parrots will give alarm calls directed at unfamiliar or familiar but less-favored people. Provided the bird is not showing other signs of more significant fear or distress, such as attempting to escape from the area, this behavior is best treated by ignoring it. If the alarming person approaches the bird, the bird may panic or act aggressively. If the owner or another favored person approaches and attempts to calm or reassure the bird, then the bird is being rewarded for screaming out alarm calls. This will teach the bird that making alarm calls works to get the owner's attention and may result in a bird that alarm calls simply as an attention-seeking behavior and not out of distress. Instead, the owner and the other people should wait until the bird has stopped screaming and then reward the bird with a delicious treat or an object to play with or attention and affection.

Pet parrots may alarm call in response to being in a new location or to changes in a familiar environment, such as new furniture or furniture that was moved. In this case "introducing" the bird to its environment is often sufficient to relieve the bird's distress. The owner should walk around the area with the bird, talking to the bird in an upbeat voice, as though this tour is the most fun thing ever to happen. The owner can touch things and gently show them to the bird. The key is for the owner to be relaxed and engaged with the environment and let the bird see that it is not threatening. The parrot will then relax and choose the level of interaction with the environment that it is comfortable with. The bird must not be pushed into interactions for which it is not ready.

If the bird is panicked by the fear-provoking stimulus or is unresponsive to the previously described approaches, then systematic desensitization and counterconditioning should be used to treat the bird's underlying fear and anxiety and

thereby reduce the problem vocalizations. After the fear-provoking stimulus has been identified and removed from the bird's environment, it is slowly reintroduced while the bird is rewarded for remaining calm and non-reactive. The stimulus is first introduced in a manner that does not cause any reaction. Gradually the level of stimulation is increased. This can be done by altering the form of the stimulus. For example, a bird that was panicked by tie-dyed t-shirts was first introduced to plain t-shirts, then t-shirts with a small area of tie-dye, then t-shirts that were tie-dyed all over. Distance from the stimulus should also be used to decrease the intensity of the stimulus. The rewards that the bird receives in the presence of the stimulus should be anything that the particular bird values highly. This can be food, toys, things to manipulate with its beak, petting, or being spoken to. Clicker training can also be a useful adjunct to a desensitization and counterconditioning protocol. In more extreme or refractory cases adjunct drug therapy may be useful.

Problems can also arise from learned vocalizations—words, phrases, and sounds that parrots learn to mimic. Parrots may accidentally or purposely be taught words or phrases that their owners would prefer they do not say. These may be as innocuous as an old flame's name or as embarrassing as obscenities. It is very likely that birds that are inadvertently exposed to expletives may repeat these words because they heard them said at a high volume and/or with a high level of emotion. Parrots are often attracted to dramatic vocal displays from people and therefore may find these phrases memorable.

Many parrots are especially adept at mimicking electronic noises, such as the beeps from microwaves, cell phones, and computers. Often these sounds can become quite wearing on people who have to hear them all day long. In addition, birds often learn that making these sounds causes people to do things, like get up to check the microwave or look for the ringing phone. The people's behavior becomes rewarding for the birds and encourages them to repeat these sounds more often.

To reduce these problematic learned vocalizations owners must be prepared to be very patient. As is the case with many learned, rewarded behaviors these vocalizations can be "unlearned" by ignoring them via the process of extinction. Since parrots are so responsive to subtle body language and facial expressions from people, owners must be prepared to be absolutely poker faced in the light of whatever their birds may be saying. Owners should be taught about the phenomenon of extinction bursts, whereby the bird may repeat the undesirable vocalization at a greater frequency or louder volume in response to the lack of reaction from the owner. Owners should also be aware that the slightest encouragement will result in a resumption of the undesired behavior. This often becomes important when there are visitors at the house or other people caring for the bird. People who do not have to live with the parrot may accidentally or purposely encourage the very vocalizations the owners have been actively working to extinguish. If the bird is not responding to the attempts at extinction a mild punishment may be added to the treatment plan. The punishment to be used, a form of social isolation, takes advantage of parrots' natural gregariousness. The instant the bird begins the unwanted vocalization all people present should turn away from the bird or even leave the room, thereby "isolating" the bird for a brief (30 seconds) period. The idea is to teach the bird that the word or sound in question no longer gets a positive response; instead it drives people away.

Another situation of learned vocalizations creating problems for pet parrot owners occurs after a person in the household has had a cold. The parrot begins to mimic the person's coughs and sneezes. Often owners will present these birds to a veterinarian fearing that the bird has contracted the person's cold. These birds show no other signs of upper respiratory tract disease and their coughs and sneezes sound like human coughs and sneezes, not avian ones. If these vocalizations are worrisome for the owners ignoring them is the best treatment.

The presenting complaint for problem vocalizations is often simply that the bird is "screaming." Although careful history taking may reveal that this is a problem that involves primarily contact calls (e.g., separation anxiety) or alarm calls (e.g., when there are visitors in the house), sometimes it is difficult to pinpoint such a cause for the problem vocalizations. In many such cases the problem is primarily one of learned vocalizations. The parrot has learned that people pay at-

tention to a screaming bird. Often the owners believe that the attention they are providing is negative and should stop the screaming. This often consists of owners yelling at their birds or returning to the room where the bird is to "scold" the bird. Some owners will attempt other forms of punishment that are inappropriate and clearly ineffective if the problem continues. In cases of attention-seeking screaming the treatment is the same as for the bird that is saying unwanted words; attempt to extinguish the unwanted behavior by ignoring it. Some owners can successfully interrupt a screaming parrot by covering the bird's cage. The cage should be uncovered immediately after the bird quiets down and the bird should be given other things like toys or food to occupy its time. Another way of reducing the volume of a parrot's vocalizations, whether attention-seeking "screaming" or normal morning and evening vocalizations, is by teaching the bird to whisper. Reward the bird with attention, food, or toys for speaking softly. This approach allows the bird to engage in a normal behavior but modifies that behavior into a form that is more acceptable for life in captivity.

In rare cases parrots' screaming becomes a stereotypic behavior. Like all stereotypic behaviors this can be thought of as an indication of inadequate husbandry and a welfare problem. The bird's husbandry situation, including but not limited to feeding, water source, caging, cage location, availability of toys, perch variety, light cycle, and contact with other birds/people, should be addressed. Some of these birds might benefit from treatment with a psychotropic medication. Drug choices would be similar to those used to treat psychogenic feather picking.

REFERENCES

Farabaugh, S.M., and R.J. Dooling. 1996. "Acoustic communication in parrots: Laboratory and field studies of budgerigars, *Melopsittacus undulates.*" In *Ecology and evolution of acoustic communication in birds,* ed. D.E. Kroodsma and E.H. Miller, pp.97–117. Ithaca, NY: Cornell University Press.

Fernandez-Juricic, E., M.B. Maretlla, and E.V. Alvarez. 1998. Vocalizations of the blue-fronted amazon (*Amazona aestiva*) in the Chancani Reserve, Cordoba, Argentina. *Wilson Bulletin* 110 (3):352–362.

Forshaw, J.M. 1989. *Parrots of the world,* 3rd (rev.) ed. London: Blandford.

Hurnik, J.F. 1995. *Dictionary of farm animal behavior,* 2nd ed. Ames: Iowa State University Press.

Pidgeon, R. 1981. Calls of the galah *Cacatua roseicapilla* and some comparisons with four other species of Australian Parrots. *Emu* 81:158–168.

Rowley, I. 1990. *Behavioral ecology of the galah, Eolophus roseicapillus: In the wheatbelt of Western Australia.* Chipping Norton, NSW: Surrey Beatty.

Snyder, N.F.R. 1987. *The parrots of Luquillo: Natural history and conservation of the Puerto Rican parrot.* Los Angeles: Western Foundation of Vertebrate Zoology.

20
Parrots and Fear

Liz Wilson and Andrew U. Luescher

Fear is a critical issue with parrots, especially when trying to establish a relationship of trust in a companion animal situation. Fear is also likely a major cause of stress in companion psittacine birds. Parrots are, after all, small prey animals and humans are large predators.

Fear can be caused by a variety of stimuli in the captive environment. There is the low-grade fear generated by a caged bird that is safely out of reach but watched constantly by an intently predatory cat. There is the fear generated when a cage-bound parrot is asked to leave the sanctuary of its cage space; the fear that is generated when a shy parrot is required to step onto the hand of a stranger; the fear caused to many psittacine birds by the proximity of a hyperactive child. Additionally, there is an anxious parrot's fear when a human shows trepidation when reaching for it, and the fear caused by something new being thrust into a parrot's personal space.

In other words, fear can be the result of an endless variety of things, many of which humans do not perceive as frightening. It is undoubtedly difficult for a predator to perceive the world as prey animals do. Unfortunately, many owners fail to comprehend the validity of parrots' fear responses. As a result, instead of being patient and reassuring, they become irritated with frightened birds, apparently believing that the birds will "get over" their fear if the human forces the issue sufficiently. This bullying tactic is ineffective; indeed, it can increase the birds' fear exponentially. Instead, humans must be sensitive to a parrots' fears and, depending on the stimulus, adjust the environment to avoid frightening parrots or to gradually desensitize the birds to the stimulus.

Additionally, psittacine birds tend to be neophobic, which is understandable for prey animals; parrots undoubtedly survive longer in the wild if they approach new things with extreme caution. In the captive situation, this type of fear manifests as terror of a new toy placed in the cage, the owner's new hairdo, or a new picture on the wall near the bird's cage.

FEAR-BASED AGGRESSION

Fear manifests itself in the basic *fight or flight* format, and parrots respond instinctively to a perceived threat by attempting to fly away. If flight is impossible due to clipped wings and/or being trapped in a cage, the alternative is to fight, and the birds will respond aggressively, which usually manifests as biting.

Fear-based biting falls into the category of *the best defense is a good offense*. This situation will be worsened if humans respond aggressively to this behavioral strategy. Aggression begets aggression, and trying to get the fear-based biter to back down will only instill more fear and, hence, more aggression. Instead, people need to study the situation and again look for techniques to gradually desensitize the bird to the perceived fear stimulus, or avoid the situation entirely.

Case Study: The "Suddenly Mean" Grey

Normally sweet and mild tempered, Lily, a 9-month-old African Grey hen (*Psittacus erithacus erithacus*) abruptly became hostile when her owner's friends tried to handle her. She became especially antagonistic with the owner's new boyfriend, striking quickly and biting hard.

Lily the Grey was biting from fear-based aggression. Frightened by unfamiliar people, she needed to be better socialized. If not identified and handled properly, a shy parrot like Lily can blossom into a determined fear biter. Lily's person needed to reassure her that she was safe when interacting with others.

Introducing her to other people in neutral territory with patience and sensitivity, the owner taught Lily that new people are fun and interesting. Initially, she only expected Lily to step onto the outsider's hand politely, and then step immediately back onto her trusted caretaker's hand. Lily's good manners were then rewarded lavishly with smiles and praise. Each time Lily did this successfully, she discovered that positive things happened when she was compliant with new people. As a result, Lily gradually learned to enjoy interactions with strangers.

"PHOBIC" PARROTS

According to human psychology, a phobia is defined as "any unfounded or unreasonable dread or fear."[1] Indeed, it is quite logical for a wild parrot to be afraid of a predator, and blatant terror at a human's approach would be expected in untamed psittacine birds. However, this is not the case with domestically raised companion parrots. When there is no precipitating incident and the bird abruptly acts terrified of people, noises, or shadows, the use of the term "phobic" would appear appropriate.

Dealing with the "phobic" or neurotically terrified parrot can be tremendously exasperating. The classic history involves an excitable young bird that abruptly reacts to specific people as if they were deadly predators. This is especially disturbing when the primary object of terror is the previously loved owner, and the parrot flails around its cage, screaming and trying to escape when the owner approaches. Particularly distressing to the avian veterinarian is the bird that demonstrates severe anxiety or phobia as a direct result of a veterinary visit.

People are contacting parrot behavior consultants about increasing numbers of "phobic" birds, but this may indicate either an increase in this phenomenon, increased recognition of the problem, or an increase in the use of these terms. Certainly, there is much discussion on the Internet about this behavior, and the term "phobic" is increasingly bantered about.

Unfortunately, many people perceive the word "phobic" as a synonym for the word "fear," which is totally inaccurate. A truly phobic bird is not simply afraid of new toys or new people. Despite being domestically bred and hand-raised by people, such a bird acts like a wild parrot upon the approach of a deadly predator. A phobic parrot is hyperreactive to direct eye contact, often going into what appears to be a full-blown panic attack if people stare.[2] It is hyperreactive to sound, movement, and especially human hands. A phobic parrot has an invisible line around its territory, which identifies its comfort zone. Once invaded, the bird will thrash wildly in a frenzied flight response. As a result, broken blood feathers are common, and serious soft tissue damage can result to keel and wing tips. In extreme cases, parrots can actually pulverize their metacarpals and phalanges in repetitive frantic efforts to flee (L. Clark, personal communication, 1998).

Nervous psittacine birds are frequently apprehensive of new things but unruffled during handling by trusted humans. These birds are not phobics. Confusing the issue further, there appear to be degrees of phobic behaviors, ranging from mild to severe, with a gray area between a bird that is simply very frightened and one that is borderline phobic.

Generally, aggressive birds are not truly phobic (J. Doss, personal communications, 1997–1998). Aggression and avoidance behaviors are two responses to the same stimulus.[3] An apprehensive parrot that views itself as being in jeopardy or vulnerable can either flee or attack. Since fear is excessive in a phobic parrot, a truly phobic parrot would always try to escape.

Phobic behaviors are more likely in certain species, including *Poicephalus* (i.e., Meyer's [*P. meyeri*] and Senegal Parrots [*P. senegalus*]); small cockatoos like the Rose-breasted (*Eolophus roseicapillus*), Citron-crested (*Cacatua sulphurea citrinocristata*), and Triton (*C. s. triton*); Eclectus Parrots (*Eclectus roratus*) and African Greys (especially the Congo [*Psittacus erithacus erithacus*]). It is not surprising that these species also are prone to feather destructive behaviors (FDB).

As a rule, phobic behaviors are seen more frequently with juvenile or adolescent parrots. Nevertheless, it is important to make a distinction between an adolescent parrot demonstrating normal pubescent challenges and the phobic. It is a hallmark of psittacine adolescence for young parrots to balk at compliancy by running away from hands that request the birds step up, refusing to exit the cage, or throwing themselves around the cage when people draw near.[4]

Theories abound about the etiology of phobic behaviors. Infrequently, owners describe a specific incident that appeared to trigger this behavior, but this probably is a stressor, not the actual etiology. The potential for phobic behaviors in high-strung species is likely to increase if neonates are maintained in too much light—for example, in glass aquariums under neon lighting in a pet store. Indeed, aviculturists note that neonate psittacine birds actually gain weight faster if kept in the dark.[5] This overexposure to light when parrots are very young appears to predispose parrots to fear-based behaviors. Linden suggests eliminating the use of fluorescent lights around phobics, due to the increased sensitivity of avian vision.[6] Rearing parrot chicks alone in a restricted environment with little handling also contributes to exaggerated emotional responses later in life.[7]

Physical and psychological abuse such as traumatic capture and restraint techniques such as overly aggressive toweling can predispose a parrot to phobic behavior.[8] Indeed, overly aggressive toweling is considered a direct cause of "fear-induced behavioral disease."[9] However, ethologists agree that aggressive handling or "punishment" is not the only reason that parrots become phobic (A. Luescher, J. Oliva-Purdy, L. Seibert, personal communications, 2003). There is no history of abuse with most of these cases.

Case Study: The Non-Phobic Phobic

Care must be taken to accurately diagnose phobics, since they are handled so differently from the more common problem behaviors seen in companion parrots. The first author (Wilson) worked with a "phobic" Yellow-naped Amazon (*Amazona ochrocephala auropalliata*) that turned out to have an idiopathic medical problem that predisposed the bird to falling from the hand because it could not grip properly with its feet. Multiple falls taught the bird a direct correlation between handling and pain. The result was a dramatic fear response when people approached. Interestingly enough, the Amazon's screaming and flailing was eliminated by the use of the dopamine antagonist haloperidol (Haldol™, Henry Schein) (D. Kupersmith, personal communications, 1997–1998).

CLASSICAL CONDITIONING AND THE FEAR RESPONSE

Birds can learn by pairing neutral and unpleasant stimuli. An example would be association of the owner's hand with restraint or the bad taste of a medication that the owner forced down the bird's throat. Another example would be fear shown when scolded because of previous punishment following scolding. Classical or Pavlovian conditioning results in the previously neutral stimulus becoming aversive, that is, evoking a fear response.

Owners of high-strung birds must learn to relax prior to approaching their animals. Movements must be deliberate and calm so they do not heighten the parrot's anxieties. Hyper owners often exacerbate a difficult situation, pushing an already apprehensive bird into a full-blown phobic state. This is especially true in dramatically frightening situations, such as natural disasters and veterinary office visits.

There have been multiple episodes in California with psittacine birds responding to the horror of an earthquake by becoming phobic with the owner. There have also been multiple situations where sensitive parrots become phobic with their owners after a traumatic visit to the avian veterinarian. In these situations, the suspicion is that the frightened bird is transferring its fear of the situation to the owner (S. Blanchard, personal communications, 1996). When parrots are traumatized, it is a natural inclination for the human to rush over to reassure the bird, hysterically worried about the animal's safety. As a result, the person's high anxiety terrorizes the bird even more, and its fear is transferred directly to the owner. This unfortunate devolution can cause a parrot to become phobic with the person it used to trust above all.

THE VETERINARY EXAM ROOM: ADVICE TO THE CLIENTS

Many psittacine birds, especially youngsters, react very negatively to visits to the veterinary office. It is important for clients to understand that they will make the situation worse if they are distressed by necessary procedures. As a result, they could not only terrify their animals more but also do serious harm to their bond with their parrots. Consequently, many experienced avian veterinarians suggest—or even insist—that procedures be done away from the owners. However, care must be taken not to give the impression the veterinarian has anything to hide, nor should the clinician automatically remove the bird from the exam room without discussion with the owner. If clients choose to be present, they should be counseled against petting their birds while under restraint, as serious bites can result. The owner should also not tell the parrot "It's okay," since being under restraint is NOT okay as far as the bird is concerned. That phrase should only be used to reassure a bird when something is intimidating but not actually dangerous (such as carrying a large object through the room). Using it when a bird is under restraint risks negating the potential of this phrase to reassure since it becomes associated with an aversive event.

To prevent any connection between owners and traumatic office visits, seriously upset parrots should be returned immediately into their carriers, *not* into the arms of their humans. Clients can then verbally reassure their birds calmly, without any physical contact. Once home, the owners should open the carrier door and walk away. Continuing to reassure in a soft voice, they allow the birds to climb out on their own. Clients should continue to soothe the birds verbally and observe from a distance. They should not approach the birds until the parrots' body language relaxes.

OPERANT CONDITIONING AND THE FEAR RESPONSE

A fear reaction can become conditioned through avoidance conditioning or negative reinforcement (see chapter 16). This is especially true if the owner either retreats (if the owner was the threat) or removes the bird from the frightening stimulus and/or shelters the bird. The removal of the threatening stimulus is the reinforcement for the fear response. Behavior conditioned that way becomes very reliable and resistant to extinction.

Birds may also learn to exhibit a fear response in situations where they are not frightened, because they learned that they can manipulate or control a situation. For instance, by acting terrified and quivering, running away, or flailing about, a bird invariably makes humans withdraw rather than allowing the bird to injure itself. In this way, a bird may prevent being picked up and put back into the cage. Therefore, exhibiting a

fear response can be a clear manifestation of a *refusal to interact*.

On the other hand, birds rarely learn to exhibit a fear response through positive reinforcement. Therefore, giving food treats to a frightened bird is very unlikely to condition fearful behavior and is always appropriate (although if too frightened the bird may not take them), and the bird will learn to associate the frightening (but in fact harmless) situation with something pleasant.

It is important to go through a careful diagnostic process to determine the extent to which learning contributes to the performance of fearful behavior. Videotapes can be especially valuable with these types of cases, as the parrot's behavior and body language can be observed when it is in its own environment. It is impossible to judge a parrot's level of fear in its own environment by observation in an alien setting such as a veterinary exam room. Indeed, fear behaviors can change tremendously in a parrot's own environment when a stranger enters the space. For more information regarding the use of videotapes, see chapter 16.

Case Study: The Umbrella That Was "Phobic" about Hands

This situation is exemplified by a consultation the first author (Wilson) did a few years ago, with a seven-year-old male Umbrella Cockatoo (*Cacatua alba*) that had become "phobic about hands." The bird was also "terrified" of the owner's new boyfriend. Upon questioning, it turned out that the cockatoo would take food from people's hands but ran away when humans asked it to step up on command. In this situation, the intelligent bird had learned that people would not press the issue if the cockatoo acted afraid, thus enabling the bird total freedom to do as he pleased.

Working with the bird away from its own territory, the owner used positive reinforcement to convince the cockatoo that following commands was a good thing, and the owner's problems with the bird were resolved.

Fear reactions can also be enhanced through learning if the fear-evoking stimulus is of short duration or if the bird can escape the stimulus. In these cases, from the bird's point of view, the fear or escape reaction appears "successful" in avoiding the expected harm. Fear reactions conditioned in this way are very persistent.

REHABILITATION OF THE PHOBIC OR NEUROTICALLY FRIGHTENED PARROT

Rehabilitation of phobic birds can be a painfully slow process, but phobics can be helped, with experience and exquisite patience.[10] However, misinterpretation and mishandling of birds with excessive fear behaviors can reinforce terrified and frantic behavior. The use of anxiolytic drugs is often indicated to speed up the process and reduce the anxiety to a level at which the bird is capable of learning. The owner has to find a way to give the drugs in a non-traumatic way or application of the drugs itself will increase the level of fear.

The first task of rehabilitation is to begin to reestablish a relationship of trust. Blanchard suggests the owner bring a chair as close to the cage as possible without frightening the bird and sit there daily. Reading aloud quietly or singing (even badly) yields a positive reaction from the phobic psittacine bird (J. Doss, personal communications, 1997; S. Blanchard, personal communications, 1997).[11] This procedure uses the phenomenon of habituation: an animal will stop reacting to a neutral stimulus, that is, a stimulus that does not have any pleasant or aversive consequences, through prolonged exposure. No direct eye contact should be made but instead one should use what Blanchard calls "soft eyes," where the owners look at the bird very briefly, then turn their eyes and face away (looking away becomes a negative reinforcement for being relaxed; see chapter 16). This procedure often reassures the frightened bird.[12] Gradually the chair can be moved closer and closer to the cage, and the owner can look for increasingly longer times at the bird. This procedure is called systematic desensitization and will likely be more expedient once the bird can be rewarded for staying relaxed.

Food treats work well, if the parrot is not too frightened to take treats from the owner. The parrot can also be provided with its favorite food in its cage only during these sessions. In this way, the times during which the owner sits by the cage become associated with something very pleasant (counterconditioning).

Phobics are often terrified of strong light and are often more comfortable in lower light. An insufficient dark period can also increase arousal and reactivity, and owners should be recommended to place the bird in a different cage for the night in a dark, quiet room. Frightened parrots are also easily alarmed by sounds, but soft music often soothes them more than total silence.

Allowing a phobic bird to regrow its wing feathers frequently helps in building its self-confidence. Owners should be carefully instructed on techniques as to how to keep the bird safe while flighted (J. Doss, personal communications, 1997). In some cases where fearful parrots are flighted, trimming of the wings may become necessary, however (see later).

Rehabilitation should also entail letting the bird choose when and how it wishes interaction. Getting "in the bird's face" and forcing the issue will only make things worse. The bird needs to progress at its own speed and cannot be hurried.

Because rehabilitating a phobic parrot can be such a slow process, it is recommended that clients start keeping a daily diary. By describing the signs of a parrot's fears in great detail, as well as recording the miniscule signs of progress, owners are better able to see that actual progress is happening, albeit slowly. These notes can greatly assist clients later, when frustration mounts due to the agonizingly protracted rehabilitation process.

Learned fears can be unlearned, although in birds this may take a very much longer time than, for example, in dogs. Treatment of fear can be achieved through systematic desensitization, counterconditioning, and response substitution. The use of anxiolytic drugs as an adjunct to the behavior modification technique may prove useful or even necessary.

SYSTEMATIC DESENSITIZATION

This is a technique used to reduce or eliminate a response (e.g., fear or aggression) to a stimulus. The animal is trained to quiescence. In a parrot that may mean sitting quietly on a T-stand or the owner's hand. The stimulus is then introduced at a low intensity (e.g., recording of a noise at low intensity, stranger from a distance) and the animal is rewarded for quiet behavior. Once the animal has habituated to the stimulus at low intensity, the intensity is increased gradually, and the procedure repeated. The increase in stimulus intensity has to be so small that no fear response is ever elicited.

Although being in full flight may generally increase a bird's self-confidence, it may be necessary to at least temporarily clip a bird in order to desensitize it to a frightening stimulus and prevent self-reinforcing precipitous escape reactions.

Systematic desensitization can only be used if the stimulus can be identified, reproduced, and its intensity controlled. The handler has to be able to present the stimulus initially at low enough an intensity that the bird does not react. Furthermore, the naturally occurring stimulus has to be avoided until behavior modification has been completed. If these conditions cannot be met, drug desensitization can be useful. In this procedure, an anxiolytic drug is given at a dose that allows the bird to function normally and without fear. The dose is very gradually reduced, which is the equivalent of increasing the intensity of a threatening stimulus slightly. The bird needs exposure to the stimuli he should be comfortable with throughout the treatment. If the drug dose is reduced gradually enough, the bird never shows fear and can eventually be taken off drugs altogether.

COUNTERCONDITIONING (IN CLASSICAL CONDITIONING)

This refers to a procedure to change the meaning of a previously conditioned stimulus. For example, a previously fear-evoking but harmless stimulus such as the sound of the vacuum cleaner when always paired with food becomes a conditioned stimulus for food. Fearful behavior (the previous conditioned response to the stimulus) is replaced by a pleasant emotional response.

RESPONSE SUBSTITUTION (OFTEN INCORRECTLY CALLED "COUNTERCONDITIONING")

This refers to changing the meaning of a discriminatory stimulus (i.e., the fear-evoking situation). The aim is to replace undesirable behavior with desirable behavior in a given situation. This is achieved by controlling the contingencies so that the undesirable behavior is no longer successful and the desirable behavior is reinforced.

The situation in which undesirable behavior usually occurs becomes a discriminatory stimulus for *desirable* behavior. The desirable behavior should be incompatible with the undesirable behavior (e.g., bird stepping up instead of biting).

Response substitution is often used in conjunction with desensitization (e.g., training for quiescence instead of fearful or aggressive behavior,

while exposing the bird to increasingly intensive stimuli).

TRAINING

Clicker training is another way of increasing the bird's self-confidence and reducing its fear, especially of the owner. It can be done hands-off from a distance in a non-threatening way. Clicker training allows for consistent and thus predictable, stress-free interaction between bird and owner. It allows for efficient communication between bird and owner and provides the bird with the ability to predict and control its environment, thereby increasing self-confidence and well-being. Most birds really enjoy being trained that way. The only problem might be how to give food treats as rewards to a frightened parrot.

PREVENTION

The methods used to encourage a psittacine bird to develop its full capability as a companion animal are the same ones used to prevent the development of high-strung or phobic personalities. The development of these skills begins in babyhood with the aviculturist and hand feeder and continues with the future owners. These techniques include

- the nurturing of self-confidence and individual potential during early development
- normal fledging, then gradual clipping prior to sale (if necessary). This enhances a young bird's self-confidence[13]
- abundance feeding and gradual weaning based on the bird's development, not the human's convenience
- the establishment of clear and consistent behavioral guidelines in the new home[14]
- the encouragement of self-sufficiency through independent play

For more detail on these subjects, see chapter 11.

CONCLUSION

Anxious parrots need to learn that they are safe and can trust the humans around them to keep them secure. Only through infinite patience can pathologically frightened parrots be rehabilitated, and trying to bully a frightened bird through its fear will make the situation exponentially worse. When working with cases of neurotically terrified birds, often the true function of the clinician is to support the owners while they make the painstakingly slow journey back to a trusting relationship with their beloved companion parrots.

REFERENCES

1. American Psychiatric Association. 1994. *The diagnostic and statistical manual of mental disorders,* 4th ed. Washington, DC: APA, p. 443.
2. Blanchard, S. 1998. "Phobic behavior in companion parrots." Proc Ann Conf Int Avicult Soc, Orlando, FL.
3. Dodman, N.H. 1998. "Pharmacologic treatment of aggression on veterinary patients." In *Psychopharmacology of animal behavior disorders,* ed. N.H. Dodman and L. Schuster, pp. 41–63. Malden, MS: Blackwell Science.
4. Wilson, L. 1998. "Phobic psittacines: An increasing phenomenon?" Proc Ann Conf AAV, pp. 125–131.
5. Silva, T. 1991. *Psittaculture: The breeding, rearing and management of parrots.* Ontario Canada: Silvio Mattacchione & Co, p. 63.
6. Parrot Education and Adoption Center. 2002. "Ask the Experts" roundtable discussion. San Diego, CA.
7. Sheehan, K.L. 2001. The effects of environmental enrichment and post-natal handling on the development, emotional reactivity and learning ability of juvenile nanday conures (*Nandayus nenday*). MS thesis, Purdue University.
8. Wilson, L. 1998. "Phobic psittacines: An increasing phenomenon?" Proc Ann Conf AAV, pp. 125–131.
9. Speer, B. 2001. "The clinical consequences of routine grooming procedures." Proc Ann Conf AAV, pp. 109–115.
10. Wilson, L. 2000. "Behavior problems in pet parrots." In *Manual of avian medicine,* ed. G. Olsen and S. Orosz, pp. 124–147. Philadelphia: Mosby.
11. Leinneweber, T. My ms. duncan, African ark. Unpublished.
12. Blanchard, S. 1992. Soft eye, evil eye. *Pet bird report* 92/2 (2):1–5.
13. Cravens, E. 1996. The progressive wing clip method. *Birdkeeping Naturally*.
14. Wilson, L. 1995. "Behavior problems in adolescent parrots." Proc Ann Conf Assoc Av Vet, pp. 415–418.

21

Problem Sexual Behaviors of Companion Parrots

Fern Van Sant

INTRODUCTION

Psittacine species have become popular as companion animals because they demonstrate many kinds of social behavior that humans find familiar and enjoyable. Such endearing traits as beauty, intelligence, and mimicry have led humans to adopt them as members of their family. Recognizing that some of these traits are innate and genetically determined will allow for a new and better understanding of companion psittacine behavior and enable us to better predict responses of different species to the conditions of pet bird care. Developing an appreciation for how and why innate behaviors can be triggered by specific actions or conditions will hopefully lead to better and healthier lives for captive psittacine birds.

Understanding innate behaviors of companion psittacines requires an appreciation for the intricate physiologic and hormonal events that adapt a species to an environmental niche. Seasonal events such as migration and molting have been observed, investigated, and found to be initiated by environmental events and driven by endocrine mechanisms.[1–3] Observations of psittacine species in the wild and the experience of aviculturists and pet bird owners support a similar pattern of environmental triggers capable of inciting reproductive behaviors. Recent advances in neurophysiology are unraveling the intricate processes of initiation and expression of innate behaviors in response to environmental stimuli. Although this research has focused specifically on the mechanisms of context-driven song, it is allowing for a completely novel view of how innate potential can lead to the expression of specific behaviors in certain situations.[4–6]

Reproductive behaviors observed in the wild, such as pair bonding, courtship regurgitation, cavity seeking, nest building, territorial aggression, and copulation, are often displayed in a home setting, though with human "flocks." Females of some species lay large numbers of eggs over extended periods of time to a point of complete physical collapse and failure. The reproductive drive can also lead to behaviors that render the bird difficult or impossible to live with. These behaviors often include incessant screaming, sudden aggression toward favored (or not favored) humans, and destructive attempts to excavate nests in closets, couches, and drawers. As many species are represented in the pet trade, there exists extreme variability as to when behaviors will start, which will be displayed, and how long they may continue.[7]

In the wild, the expression of these largely reproductive behaviors would be regulated by environmental conditions, pair bond formation, and the social hierarchy of the flock. Environmental cues such as photoperiod, temperature, rainfall, available food supply, the presence of nesting material, or the presence of a mate can stimulate reproductive activity in birds.[3, 8, 9] Pair bond formation is enhanced with regurgitation, copulation, nest-site inspection, feeding, and mutual preening.[10] When favorable environmental conditions are present, opportunistic breeders can become active. Other species may not even breed on a yearly basis. The hypothalamic-pituitary-gonadal (HPG) axis, responsible for controlling reproductive development and subsequent reproductive behaviors, is triggered when environmental conditions are appropriate for the species.

Behaviors that enhance the pair bond are also recognized as triggering cues for reproductive activity.[10] In other words, the hormones flow when triggered by favorable conditions. In the case of companion psittacine birds, under constrained circumstances, many of the conditions of pet bird care are capable of triggering reproductive behaviors.

Unfortunately, as companion birds, parrots are not subjected to the normal limiting factors of their native environment and behavioral interactions with a flock. In fact, pair bonded owners often indulge their birds, providing them with several of the environmental and behavioral cues that can trigger the HPG axis. Owners often feed a varied, nutrient-rich diet daily (with possible increases in fat and protein), provide a nest (cage) and nesting material (newspaper), and, inadvertently, provide themselves as a perceived mate. They sometimes feed the bird warm, soft food, much as might occur during courtship feeding. Owners encourage the pair bond formation by "preening" the birds with petting (often including the tail and back areas) and allowing excessive preening to their person. In short, the owners inadvertently encourage reproductive behavior over a long period. The abundance of these environmental cues and pair bond activities in a home setting may encourage the early development of both clinical and behavioral problems, stemming from the reproductive drive.

Attempting to explain the sexual behaviors of companion psittacine birds without understanding their biology is impossible. With continued investigation, we are likely to find that the biological niche that supports the existence of a species also directs the timing of sexual behavior and reproduction. That said, it is possible to piece together what we have observed throughout the last 30 years and overlay that information with general reproductive biology, avian science, and psittacine biology. We will then begin to interpret behaviors carefully.

This discussion will identify and address significant clinical and behavioral problems that appear to develop over time because of chronic hormonal stress from the abundance of environmental cues and pair bond enhancing behaviors provided in many homes. Clinical conditions include those obviously related to reproductive physiology such as chronic egg production, egg peritonitis, and yolk embolis [11, 12] An effort will be made to explain many conditions of feather loss and feather-destructive behaviors that seem to be the result of abnormal, long-term, hormonal stress.[13] Other clinical conditions including degenerative changes of pelvic and abdominal muscle that may result in herniation or prolapse are typical of chronic hormonal stress or overproduction. Chronic egg laying may drain calcium stores, predisposing the hen to dystocia and osteoporosis.[10] Dramatic and abnormal conditions of bone are frequently seen in female birds demonstrating reproductive behaviors over protracted periods of time.[10]

By carefully examining the many complicated interactions between psittacine birds and their various natural environments, we will be better able to interpret social and sexual behaviors of captive companion psittacine birds. This improved understanding will lead to more effective medical intervention when necessary and hopefully improved preventative care.

PSITTACINE BEHAVIORAL BIOLOGY

Psittacine species are thought to derive from an ancient class of birds. It is considered likely that these birds have a more than 30-million-year history, with their roots in the ancient landmass of Gondwanaland. As landmasses slowly drifted and continents formed, the evolutionary processes that drove speciation slowly produced the three families and 332 species of the order Psittaciformes that we now know.[14, 15]

Of the 332 species known today, there are clear distinctions between psittacine birds based on geographical distribution. Neotropical species (from Central, South, and rarely North America) account for nearly two-thirds of all psittacine species. At first glance, they appear to be a diverse group of birds, but Neotropical species share many physical and behavioral traits and represent only one subfamily (Psittacinae). In contrast are the 109 species from Australia, New Zealand, and the Philippines that represent all three subfamilies of psittacine species (Loriinae, Cacatuinae, and Psittacinae). This incredible diversity of species is thought to result from the relatively long isolation of these geographic areas as well as the absence of pressure from mammals. Only 34 species are found in Africa, India, and Southeast Asia.[14–16]

If any single evolutionary tendency of these birds were to be singled out, it would have to be their flexibility to adapt to an impressive range of habitats. In order to understand the needs and behaviors of companion parrots, we must acknowledge the individual adaptations that species have made to survive in their distinctive environments. Viewing psittacine species from the perspective of evolution offers insights into many of the unique adaptations and behaviors that we recognize as characteristic of parrots. Most psittacine species display an uncanny ability to learn, socialize, and adapt. Some of these behaviors have been studied extensively.[17–19] Other physical and behavioral traits such as feather color, vocalizations, food preferences, learning abilities, photoperiod responsiveness, and breeding behavior may reflect adaptations to very different climates and environments over millennia. Once developed, an evolutionary perspective may offer a better understanding of many attributes and behaviors that owners and behaviorists have found puzzling or difficult.

Innate Behaviors

Innate, or "hardwired," behaviors are inherited, genetically driven, and species-specific like songs and nest design. These are observed in individuals raised independently of conspecifics. Learned behaviors are those acquired by impressionable individuals. These behaviors include imprinting, flying, food identification, and navigation. As a member of a flock, each individual bird must learn a complex set of vocalizations and body signals to maintain cohesiveness. Individuals in a flock manifest an innate ability to conform.[15, 20] Innate and learned behaviors support the group dynamic and facilitate social order. Although the mechanisms of expression of innate and learned behaviors at a molecular level remain poorly defined, ongoing research by Erich Jarvis at Duke University is identifying the roles of specific parts of the brain that direct certain innate behaviors under a set of external conditions.[4–6] He is also unraveling the ways that complex behaviors, both innate and learned, are triggered and expressed in an individual.

Reproductive Behaviors

Many of the commonly observed and commonly misunderstood behaviors of companion psittacine species are reproductive in nature and stem from activation of the HPG axis, as well as from pair bond formation.[10] These behaviors include cavity seeking (the drive to find a small dark hideaway), nest preparation (shredding of paper or other bedding), bonding (an innate drive to display an affinity for a single individual), sexual regurgitation (regurgitation of food to a bonded bird or human), and even copulation (birds of either sex displaying receptive postures or actual copulation). The seasonally aggressive behaviors of many male amazon parrots are another example of innate sexual behaviors demonstrated seasonally and apparently triggered by environmental conditions. Some clinical presentations, such as cloacal prolapses in male cockatoos, which seem to be linked to abnormal eating habits, may be made worse by chronic reproductive stimulation (F. Van Sant, personal observation, January 2004).

Reproductive behaviors may best be understood by defining the events that trigger them and the general context of the biology in which they occur. In short, what are the environmental cues and other triggers that stimulate reproductive behavior in a particular species? And what are their biological effects? If we can appreciate the influence of environment and pair bond formation in wild species, we will better understand the quirky reproductive behaviors and personalities of companion birds. Further, we may be able to use this information to help modify problem reproductive behaviors of companion psittacines.

Endocrine Regulation of Reproductive Development and Behavior

The set of innate and learned behaviors that drive reproduction and the physiologic mechanisms that underlie the process are complex. Reduced to simplest terms, common themes emerge. In birds, specific, and usually age-related, changes signal reproductive competency. The physiologic regulation of these events is controlled by the hormonal centers of the brain and the ovaries through the HPG axis, and it is these endocrine pathways that regulate reproduction.[10] Similar mechanisms in the male result in the production of testosterone, the hormone that directs the reproductive drive of males.[21] The HPG, responsible for controlling reproductive development and expression of behaviors, is triggered by various environmental conditions appropriate for the species.[3, 8, 9]

Pair bond enhancing behaviors can trigger reproductive activity as well.[10]

As in mammals, the HPG axis in birds regulates reproductive events, with several differences in birds. Because the capacity for flight demands that weight be minimized, females have only one active ovary. Birds further minimize their weight by maintaining inactive and atrophied gonads during most of the year. Only when conditions are appropriate for breeding will the HPG axis stimulate activation of the ovary and testes.[3, 22] During breeding season, these organs may weigh many times more than the inactive gland.[22] This adaptation necessitates a mechanism for effectively signaling the body that breeding season has arrived. For example, in temperate climate zones, day length is a common trigger.[2]

Species Variation

Matching reproductive activity to appropriate environmental conditions benefits the survival of the species. Environmental triggers help ensure that food and other resources are available to make reproductive activity successful. Along these same lines, when conditions are such that food and water are scarce, the biologic behaviors that promote and sustain reproduction are not triggered.

In some species, the initiating events are minimal and the response is swift. In others, there is a snowball effect that requires a complex synchrony of events that build progressively and cumulatively to nesting and oviposition. Cockatiels, Budgerigars, and other small psittacines native to harsh, water-limited environments respond swiftly to rainfall.[14, 15] The hormonal cascades that drive reproduction are initiated quickly by the hypothalamus. Pairing, courtship, nesting, and ultimately oviposition are driven rapidly by the HPG axis. Gestation is short and the young mature to independence quickly.

In contrast, many species of Neotropical parrots, particularly macaws and amazon parrots, have a low rate of reproduction.[23, 24] Research conducted by Charles Munn demonstrates that the macaws of Peru maintain stable pair bonds. For these species food is rarely a limiting factor, but nest cavity availability appears to be the ultimate limiting factor. When food is present, then nest cavity availability becomes the most important factor in stimulating reproductive behavior.

Finding, excavating, and preparing a cavity elevates sexual hormones in these birds, preparing birds for copulation and oviposition.[24, 25]

Studies by Millam with another Neotropical species, Orange-winged Amazon Parrots (*Amazona amazonica*), have shown that testosterone production builds and peaks as cavities are excavated.[26] The increased levels of testosterone may drive the sexual regurgitation (courtship feeding) that acts to nourish the female and provides the nutrients necessary to support ovulation.

ENVIRONMENTAL CUES FOR REGULATION OF SEXUAL BEHAVIOR AND MIGRATION

Once an understanding of parrots' natural response to environmental cues is developed, it becomes possible to look at many of the "quirky" behaviors they may exhibit in captivity. For example, companion psittacine birds demonstrate the same sexual behaviors seen in their wild counterparts but necessarily adapt them to the conditions found in the typical home. Companion parrots will shred their bedding and cage liners, nest in food dishes, woo their images in mirrors, and excavate cavities under furniture and in drawers. Companion birds will court and then copulate with toys. Females of certain species can produce an alarming number of eggs over months or even years.

It is imperative that the role of "normal" development be considered. As social species, parents, other adults, conspecifics in the flock, and even the competition of nest mates provide many behavioral mechanisms to moderate drives.

Innate drives are also tempered by environmental factors. In arid areas, the limiting factor of water exerts a powerful influence on the ability to survive. In moderate tropical climates, environmental factors can seasonally affect food supplies and habitat. In the stable home environment with regular and plentiful food supplies, it then becomes a distinct possibility that innate drives will go unchecked and often escalate. In the absence of limiting factors and plentiful attention, the home setting may contribute to behavioral or clinical problems. When these conditions are coupled with a lifestyle that is devoid of intense physical activity in animals that have evolved specifically to fly, there is little wonder that problems arise.

Seasonal Breeding

In tropical and subtropical locations, avian species have adopted several triggers to signal breeding season such as cessation or arrival of seasonal rains.[15, 16] Defining and understanding different triggers to reproductive behavior and their effect on different species is necessary before we can attempt to modify the behavior of companion psittacines. Equally important is an understanding of how the process needs to be self-limiting and turn itself off.

With rare exceptions, psittacine species are diurnal. Although these species, distributed among five continents, have established themselves in a wide array of environmental niches, most species can be relied upon to demonstrate regular patterns of moving and feeding through specific areas. The pineal gland contains photoreceptors that sense light independently and through visual pathways, and it is important in maintaining the circadian rhythms of psittacines.[27] It appears that the pineal gland may also play an important role in mediating seasonal breeding.[27]

Molting

The process of molting involves an orderly replacement of an individual's feathers and usually occurs as an annual event. Molting typically involves cessation of breeding activities and regression of the gonads. Although the mechanism of molt is poorly defined, it is thought to be mediated by the pituitary, thyroid, and adrenal glands. Molt can be forced in several species by the administration of thyroxine, prolactin, and progesterone. Sudden environmental events such as decreased day length and restricted food and water can also precipitate a molt.[2, 16]

Seasonal Migration

Seasonal migration to follow food supply is seen in a few parrot species. The Great Green Macaw (*Ara amigua*) seasonally migrates from coastal lowlands in Costa Rica to higher elevation forests in Nicaragua.[13] Two species of grass parakeets migrate over the Bass Straits of Australia across 120 miles of open water to Tasmania to breed each year.[15] The Patagonian Conure (*Cyanoliseus patagonus*) migrates during harsh winters to warmer areas of Uruguay. Species living at high altitudes in the Andes migrate vertically to lower

altitudes during winter.[28] Thick-billed Parrots (*Rhynchopsitta pachyrhyncha-pachyrhyncha*) used to migrate from northwestern Mexico to southern Arizona where they found abundant piñon pine nuts.

Light changes may trigger seasonal migrations. Fluctuating seasonal photoperiods, subtle changes in light wavelengths, or temperature fluctuations seem to initiate hormonal events directing migration. Corticosterone and prolactin, triggered by changes in the pituitary gland, are integral in the hormonal regulation of migration.[2]

NORMAL SEXUAL BEHAVIORS OF WILD PSITTACINE SPECIES

An understanding of normal sexual behaviors of wild psittacine birds is essential if we are to understand, and in turn prevent, the development of problematic sexual behaviors in companion parrots. Part of the solution is to recognize reproductive behaviors and environmental triggers in the wild, then to recognize those behaviors as expressed in a home setting.

Formation of Pair Bonds

Most psittacine birds are monomorphic and many form stable pair bonds. The pair bond offers a distinct advantage in undertaking the all-consuming commitment to hatching and rearing altricial young. Birds using this reproductive strategy are typically ready to breed without the need for elaborate courtship rituals. When environmental cues such as climate and available food supplies trigger the HPG axis, the birds are primed for reproductive behavior and courtship rituals can ensue, in greater or lesser degree. Although stable pair bonds are common among all avian species, these adaptations are well suited to the tropical and subtropical distribution of psittacine birds and reflect the huge biologic investment required to raise altricial young.[1, 16]

Vocalization

Specific vocalizations signaling sexual readiness have been observed in many species of parrots. Cockatiel males court females with shrill whistles and ready females answer with incessant chatter. Orange-chinned Parakeet (*Brotogeris jugularis*) pairs exhibit a back-and-forth chatter so well coordinated, it sounds like it is coming from a single bird.[15] Some cockatoos begin their courtship with loud vocalizations that grow progressively quieter as the pair mates, the female lays eggs, and the pair begins the work of incubation.[28] Budgerigar males woo hens with a warble that continues in four-minute bursts that may continue for hours. In Budgerigars, specific areas of the brain have been identified as similar to the well-studied song nuclei of passerines. The warble of the male Budgerigar seems to be a learned testosterone-driven behavior.[29]

Courting Behavior

Because many psittacine birds maintain stable pair bonds, courting behaviors usually involve a variety of simple moves like hopping, bowing, strutting, or tail wagging.[14, 15] Excited or aroused psittacine birds may exhibit pinning of the pupil and blushing. Macaws and Palm Cockatoos (*Probosciger aterrimus*) can display a rush of color in their facial skin. Many Australian and Indonesian birds have impressive crests that can be used in very demonstrative ways. Head bowing, an invitation for mutual preening, is often intensified during breeding and courtship and seems to convey sexual signals. Physical contact intensifies dramatically during breeding season. Although social preening is common among parrots, there are many nomadic species that reserve physical contact for breeding and fighting. For species that usually maintain a discrete critical distance between individuals, the physical contact of courtship is a powerful mechanism to synchronize males and females for successful breeding.[15, 16, 28] In a home setting, psittacine owners may inadvertently excite their birds through excessive physical contact, thereby encouraging reproductive behavior.

Courtship Feeding

Some species of parrots, particularly macaws and amazon parrots, will use courtship feeding, motivating the hormonal cascades that culminate in egg laying by both stimulating hormonal changes and providing the caloric abundance that contributes to egg production.[15, 24] It is notable that many psittacine owners feed soft, warm food to their parrots, inadvertently mimicking courtship feeding and encouraging reproductive behaviors.

Nesting

There is amazing variability among the 332 species of parrots as to how they claim and possess a nest site, and in their willingness to defend it. In the Neotropics, nest cavities are a limiting factor to breeding. Because the cavity plays such a key role in successful breeding of Neotropical species, it is not surprising that pairs of birds will incorporate a great deal of care and effort to prepare it. Large cockatoos, specifically Black Palms, have been observed drumming with sticks in displays that appear to claim territory and woo mates.[14, 15] In a home setting, birds may seek cavities, such as under a chair or in a closet, or they may use their cage as a nest.

Work done in Peru by Charles Munn identified nest cavities as the primary limiting condition for reproduction in Scarlet (*Ara macao*) and Green-winged Macaws (*Ara chloroptera*).[24, 25] When artificial cavities were provided high in the canopy, pairs of macaws quickly set up housekeeping. Biologists have noted that several species of macaws and amazons have established stable shared ownership of nest sites.[24]

A few species of parrots (most notably Monk Parakeets [*Myopsitta monachus*]) are colony breeders that construct elaborate nests. Eclectus Parrots have been observed breeding in colonies. Several males may work together to support a nesting female.[28, 30]

Several species of lovebirds (*Agapornis* species) transport leaf litter, bark, and twigs for elaborate nest construction. Peach-faced Lovebirds (*Agapornis roseicollis*) tuck long pieces of nest material across their back secured by the feathers of the lower back. Lovebirds with white eye rings carry nest material in their mouths. Other species carry small pieces tucked under their body feathers.[15] William C. Dilger investigated these behaviors three decades ago, finding that both the method of carrying material and nest design had a clear genetic basis.[31] In a home setting, birds may shred newspaper as a substitute nest material.

Copulation

Clear differences are observed in the physical posture assumed during copulation in Neotropical and old world birds. To achieve the cloacal contact of copulation, Neotropical males will mount the female with one foot holding on to a perch. In contrast, the males of old world species will mount the back of the hen with both feet. Copulation usually lasts about a minute. Lovebirds have been observed copulating for up to six minutes. To achieve internal fertilization, breeding must be timed to imminent ovulation. Oviposition, or laying, usually follows ovulation by roughly 12–24 hours. Generally a clutch of determinate size will be laid before incubation begins.[14, 15, 32]

Laying of Eggs

Most large parrots lay small clutches of one to three eggs. Parrot eggs are relatively small and are incubated for a fairly long period of time. The very altricial young are tiny and helpless at hatch. The value of a strong, well-protected nest is untold considering the substantial investment in time and energy that large psittacine birds devote to their offspring. Female macaws assume the duty of incubation while the male ensures that she is fed and protected. Cockatoos share incubation duties. Many smaller nomadic parrots use a different strategy, producing large clutches with relatively short incubation times. Young develop quickly, fledge, and mature to independence.[14, 15, 28]

Thermo-regulation is crucial in ensuring successful incubation.[33] In hot, humid, tropical areas, it can be assumed that adaptive physiologic mechanisms maintain stable body temperatures in a brooding parent. Thermo-regulation of avian species has been investigated and seems to be controlled by the dorsal hypothalamus and peripheral receptors. The propatagium of the thoracic limb has long been considered to be a principal site of thermo-regulation in flight and at rest. Other sites likely to play a role in critical thermo-regulation are legs, abdomen, and possibly feet.[26, 33]

CLINICAL PRESENTATIONS

The clinical implications of feather picking and other feather-destructive behaviors have been the focus of a great deal of attention by avian veterinarians, parrot behaviorists, and bird owners. By default, many of these conditions are dismissed as "normal" because systemic pathology cannot be diagnosed.[34] There is no single predisposing cause but rather a very complex mesh of genetic, environmental, and medical factors. Several clinical presentations of feather loss seem to regularly occur in concert with hormonally driven behaviors. In many instances, reversal of hormonal drives will be followed by regrowth of healthy skin and feathers. In principle, it follows that chronic reproductive behaviors are hormonally driven. In nature, parrots are "turned on" to breed by a set of well-defined environmental factors including seasonal changes, abundant food, available mates, and available cavities. The conditions of abundant food, bonded owners, cages that may trigger cavity-nesting behavior, and considerable physical contact seem to initiate breeding behaviors that may subject the bird to chronic reproductive stimulation. Without the naturally occurring environmental pressure of dwindling food supplies, changing environmental conditions, and competition for resources that limit breeding behavior in wild populations, breeding behaviors and hormonal activation persist unchecked. When these behaviors continue in an unrelenting fashion, the physiologic occurrences timed to occur during non-breeding season, such as molting, do not occur.

Molting follows breeding in the lives of most birds. Because both events are physically taxing, timing is important. Large psittacine birds have been observed to have a one- or two-year molt cycle synchronized with gonadal cycles. Large parrots reproducing year-round in avicultural situations have been noted to not molt in the same manner as non-breeding or free living conspecifics.[35] Delayed molts and failure to molt are common complaints of companion parrot owners. Also common are sets of clinical signs that have been observed to occur in companion parrots showing chronic breeding behavior.

Neotropical Parrots

Mature bonded female amazon parrots commonly demonstrate chronic breeding behaviors such as posturing, shredding, and cavity seeking. Birds with these signs are typically well nourished and often obese. Feather loss over the trunk, legs, back, and patagium are common. Many seem pruritic. New growth is sparse and often removed by the bird as pinfeathers erupt. Environmental changes are less rewarding in these birds as it appears that the owner has become the bonded mate and the cage has become the perceived nest. Endoscopic exams of these birds usually reveal a mature but abnormal ovary.[36] Lacking is the usual cascade of developing oocytes. Instead, a solitary, mature follicle is usually found. Therapy with leuprolide acetate (Lupron®) by itself is often insufficient in restoring the normal cascade.

Lupron® can shut down the reproductive cycle briefly, but if reproductive triggers remain unchanged, clinical symptoms can reappear. Successful therapy can be achieved with weight loss. Individual birds seem to have a weight threshold under which chronic breeding behaviors cease. This clinical recommendation is supported by observations of wild amazon parrots that describe a weight increase triggered by food availability and male regurgitation and feeding preceding ovulation.[15, 26]

Female macaws may demonstrate cavity seeking and protracted egg laying. In this context, Lupron® is a very useful therapeutic tool, providing a means to diminish both. A less common but very significant presentation in bonded female macaws is an inflammatory process of the medial leg. These birds exhibit agitation and foot stomping. Close exam of the medial vascular pattern of the legs will usually reveal dilation and inflammation of the vessels. The legs are often hot. This condition may develop into a crusty dermatitis. Therapeutic Lupron® coupled with HCG and a non-steroidal anti-inflammatory are helpful. Discontinuing any warm food is imperative as that practice seems very capable of mimicking mate regurgitation and inciting hormonal stimulation.

Male amazon parrots have been observed to demonstrate seasonal aggression, territorial displays, and recurring focal inflammatory lesions of the feet. These conditions can be successfully treated with Lupron® and HCG. Cool water baths to the legs are helpful.

Examining the cooling mechanisms of parrots may provide insights into clinical presentations of inflamed legs and feet. Thermo-regulation is a critical component of successful incubation. Hormonal regulation of vascular channels is well defined in mammalian and avian physiology and could be assumed to be a critical factor here.

African Parrots

African Grey Parrots frequently demonstrate signs of breeding behavior. These can occur year-round, especially when there is a bonded owner. Warm food and abundant food will often trigger regurgitation behaviors. Commonly coupled with these behaviors is feather picking of the trunk and legs. Control of calories, especially those obtained from rich simple carbohydrates like pasta and cookies, is very helpful. Of serious consequence is the tendency of African Grey Parrots to develop severe non-responsive dermatitis of the patagium. When closely monitored, these conditions appear to start with the loss of down and contours of the wing web. Superficial vessels usually appear dilated. If allowed to continue, secondary opportunistic yeast and bacterial infections may develop. Control of chronic dermatitis can be difficult, but early intervention and environmental and behavioral corrections that focus on decreasing hormonal stimulation are usually successful.

Considering the critical distance observed between African Grey Parrots in the wild and in aviary situations, the role of physical affection demonstrated by frequent petting and body contact with an owner should be considered to be a powerful predisposing factor.

Indonesian/Australian Parrots

Three species of companion cockatoos commonly demonstrate clinically significant changes that may relate to hormonally driven behaviors. Umbrella Cockatoos, Moluccan Cockatoos (*Cacatua moluccensis*), and Goffin's Cockatoos (*Cacatua goffini*) are frequently presented for feather loss, feather picking, and dermatitis. Female cockatoos are commonly handled and cuddled by adoring owners. Lavishing physical attention to the bird's head, crest, and trunk usually elicits posturing and often orgasmic-like shuddering. In many cases, these birds exhibit these behaviors for years. Clinical impressions of these birds seem to reveal a progressive and serious pattern of degenerative changes including dermatitis, loss of cloacal tone, and anemia. The availability of an estrogen panel assay at the University of Tennessee Clinical Endocrinology Service made possible quantification of hormonal levels in these species. Therapeutic Lupron®, HCG, and a concerted change in the birds' environment result in dramatic recovery.

It now seems very likely that the role of intense physical contact is capable of eliciting hormonal responses, starting early and continuing progressively for years. The perception that "no amount of attention is ever enough for the social cockatoo" has been difficult to overcome. The missing piece of information is the naturally occurring environmental conditions that serve to make these behaviors seasonal rather than constant. In the case of the Goffin's Cockatoo, seasonal shifts in the Tanimbar Islands are dramatic. As the islands are located in the geographical rain-shadow of Australia, there is a distinct periodicity to rainfall. Nine months of the year bring regular rainfall and abundant water. For three months of the year rainfall amounts drop precipitously. Inherent in this pattern is an environmental shift that is not conducive to reproduction and challenging for survival. For birds as companions, these conditions, or seasonal stresses, never occur and breeding behaviors continue in an unrelenting fashion.

Male Moluccan Cockatoos, particularly those that have endured sedentary life and seed diets for ten or more years, have a high incidence of self-mutilation over the sternum. Considered a behavioral problem by many or the result of abject boredom, perhaps this should instead be investigated as a physiologic event. Building on the experience of successful clinical intervention of these cases where lifestyle changes including diet and exercise have been used in concert with Lupron® and symptomatic medicine, it might be possible to hypothesize underlying factors involving vascular changes, tissue perfusion dependent on physical conditioning, and even chronic hormonal stress.

THERAPEUTIC REMEDIES

Avian veterinary medicine has become adept at developing effective therapeutic modalities for the most common manifestations of hormonal dysfunction. Experienced clinicians routinely handle medical emergencies related to ovulation. Protracted egg laying, as is commonly exhibited in Budgerigars, Cockatiels, and Umbrella Cockatoos, is routinely treated with Lupron®, a gonadotropin-releasing hormone (GnRH) agonist, that acts by down-regulating pituitary GnRH receptors.[7, 37] These therapies, though effective in the short term, may become inadequate as a long-term solution. When faced with the recurrent nature of these problems, many companion psittacine owners become impatient with the need for return visits and expensive injections.

Based on Millam's research, recommendations to restore Cockatiels to a short-day photoperiod as a remedy to chronic egg laying became common.[38] Other management-based recommendations, such as removal of the nest box and separation from the male, also became common-

place. Many veterinarians counseled clients about the role of physical contact in hormonal stimulation. But explanations about the mechanics of how to prevent recurrence are often poorly received and viewed as undesirable or impossible. Reinforcing these recommendations with interesting information about the bird's origins and adaptations has proven to be an extremely useful tool.[37]

Adjust Photoperiod

If there is one single positive change that companion bird owners can make, it is returning the bird to a regularly recurring photoperiod. Whether in the wild or in captivity, most birds demonstrate a remarkable periodicity to their days. Restoration of a regular recurring day and night cycle usually results in a happier and healthier companion bird. Ideally the photoperiod would begin at dawn when most birds, covered or not, sense the new day and begin to stir. As most birds are from equatorial and subequatorial latitudes where day length is roughly 12 hours year-round, establishing a routine that follows a 12-hour day with a 12-hour night is ideal. Birds have in their brains a finely tuned, light sensitive pineal gland. This gland is likely the mechanism by which birds set their circadian rhythm. There is some evidence to support the theory that seasonal shifts are sensed by the rate of change of day length (like those that occur in spring and fall) rather than just keying off of a single day length. Many owners initially anticipate a hardship or a loss of interactive time but instead find that the bird adapts within days to the new routine and quickly demonstrates that the change is a benefit.

Control Shredding

One of the easiest remedies to derail reproductive drives is also one of the most powerful. Shredding of paper, cardboard, or other bedding material seems to mimic the intrinsic behaviors of nest preparation. Typically regarded as benign, playful activity, shredding instead seems to promote reproductive activity, boosting hormone levels.[9, 15, 26] As most cages are equipped with grates that prevent access to the cage floor, this behavior is usually easy to control. In cases where a grate is not provided, all liners can be removed and the cage tray simply rinsed daily. In many cases, this behavior may be one of the earliest warning signs of reproductive activity. Preventing access to shredable substrate may quickly defuse reproductive activity.

Curtail Cavity Seeking

As reproductive drives escalate, many companion birds begin to roam and explore, seeking a cavity. The perceived cavity may be a closet, a drawer, or a box. Many birds have attempted to set up housekeeping under a chair or a couch. Owners have found chair stuffing excavated and carpets ripped up by companion parrots driven to find a suitable nest site. Cavity seeking should be viewed as a serious escalation of hormonally driven behavior. Many Neotropical species will become very territorial and fiercely guard their homestead. Cavity seeking is often a sign of imminent ovulation in the female. Millam investigated the importance of this hormonal drive in the cascade of physiologic changes that lead to oviposition. His studies demonstrated that testosterone levels crescendo to their peak levels in male Orange-winged Amazons during cavity exploration.[26] This information dovetails perfectly with the observed importance of cavity availability to many Neotropical species, including amazon parrots and macaws. Curtailing this behavior by not allowing the bird to wander is a simple and powerful solution. Female birds that are permitted or encouraged to establish ownership of a "cavity" will often begin a long stint of unrelenting egg production. Often these female birds will lay several lifetimes worth of eggs and become quite stressed and—eventually—quite ill from the physiologic demands of egg production and incubation.

Watch Physical Contact

The role of physical contact, usually in the form of affectionate petting, can become extremely important in inciting and fueling hormonal behaviors. Physical contact seems most powerful in cockatoos, Cockatiels, and Budgies. Cockatoos in fact have been recommended and sold as companion birds that will thrive on attention and probably suffer derangement without it. Many birds train their owners early on in the best techniques to cuddle and adore them. These birds delight in having their crests stroked and will often elicit attention by lowering their head. Many female cockatoos demonstrate orgasmic panting and shaking while caressed by owners. The sig-

nificance of this behavior is often missed by owners, who may interpret it as anything from a seizure to a sinus infection. Owners who have been warned about the risks of behavioral problems and feather picking that may result from a lack of attention are often devastated to see these behaviors develop in their companion birds.

The role of physical contact in most adult birds is reserved for courting and breeding behaviors. It is not surprising to find that species that crave physical attention as companion birds are the same ones that incorporate more physical contact into their courtship rituals. Indeed, the crest of cockatoos has been conjectured to be an important lure. The bowing and head-lowering behaviors commonly demonstrated by cockatoos are likely signals between the male and female. These signals probably serve to synchronize the behaviors of the female and male to time nesting, copulation, and ovulation. The remedy, of course, is to decrease physical contact with susceptible birds. As these patterns are often very difficult for pet owners to break, efforts must be made to frame the change in understandable terms. Unfortunately, most owners will only start to listen once degenerative signs develop.

Adjust Feeding

Contrasting the patterns of food gathering in wild parrots with the feeding styles of companion parrots reveals important and dramatic information. Foraging is thought to occupy a considerable part of every wild parrot's day. Even in environments such as rain forests where food is relatively abundant, parrots have been observed spending considerable time locating and foraging for food. Some biologists have hypothesized that the impressive capacity of the parrot to learn and remember may have evolved in response to the need to locate and recognize a huge variety of foods spread out over considerable distances, along with the amount of time necessary to cover these distances.[24] When this is coupled with the reasonable expectation that many parrots will be triggered to breed by seasonally abundant food supplies, the impact on companion parrots of regularly delivered meals is immense.

When contrasted with wild parrots, the accepted tradition of two or three daily meals prepared and delivered, often augmented with treats and goodies, leaves little else to do during the day but digest. Companion parrots are notorious for disrupting meal times, as they demand favorite morsels from the table. As many owners think their bird will balance its own diet and life is easier at table times when the bird is happy, many birds end up eating the foods that feel best going down. Bread, rice, pasta, sweets, and butter have universal appeal but will not nourish a parrot in a manner that will provide sustainable health.

Many simple methods can remedy these common problems. Varying the foods offered and feeding only the amounts readily consumed can simplify life and result in a healthier bird. Organic formulated diets deliver nourishing fare easily and quickly. Supplementation with organic vegetables offers variety. As birds typically feed twice a day, early morning and late afternoon, meal-feeding for a finite time (one to two hours) twice a day can have numerous benefits. Meal-feeding restores one more facet to the regular periodicity observed in wild parrots. Meal-feeding avoids a lot of waste and seems to return food to a mode of sustenance instead of entertainment. Techniques that encourage foraging are becoming more popular. Hiding morsels of food among rocks in a bowl can keep a parrot thinking and moving. Stainless steel skewers offer a handy way to hang vegetables. Careful timing of feeding can turn a loud morning or evening "power hour" into a quiet mealtime.

Provide Opportunities for Exercise

Parrots have evolved to fly. Most of the unique physiologic adaptations of a bird are geared to this very physical activity. Flight demands vigorous health. From physical structure to mechanisms of gas exchange in their respiratory system birds, including parrots, are all about flight. The drive to exercise is seen in companion birds. Many aviculturists advise allowing a young bird to successfully fledge as an important developmental milestone.[39] Certainly flight in most homes is indeed more hazardous than a physically unchallenging sedentary life, but the fact remains that real sustainable health in parrots requires exercise and physical conditioning. Flight can be taught to any bird. Taking off is innate, landing and navigating are learned. The opportunity to fly can sometimes be offered in the home, or outdoor enclosures can offer an alternative. There is no doubt that allowing flight is risky in many or most

situations and owners should educate themselves thoroughly before choosing this option. Whether exercised indoors or outdoors, clipped or flighted, physical activity is imperative for sustainable health. It is worth considering that a lack of physical exercise and the subsequent disuse (atrophy) of the poorly defined but unique cardiovascular adaptations that allow for flight might predispose an individual to untoward effects of chronic hormonal stimulation of the circulatory system.

Use Clicker Training

Clicker training has emerged as a very easy and rewarding way to enhance life and learning in many animals. When the clicker is used with a food reward to develop new lines of communication between a parrot owner and a bird, the capacity of the bird to learn can be astounding. Most owners can be trained to teach simple behaviors quickly and easily. The real beauty of this technique is that it offers redirection of attention toward learning and exercise. Clicker training has the potential to replace quality-shared time between an owner and a parrot with skills and learning instead of cuddling. In this way, inappropriate and generally unintended overbonding with a companion bird with its attendant reproductive behavioral cues can be reduced or eliminated.

Address Problematic Bird Husbandry

In many homes, owners have adopted the notion of consistent cage arrangement, a wide variety of foods chosen by preference instead of nutritive value, and quality time usually consisting of late nights and cuddling. Unfortunately, these well-intended practices have likely contributed in a major way to undermining the chances of a long-term successful pet relationship. However, sustainable health may be possible using knowledge gained from the natural history and innate behavioral tendencies of companion parrots. Changing environmental conditions, minimizing pair bond formation, and recognizing and addressing reproductive behaviors early could change the lives of birds—and their owners—dramatically.

CONCLUSION

Reproductive problems are common in avian veterinary medicine and frequently recur after medical intervention. While many of these disorders are perceived as behavioral problems, birds are likely being cued reproductively by environmental conditions present in the home that activate the HPG axis. Understanding the pathophysiology of these reproductive behaviors provides a likely means to prevent chronic hormonal stimulation. Individual species have their own triggers for reproductive activity, and environmental manipulation and attention to husbandry issues/pair bond formation may remove these triggers. Prevention, rather than intervention, may be the key. Enhancing our view of individual species with a renewed appreciation for their natural history and innate behaviors will be necessary for success.

REFERENCES

1. Short, L.L. 1993. *The lives of birds.* New York: Henry Holt and Co.
2. Meyer, D.B. 1986. "Pineal gland." In *Avian physiology,* ed. P.D. Sturkie, pp. 501–505. New York: Springer-Verlag.
3. Johnson, A.L. 2000. "Reproduction in the female." In *Sturkie's avian physiology,* 5th ed., ed. G.C. Whittow, pp. 569–596. San Diego: Academic Press.
4. Jarvis, E.D., C. Scharff, M. Grossman, J.A. Ramos, and F. Nottebohm. 1999. For whom the bird sings: Context-dependent gene expression. *Neuron* 21:775–788.
5. Jarvis, E.D., and C.V. Mello. 2000. Molecular mapping of brain areas involved in parrot vocal communication. *J Comp Neurol* 419:1–31.
6. Jarvis, E.D., S. Ribeiro, J. Vielliard, M. DaSilva, D. Ventura, and C.V. Mello. 2000. Behaviorally-driven gene expression reveals hummingbird brain song nuclei. *Nature* 406:628–632.
7. Ottinger, M.A., J. Wu, and K. Pelican. 2002. Neuroendocrine regulation of reproduction in birds and clinical applications of GnRH analogues in birds and mammals. *Semin Avian Exotic Pet Med* 11 (2):71–79.
8. Speer, B.L. 2003. "Sex and the single bird." Proc Annu Conf Assoc Avian Vet, pp. 331–343.
9. Millam, J.R. 1997. "Reproductive physiology." In *Avian medicine and surgery,* ed. R.B. Altman, S.L. Clubb, G.M. Dorrestein, and K. Quesenberry, pp. 12–28. Philadelphia: .W.B Saunders.
10. Pollock, C.G., and S.E. Orosz. 2002. Avian reproductive anatomy, physiology and endocrinology. *Vet Clin North Am Exotic Anim Pract* 5:441–474.
11. Joyner, K.L. 1994. "Theriogenology." In *Avian medicine: Principles and application,* ed. B.W. Ritchie, G.J. Harrison, and L.R. Harrison, pp. 748–804. Lake Worth, FL: Wingers Publishing.
12. Romagnano, A. 1996. Avian obstetrics. *Semin Avian Exotic Pet Med* 5 (4):180–188.
13. Rosskopf, W.J., and R.W. Woerpel. 1996. "Feather picking and therapy of skin and feather disorders." In *Diseases of cage and aviary birds,* ed. W. Rosskopf and R. Woerpel, pp. 397–405. Baltimore: Williams and Wilkins.
14. Forshaw, J.M., and W.T. Cooper. 1989. *Parrots of the world,* 3rd (rev.) ed. Willoughby, NSW, Australia: Weldon Publishing.
15. Sparks, J., and T. Soper. 1990. *Parrots: A natural history.* New York: Facts on File, Inc.
16. Coyle, P.G., Jr. 1987. *Understanding the life of birds.* Lakeside, CA: Summit Publications.
17. May, D.L. 1996. The behavior of African grey parrots in the rainforest of the Central African Republic. *Psittascene* 8:8–9.
18. Pepperberg, I.M. 1994. Numerical competence in an African grey parrot. *J Comp Psych* 108:36–44.
19. Pepperberg, I.M. 1992. Proficient performance of a conjunctive, recursive task by an African grey parrot (*Psittacus erithacus*). *J Comp Psych* 106:295–305.
20. Elphick, C, J.B. Dunning Jr., and D.A. Sibley. 2001. *The Sibley guide to bird life and behavior.* New York: Alfred A. Knopf.
21. Hudelson, S.A. 1996. Review of the mechanisms of avian reproduction and their clinical applications. *Semin Avian Exotic Vet Med* 5 (4):189–198.
22. Johnson, A.L. 1986. "Reproduction in the male." In *Avian physiology,* ed. P.D. Sturkie, pp. 432–451. New York: Springer-Verlag.
23. Powell, G., and R. Bjork. 1996. *Ara ambigua*: Preliminary observations on the Costa Rican population and their lowland forest habitat and on their conservation. Washington, DC: RARE Center for Tropical Conservation.
24. Munn, C.A. 1994. Macaws: Winged rainbows. *National Geographic* 185 (1):118–140.
25. Munn, C.A. "Macaw biology and ecotourism" or "When a bird in the bush is worth two in the hand." In *New world parrots in crisis, solutions from conservation biology,* ed. S.R. Bessinger and N.F.R. Snyder, pp. 47–72. Washington DC: Smithsonian Institution Press.
26. Millam, J.R. 1999. Reproductive management of captive parrots. *Vet Clin North Am Exotic Anim Pract* 2:93–110.
27. King, A.S., and J. McLelland. 1984. *Birds: Their structure and function.* London, UK: Bailliere Tindall.
28. Arndt, T. 1986. *Parrots: Their life in the wild.* Bromlitz, Germany: Horst Muller-Verlag Walsrode.
29. Nespor, A.A., M.J. Lukazewicz, R.J. Dooling, and G.F. Ball. 1996. Testosterone induction of male-

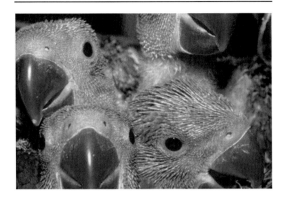

Figure 11.2. Healthy neophytes, such as these Alexandrine chicks, have bright eyes and appear inquisitive during their busyness. (Photo by Alice J. Patterson, courtesy of Santa Barbara Bird Farm.)

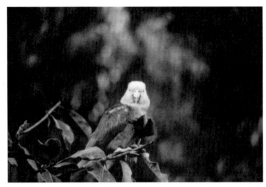

Figure 11.6. The naturalized Double Yellow-headed Amazon, a proven male, keeps lookout for his fledglings amid the trees at the Santa Barbara Bird Farm, where the wild flock's daily activities are noted. (Photo by Harry A. Linden, courtesy of Santa Barbara Bird Farm.)

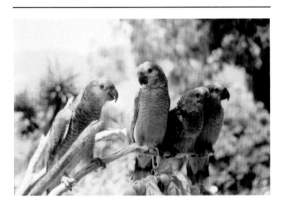

Figure 11.10. The author's one-year-old Blue-fronted Amazon, Bucket, meets his prospective mate, Bonnet, for the first time as she sits on a perch with her clutch mates. Fifteen years later, they are still together. (Photo by Margaret Ames, courtesy of Santa Barbara Bird Farm.)

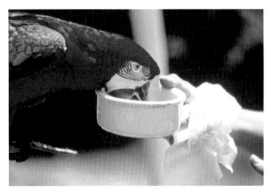

Figure 11.11. Rosie, a one-year-old Green-winged Macaw, occasionally needs encouragement to eat foods selected by her caregiver. A handheld bowl and lots of verbal interaction assist her in making good food choices. (Photo by Layne David Dicker, courtesy of Santa Barbara Bird Farm.)

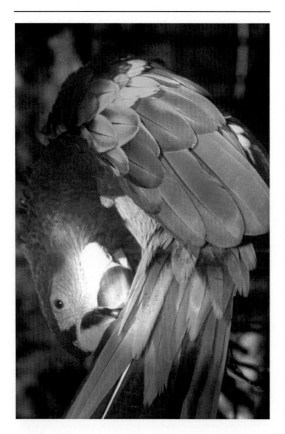

Figure 11.13. The art of preening occupies many moments in parrots' daily lives. Human caretakers can promote preening with praise and by giving parrots the baths and space necessary for expansive preening sessions. (Photo by Kelly Flynn, courtesy of Santa Barbara Bird Farm.)

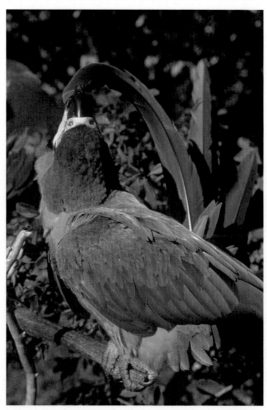

Figure 11.14. Young Blue-and-gold Macaw twists and reaches as she preens her tail feather while outdoors. (Photo by Kelly Flynn, courtesy of Santa Barbara Bird Farm.)

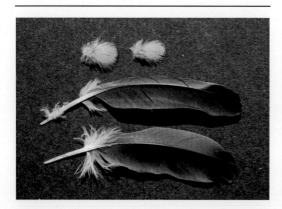

Plate 1. Feathers from an amazon parrot under normal light.

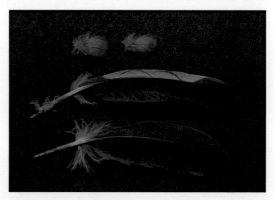

Plate 2. Feathers from an amazon parrot as seen under ultraviolet light.

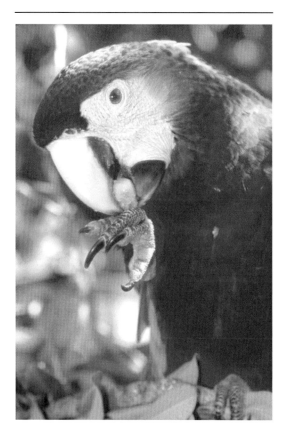

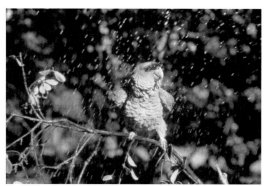

Plate 5. Our companion Lilac-crowned Amazons, like Zephie here, enjoy outdoor bathing, just like the wild flock. (Photo by Kelly Flynn, courtesy of Santa Barbara Bird Farm.)

Plate 3. The development of enough manual dexterity to lift food with one foot while balancing on a perch with the other involves skills practiced during fledging. (Photo by Kelly Flynn, courtesy of Santa Barbara Bird Farm.)

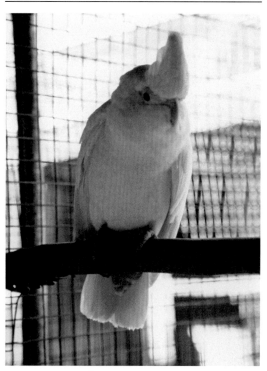

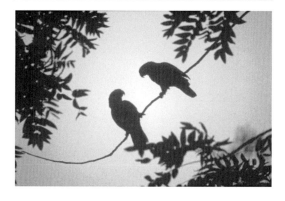

Figure 22.1. The most aggressive white cockatoo is the Red-vented Cockatoo like the one pictured here.

Plate 4. Two Lilac-crowned Amazons, ready to take off for their evening roosting site. (Photo by Harry A. Linden, courtesy of Santa Barbara Bird Farm.)

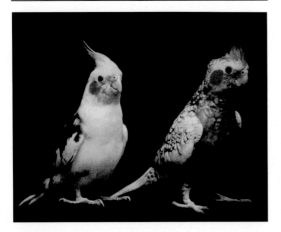

Plate 6. Cockatiels are highly social and very suitable as pets.

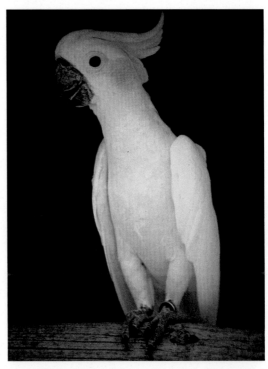

Figure 22.2. The aggressive Red-vented Cockatoo is closely followed in level of aggression by the Lesser Sulfur-crested Cockatoo like the one pictured here.

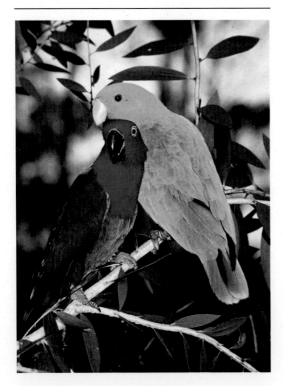

Figure 22.3. Eclectus, like those pictured here, are also capable of mate trauma.

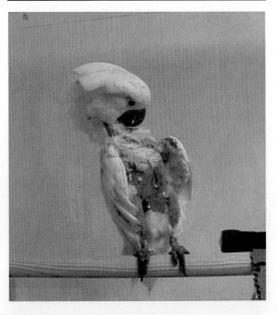

Figure 23.1. Cockatoo with feather-picking disorder.

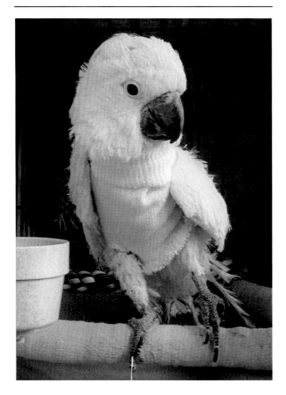

Figure 23.8. Moluccan Cockatoo wearing a sock sweater.

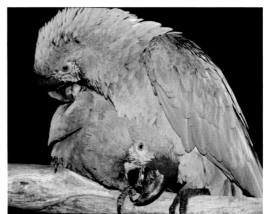

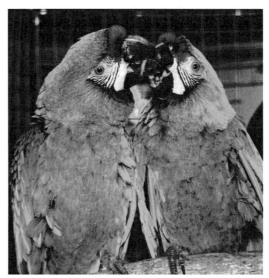

Figure 25.1a and 25.1b. A bonded pair of Military Macaws engaged in allopreening and allofeeding.

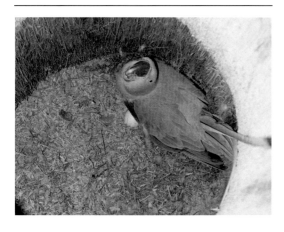

Figure 25.7. Deep, dark natural nesting cavities, such as this hollowed out palm log, are often preferred nesting sites, as demonstrated by this Alexandrine Parakeet hen on five fertile eggs.

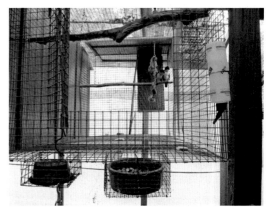

Figure 25.8. Keeping the nesting box away from high traffic areas, such as the path traveled when doing daily feeding, may increase breeding success.

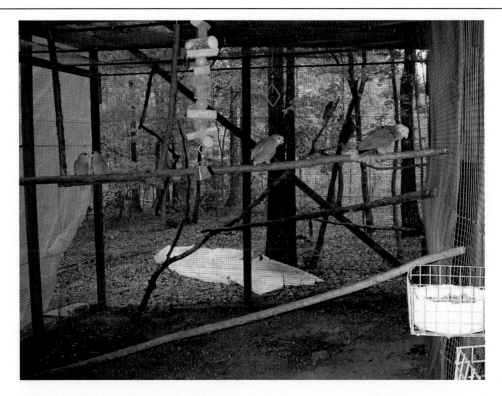

Figure 25.2. Flocking birds of the same species or genera in the non-breeding season may increase production by allowing voluntary mate selection.

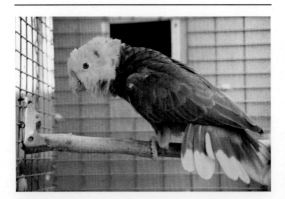

Figure 25.12. A Double Yellow-headed Amazon Parrot displaying normal territorial aggression in defense of the nest box where the hen is on eggs.

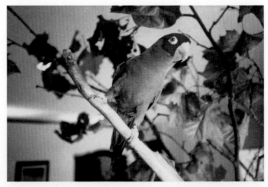

Figure 26.3. A Red-masked Conure (*Aratinga erythrogenys*).

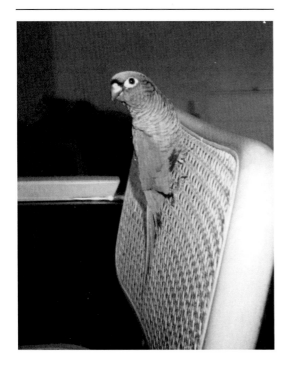

Figure 26.2. A Maroon-bellied Conure (*Pyrrhura frontalis*).

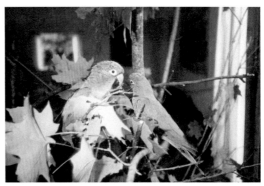

Figure 26.6. Two Sharp-tailed Conures (*A. acuticaudata*) enjoying natural branches.

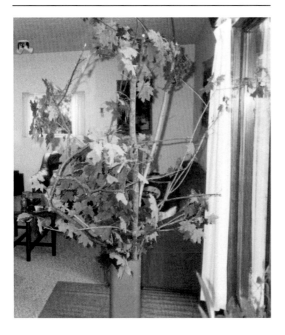

Figure 26.5. An appropriate play gym for small to medium-sized birds, made from a chimney flue and natural branches.

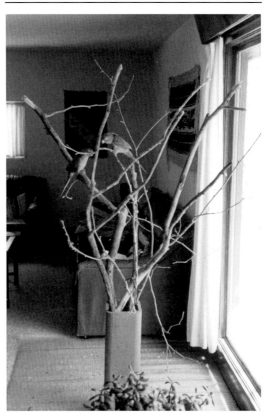

Figure 26.7. A play gym made from a chimney flue and natural branches after the birds spent some time on it.

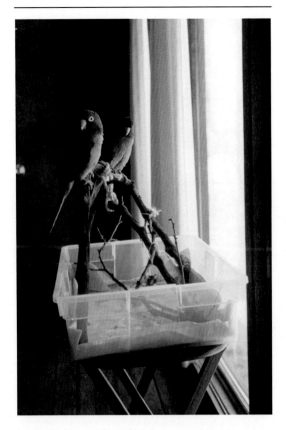

Figure 26.8. A smaller play gym made from a storage container and wild grape vines.

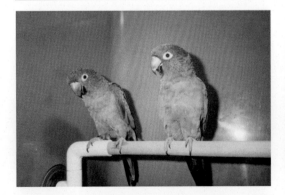

Figure 26.9. Some birds enjoy joining the owner in the shower on a commercially available shower perch.

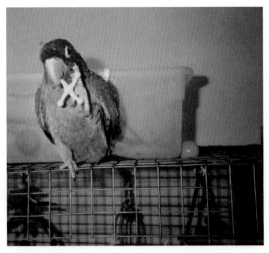

Figure 26.12. A Mitred Conure (*Aratinga mitrata*) with a "foot toy," a top commercially available for cats.

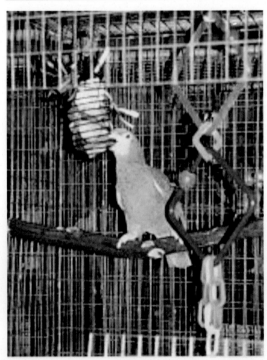

Figure 27.1. Examples of the enrichments utilized in the U.C. Davis experiments.

like vocalizations in female budgerigars (*Melopsittacus undulates*). *Horm Behav* 30 (2):162–169.

30. Sweeney, R.G. 1993. *The Eclectus: A complete guide.* Ontario, Canada: Silvio Mattacchione and Co.

31. Dilger, W.C. 1962. The behavior of lovebirds. *Sci Am* 206:88–98.

32. Millam, J.R., B. Zhang, and M.E. el Halawani. 1996. Egg production in cockatiels (*Nymphicus hollandicus*) is influenced by number of eggs in nest after incubation begins. *Gen Comp Endocrinol* 101 (2):205–210.

33. Whittow, G.C. 1986. Regulation of body temperature. In *Avian physiology,* ed. P.D. Sturkie, pp. 221–252. New York, NY: Springer-Verlag.

34. Rosenthal, K.L. 2003. "Cytology, histology, and microbiology of feather pulp and follicles of feather pickers." Proc Annu Conf Assoc Avian Vet, pp. 27–31.

35. Cooper, J.E., and G.J. Harrison. 1994. "Dermatology." In *Avian medicine: Principles and appli-*

cation, ed. B.W. Ritchie, G.J. Harrison, and L.R. Harrison, pp. 607–639. Lake Worth, FL: Wingers Publishing.

36. Bowles, H.L. 2002. Reproductive diseases of pet bird species. *Vet Clin North Am Exot Anim Pract* 5 (3):489–506.

37. Millam, J.R., and H.L. Finney. 1994. Leuprolide acetate can reversibly prevent egg laying in cockatiels (*Nymphicus hollandicus*). *Zoo Biol* 13:149–155.

38. Shields, K.M., J.T. Yamamoto, and J.R. Millam. 1989. Reproductive behavior and LH levels of cockatiels (*Nymphicus hollandicus*) associated with photostimulation, nest-box presentation, and degree of mate access. *Horm Behavior* 23 (1): 68–82.

39. Linden, P.G. 1999. "Fledging and flight for avian companions." Proc Annu Conf Assoc Avian Vet, pp. 61–65.

22
Mate Trauma

April Romagnano

SUMMARY

Mate trauma is considered a syndrome of captive psittacine birds. It is thought to be induced by the circumstances of captivity and how they interplay with the natural behaviors of breeding psittacines, that is, their breeding seasonality. Mate trauma occurs predominately in sexually mature cockatoo pairs. It is most common in the white, or light-colored, cockatoo species. In the author's experience, mate trauma appears to be most common in domestically raised pairs, early in the breeding season, and early in the morning. Typically, the male bird is the aggressor and he most often attacks the female in the head, neck, and beak region. The beak is typically the most seriously and permanently affected, and thus needs long-term—often lifelong—therapeutic trimming and filing. Unfortunately, in addition to the cockatoos, numerous other psittacines and some passerine and rhamphastidae species also experience mate trauma in captivity. Fortunately for these species, the incidence of attacks is much lower. In a select few, the female bird is the aggressor.

This chapter will review the syndrome of mate trauma, complete with a discussion of its proposed etiologies, preventative management, and treatment. The chapter will also briefly review the anatomy and the prehensile function of the avian beak.

MATE TRAUMA

The majority of large psittacine aviculturists in America and Europe have witnessed mate or intraspecific aggression.[1–5, 7] It is generally accepted that breeding seasonality plays a significant role in the occurrence of mate aggression and/or trauma in captivity. During the breeding season, reproductively active psittacine birds become more possessive of their cages and, especially, of their nest boxes; hence, aggressive displays increase. For this reason, visual barriers on the nest box side of the cage are imperative.[7] It should be noted that mate aggression resulting in severe injury or death—also referred to as mate trauma—does not occur in the wild nor is it recognized in aviculture in Australia.[7]

The specific etiology of mate trauma is not known. However, numerous theories exist, including asynchrony of reproductive activity, territory and/or food defense, invasion of personal space, confinement in too small a cage, displaced aggression due to territorial issues, behavioral interactions with birds in nearby cages or humans outside the cage, hormonal imbalances, dietary imbalances, and so forth.[5, 7] Mate traumas appear to occur sporadically and without provocation. A productive bonded pair may suddenly experience fatal mate trauma for no apparent reason. The pair can be domestic, wild-caught, or mixed. It can be composed of young or old birds or both. The pair could be recently set up or have a proven history of many years' duration. The frequency of mate trauma is highest in breeding cockatoo species during the spring and early summer months. In the author's experience, mate trauma occurs most commonly in domestically raised pairs, early in the breeding season, and early in the morning.

This intraspecific aggression is most common in white cockatoos. In the author's experience, the White Cockatoos are more commonly affected than pink, salmon, or black cockatoos. The most aggressive white cockatoo is the Red-vented Cockatoo (Figure 22.1). This species is closely followed by the Lesser Sulfur-crested Cockatoo

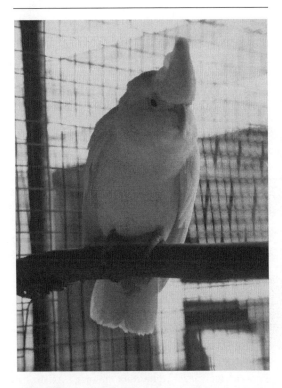

Figure 22.1. The most aggressive white cockatoo is the Red-vented Cockatoo like the one pictured here. See also color section.

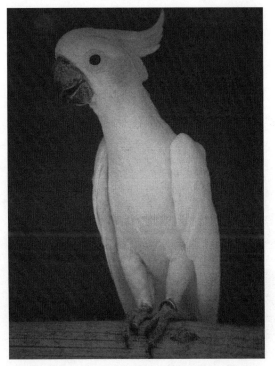

Figure 22.2. The aggressive Red-vented Cockatoo is closely followed in level of aggression by the Lesser Sulfur-crested Cockatoo like the one pictured here. See also color section.

(Figure 22.2). The Red-vented Cockatoos will often kill and then attempt to eat their dead cagemates, and thus it is safest to keep the mating pairs of this species in separate cages during the non-breeding season.

Mate trauma has also been seen in macaws, amazons, conures, Eclectus (Figure 22.3), Ring-necked Parakeets, Senegals, and thick-billed psittacine parrots. Many species of soft bills, such as toucans, turacos, doves, and finches, also exhibit intraspecific aggression. In the majority of species affected, the male attacks the female except in the case of the Eclectus Parrot, where the female is known to be the aggressor. Occasionally, individual females of different species may attack their male mates, but this phenomenon is not necessarily species specific. In the author's experience, other female psittacine birds that have been noted to attack their male cagemates are Ring-necked Parakeets, lovebirds, Senegal Parrots, and Palm Cockatoos.

THE MATE TRAUMA ATTACK

Male cockatoos are the most common aggressors. The typical mate trauma attack occurs at dawn. The etiology of these aggressive attacks is thought to be multifactorial. It is the author's opinion that it is triggered, to some extent, by hormonal changes since the majority of attacks occur in the spring and early summer. Presumably, if the male bird's aggressive advances are ignored or thwarted (i.e., disturbed by other birds or people, misinterpreted, or not fully acted out due to cage space limitations), the male tends to lash out at his female cagemate. Since the female bird can run but not escape the male's offensive aggressive advances, she is forced to defend herself. The author feels that the male becomes further enraged and increases the frequency of his attacks. Thus it appears that the male then relentlessly chases the female, attacking her whenever possible. The author has treated approximately 100 mate traumas. If the female is rescued alive, in addition to being

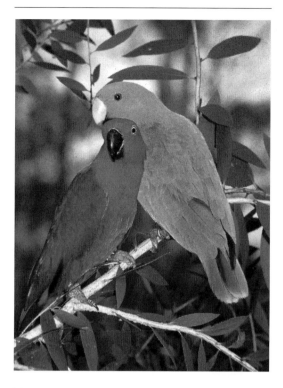

Figure 22.3.   Eclectus, like those pictured here, are also capable of mate trauma. See also color section.

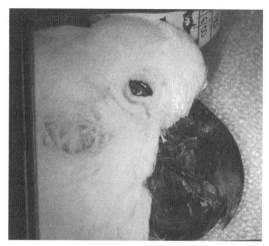

Figure 22.4.   Severe beak damage in a white Cockatoo, killed by mate trauma.

wounded and moribund, she is typically ravenous and has lost a significant amount of weight. This suggests most mate traumas are not an isolated event and are more likely a series of offensive attacks by the male. If the female is not too old, in good health, and flighted, she will initially be able to evade the male's aggressive attacks. However, without human intervention, captive females become exhausted and succumb. Attacks can occur anywhere in the cage, but are more likely to occur in areas of increased contact such as the feeding and drinking area or the nest box. These aggressive attacks essentially run the female ragged, and both prostration and starvation set in. The caged female thus becomes easy prey and is ultimately mauled by the male. Usually, after the initial mate trauma attack occurs, the male goes back for more, unless an astute aviculturist rescues the female. Most fatal attacks occur within the nest box, since it is the easiest place for the male to corner the female. If the female is not rescued, the

male will continue to attack his female cagemate until she is rendered completely moribund and finally dies.

Mate trauma is virtually unknown in Australia.[7] It is presumed that in the wild, the unresponsive female simply flies away, escaping mate aggression and trauma completely. In captivity, as previously mentioned, mate trauma attacks typically continue until prostration, death, or human intervention occurs. Male cockatoos are relentless, inflicting physical damage predominately to their mate's head, face, mouth, and beak (Figure 22.4).

Although beak trauma can also occur during parental feedings of neonatal or juvenile birds, between neonatal birds and young juvenile birds, and between weaning birds housed together in outdoor aviaries or in cages within a home, these beak traumas are often accidental or are isolated squabble incidents. Many result from parents (too aggressively) feeding their babies or their babies innocently pumping on each other's soft pliable uncalcified and unkeratinized beaks. The author has only once witnessed what appeared to be a weaning bird cagemate trauma. The mate trauma appeared to be deliberate and resulted in the death of the attacked female. This trauma occurred in a juvenile pair of unrelated Palm Cockatoos housed in a large outdoor nursery flight cage. The deliberate nature of this cagemate trauma appears to be the exception and not the rule when the involved birds are immature and not set up for breeding. The author has also witnessed this level of fatal aggression in bonded, same-sex pairs that were unknowingly set up and in groups of mate trauma males housed together. Same-sex aggression and trauma involving male cockatoos has been witnessed by other aviculturists and avian veterinarians where birds were set up in a breeding colony or known aggressive male were accidentally placed with another breeding pair or with conspecific males.

PREVENTATIVE MANAGEMENT

To best manage psittacine birds, it is necessary to consider their life stages.[3] A parrot's life stages can be divided into neonatal and juvenile, adult reproductive, and adult post-reproductive stages. The adult reproductive stage is the longest period of the bird's life and when the majority of mate traumas occur.[3]

The adult reproductive life stage is also the most aggressive stage, when birds are the most vocal and the least tame. A calmer, better pet-quality bird is characterized by the neonatal and juvenile stage and the post-reproductive stage.[3] Birds are the most affectionate and playful when young and then return partially to this state as quiet, calmer, geriatric birds, even if they spent the interim years in breeding.[3]

Various methods of mate trauma prevention have been reported.[1–5, 7] The author feels most comfortable with the simplest methods, which are non-surgical and the least invasive. These include routine bilateral wing and maxilla beak tip trimming and filing (to roundness) of known aggressive male birds.

These procedures must be performed in the pre-breeding season, that is, the fall.

Although these beak and wing filing and trimming methods are temporary, the results usually last for up to four months, getting the pair through breeding season—the prime time for mate trauma aggression.

Other more invasive mate trauma prevention methods include acrylic beak balls or rubber beak bumpers being surgically applied to the tip of the male's maxilla. These methods were explored in the 1990s and offered effective, albeit temporary (two weeks to three months), protection for female cagemates.[1–4]

The rubber beak bumpers lasted longer than the acrylic beak balls. This same author developed a modified surgical debeaking procedure for aggressive male psittacine birds.[1–4] In this procedure, the bird is placed under anesthesia and the maxilla tip is cut off with the cutting wheel of a dremel drill.[4] This procedure was found to be temporary, as the cut maxilla tip regrew in all cases but was often reduced in size. When compared to the acrylic beak balls or rubber beak bumpers, this procedure lasted the longest.[4] That author further noted that although disfigurement of the beak occurred, the process was temporary and could save pairs. Another author reported a more aggressive surgical technique that was intended to be permanent; it is called lower beak and complete mandible bisection or splitting.[5] This surgery was viewed, by that author, as a salvage procedure to be performed only when all other methods failed to protect the female from an attacking male. The author stated that he performed this surgery on only the most aggressive male cockatoos, so the pair could be kept together. However, any surgical procedure that permanently disfigures an animal is indeed controversial, as stated by that, and this, author.[5] In cases of very aggressive males, it is recommended to resort to the other preventative methods such as permanent pair separation. In some cases, the pair must be sacrificed to save the female.

Other preventative measures include removing or changing the nest box. Special nest boxes can be made with two entrances and baffled interiors. This type of nest box design may limit box attacks on females. An extension of this design is two cages attached together, side by side. Each cage has its own nest box with two entrances. The cages communicate by two entrances (or exits), one at the front and one at the back of the bi-cage setup. Other special cage designs focus on elevated escape areas for the flighted female that are less accessible to the wing-clipped males. To make these areas completely inaccessible to the clipped males they must also be skirted by cockatoo-safe sheet metal to prevent the clipped male from climbing to the female's elevated escape areas. Temporary pair separation is usually necessary and occasionally breaks the cycle of aggression. This separation can be for a minimum time of several weeks to several months or years depending on the severity of the mate trauma attack and the time needed by the female to fully recover. Permanent separation, however, is the ultimate way to break the cycle of aggression and assure the safety of the female.

Repair of the involved birds is yet another preventative measure. However, in cases of recurrent mate traumas, very severe mate traumas, or mate death the aggressive males should be retired altogether from breeding. The pair should be separated and the males placed in new homes either as display birds in zoological collections or pet birds in home situations. It is the author's experience that some of these males do indeed make good pets in single-pet homes. The surviving females with extensive beak lesions may be retired to rescue or pet bird home situations. Future owners of these severely affected female mate trauma birds must be willing to be diligent with the bird's veterinary care for life. If repair of the birds is an option, mate trauma males should be given larger, more aggressive female mates and the females given smaller, less aggressive male mates.

TREATMENT

To properly treat mate trauma, which typically involves various types of severe beak trauma, the avian veterinarian must be very familiar with the avian beak. The avian beak function and anatomy must be fully understood. The two following sections on prehensile function of the beak and anatomy of the beak will outline the vast importance of this organ to the healthy psittacine bird.

Moribund mate trauma females do best when minimally handled. A quick careful physical examination should be followed by parenteral fluid administration.

Take care to also check that the bird is not egg bound by performing gentle abdominal palpation. Only warmed fluids should be used on mate trauma birds. After their quick physical examinations, the females should be treated immediately with intravenous (IV) dextrose and crystalloid fluids, subcutaneous (SQ) dextrose and crystalloid fluids, plus a shock dose of SQ dexamethasone. If possible, the female's wounds should be very carefully and quickly cleansed. She should immediately be placed into a dark incubator where heat and oxygen are provided. Next, depending on the extent of beak trauma, soft foods, such as mixed commercial baby bird formula,

soaked commercial bird pellets, and large juicy pieces of fruit, should be offered. No water should be offered initially. A water bowl in the cage of an extremely weak bird is dangerous since the bird could drown if it falls in. The weak traumatized female should be kept quiet during her initial period of stabilization.

After the bird is stabilized, the avian veterinarian can safely work on her wounds and address her beak trauma in a conservative fashion. Please take note that in the vast majority of cases, acrylics are not indicated. The application of acrylics to an ultimately infected bite wound is a recipe for abscess formation. Wounds in the avian beak, like turtle and tortoise shell wounds, do best when managed as open wounds. The female's beak wounds should be cultured and treated with parenteral and topical antibiotics and antifungals as indicated. Careful flushing and repeat debridement over time are an important part of the slow healing process.

Despite the fact that female mate trauma victims typically have permanent grotesquely disfigured beak lesions, they learn to adapt and eat on their own quite quickly. Their lesions, however, often require lifelong beak trimming and filing by an avian veterinarian. This is because most beak traumas result in malocclusion, which over time causes horrific unnatural overgrowths of affected portions of the keratin of the upper or lower beak. In order to attempt to align the working horn, the hard keratin occlussal surface, the cutting edge or the tomium, trimming and filing is imperative for life so these birds can eat to the best of their ability. Beak trauma birds are destined to have overgrown beaks secondary to their beak trauma-induced malocclusion. It is the author's opinion that birds altered in this way are more likely to be depressed, timid, and non-confrontational but fare well if they survive the initial attack.

If these birds are subsequently kept alone as either educational or pet birds, they can still have happy and healthy lives.

PREHENSILE FUNCTION OF THE BEAK

The psittacine beak has numerous prehensile functions and hence must be in the best possible form at all times.

Since birds do not have lips and teeth and because their thoracic limbs are specialized for flight, their beaks have evolved to have significant and extensive prehensile function. The highly evolved prehensile function of the avian beak is aided by the dexterous tongue and flexible feet of the various avian species.[6]

Avian beak functions are numerous and include the procurement of food and water and the preparation of food. The beak's cutting edge, or tomium, serves to shave the bird's food versus chewing it. The beak also serves in grooming, sexual display, courtship, nest building, egg turning, evaporative heat loss (panting), locomotion, and ultimately, defense.[6]

The adult avian beak is also a formidable weapon. It is known as the rhamphotheca and is a hard keratin structure that covers the rostral aspect of the upper and lower jawbones of the bird. The upper beak is called the rostrum maxillaris and the lower beak the rostrum mandibularis.[6]

On the other hand, the growing neonatal and juvenile beak is a pliable and malleable appendage until calcification and keratinization occur. The beak of a young chick can therefore change from perfect occlusion to complete malocclusion in a day. The majority of beak problems in the very young are divided into five categories: lateral deviations of the maxilla (scissor beak), compression deformities of the mandible, prognathism (pug beak), subluxation of the premaxilla, which occurs more often in juveniles, and beak trauma, which can occur in birds of any age. The first two malformations are most common in macaws, the third in cockatoos, and the fourth in juvenile macaws.[6]

While chicks are young and the beak is still pliable and fast-growing, physical therapy and trimming and filing, along with medical treatment, are indicated post-beak trauma and extensive surgery may not be necessary. After calcification and keratinization, however, in addition to frequent clipping and filing, surgical acrylic implants or extensions may be needed to properly align a crushed and damaged beak. Hence after calcification and keratinization beak trauma repair may require rhamphothotics to correctly repair the beak's alignment and integrity. However, this is often not necessary even in the worst of trauma cases, as psittacines are very adaptable and learn to eat and drink with even the most severe of beak traumas.[6] Further, acrylic patches, or implants, applied over infected beak wounds foster bacterial and fungal abscess formation.

Physiologically the rhamphotheca is an ever-growing dynamic tissue, which contains abundant keratin and, in adults, free calcium phosphate. It takes approximately six months to replace itself in adults, making beak healing and repair a very slow process.[6]

ANATOMY OF THE BEAK

The avian beak is composed of bone, dermis, epidermis, a transitional layer, and the keratinized epidermis (horn or rhamphotheca). The rostrum maxillaris (upper beak) and the rostrum mandibularis (lower beak) are all-inclusive terms for the keratin, soft tissue (dermis), and boney structures of the indicated beak.[6]

The cancellous boney structure of the upper beak includes the premaxilla, nasal, and frontal bones. The premaxilla thickens at the tip in psittacines forming the bill tip organ, which is innervated by cranial nerve VI (deep ophthalmic nerve). This organ contains highly sensitive receptors important in food collection, eating, and preening. The lower cancellous boney beak consists of the mandible, which joins the quadrate bone.[6] It also contains a bill tip organ in certain species, such as parrots, geese, and ducks. The exact location and development of the bill tip organ varies among avian species. In parrots it is believed that the bill tip organ is most developed in the lower beak. The bill tip organ is extremely sensitive and this should be considered when manipulating the tip of both the upper and lower beak. To improve the sensory capacity of the bill tip organ, the lower beak should always be included in routine grooming of the overgrown beak.

The soft tissues of the beak include the rhamphotheca, which is divided into the harder working horn and the softer covering horn. Rostrally the rhamphotheca changes into the working horn, a hard keratin occlusal surface ending in the cutting edge, or the tomium. The maxilla's keratin is known as the rhinotheca, and the mandible's keratin is called the gnathotheca. The cere is known as the base of the rhinotheca, which remains soft. The rhinotheca joins the frontal bone via a kinetic joint, or the nasal-frontal hinge. This synovial joint is mobile in psittacines and fixed in raptors. The gnathotheca is adjoined to the mandible via connective and muscular tissue attachments.[6]

The rhinotheca grows in the cranioventral

plane and the gnathotheca grows more quickly in the craniodorsal plane. The rhamphotheca is composed of thickened layers of stratum corneum originating from the stratum germinativum. It contains abundant keratin and, in adults, free calcium phosphate. Baby birds' beaks are pliable because the free calcium phosphate has not yet been laid down, or calcified.[6]

CONCLUSION

Mate trauma is a syndrome induced by the confines and limitations of captivity. It apparently does not occur in the wild, and given this fact, the author feels aviculturists and avian veterinarians should go above and beyond to treat these abused birds to the best of our collective abilities. We, as avian veterinarians, should also attempt to address the emotional healing of these wounded birds and fight for their future protection from repeat abuse situations by encouraging their removal from breeding in captivity when necessary. Further, the author feels we, as avian veterinarians, should also educate new, and remind old-time, aviculturists of the horrors of mate trauma and the importance of an intact, fully functional *prehensile* beak appendage.

ACKNOWLEDGEMENTS

The author would like to thank Dr. Scott G. Martin and Dr. Tarah Hadley for their expert editorial comments and advice.

REFERENCES

1. Clubb, K., S. Clubb, A. Phillips, S. and Wolf S. 1992. "Intraspecific aggression in cockatoos." In *Psittacine aviculture, perspectives, techniques and research,* ed. R.M. Schubot, K.J. Clubb, and S.L. Clubb, pp. 25-1–25-5. Loxahatchee, FL: Avicultural Breeding and Research Center.
2. Clubb, S.L. 1997. "Avicultural medicine and flock health management." In *Avicultural medicine and surgery,* ed. R.B. Altman, S.L. Clubb, G.M. Dorrestein, and K. Quesenberry, pp. 101–116. Philadelphia: W.B. Saunders Co.
3. Clubb, S.L. 1998. Captive management of birds for a lifetime. *JAVMA* 212 (8):1243–1245.
4. Clubb, S.L. 1998. Management of psittacines to reduce mate aggression and trauma. *PAAV,* pp. 133–138.
5. McDonald, S E. 2000. Beak altering procedures to disarm aggressive male cockatoos. *Exotic DVM* 2.2:29–31.
6. Romagnano, A. 1998. "Beak malformations and corrections." ABVP Symposium, pp. 37–40.
7. Styles, D. 2001. "Captive psittacine behavioral reproductive husbandry and management: Socialization, aggression control, and pairing techniques." PAAV (Speciality Advanced Program), pp. 3–19.

23
Feather-Picking Disorder in Pet Birds

Lynne M. Seibert

Feather picking is one of the most common and challenging behavior problems of captive psittacine birds. It has been described as an exaggeration of normal preening behavior. However, the normal preening patterns of most psittacine species have not been studied, and normal birds may spend a significant portion of their daily time budget engaged in preening behavior (Spruijt et al. 1992). Regardless of the duration, in the course of normal preening, no damage to the feathers or skin should occur.

Rosskopf and Woerpel (1996) define feather picking as a condition in which the bird damages its feathers or skin or prevents the normal growth of feathers. Feather picking in birds is associated with feather chewing or removal, with or without self-inflicted soft tissue damage (Galvin 1983; Nett & Tully 2003). Soft tissue damage to skin or muscle occurs in some birds, with a higher incidence in cockatoo species (Rosenthal 1993) (Figures 23.1, 23.2, and 23.3). The term "feather-picking disorder" will be used in this chapter to describe the syndrome involving a variety of self-directed feather and soft tissue destructive behaviors with no apparent underlying medical etiology.

Clinical signs vary widely, ranging from mild localized feather damage to completely denuded areas and soft tissue excoriations. Chewed feathers have an irregular appearance, with the ramus of the feather shaft split longitudinally. Damage is inflicted to areas of the body that are accessible to the bird, with normal, unaffected head and crest feathers (Harrison 1986). The distribution of feather loss or damage is highly variable. According to Rosenthal (1993), the inner thighs and sternum are often affected. Nett and Tully (2003) report that the most commonly affected sites are the chest, under the wings, and over the rump, with feather chewing primarily affecting primary feathers. According to Perry (1994), the condition often lacks bilateral symmetry, especially in the early stages.

SPECIES PREDISPOSITIONS

African Grey Parrots (*Psittacus erithacus*), macaws (*Ara* spp.), cockatoo species, conure species, Eclectus Parrots (*Eclectus roratus*), and Grey-cheeked Parakeets (*Brotogeris* spp.) are reportedly predisposed to feather-picking disorder, while it is less common in Budgerigars (*Melopsittacus undulatus*), Cockatiels (*Nymphicus hollandicus*), and amazon parrots (*Amazona* spp.) (Rosskopf & Woerpel 1996). Jenkins (2001) includes Monk Parakeets (*Myiopsitta monachus*) as being predisposed to feather-picking disorder. According the Rosskopf and Woerpel (1991) and Briscoe et al. (2001), African Grey Parrots are the most commonly presented species for feather-picking disorder.

DIAGNOSIS OF FEATHER-PICKING DISORDER

Feather damage, removal, or loss may result from a variety of medical, environmental, or behavioral causes (Harrison 1994; Welle 1999). Self-trauma to feathers or skin is a non-specific symptom that has many possible etiologies. Medical disorders, nutritional deficiencies, toxin exposure, and environmental irritants should be considered in any case of feather picking, and primary medical problems and medical complications resulting from self-inflicted trauma need to be addressed.

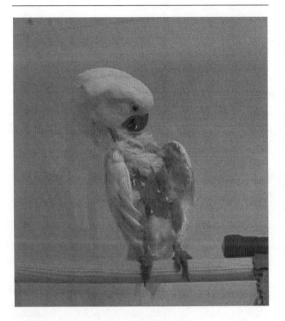

Figure 23.1. Cockatoo with feather-picking disorder. See also color section.

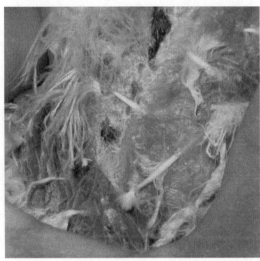

Figure 23.2. Self-inflicted soft tissue lesions in a Moluccan Cockatoo with feather-picking disorder.

All birds with feather abnormalities warrant a thorough history and physical examination, with appropriate diagnostic testing (Rosskopf & Woerpel 1996; Welle 1999). Any treatment plan should address both the physical and mental needs of the patient.

Medical differentials that should be considered include endoparasitism, systemic diseases, infectious diseases (circovirus, polyomavirus), malnutrition, and neoplasia. Giardia has been associated with feather picking, particularly in Cockatiels (Fudge & McEntee 1986). Less common causes of feather picking include ectoparasitism, primary infectious dermatitis or folliculitis, and endocrine imbalances (Rosenthal 1993).

The influence of pruritis, allergies, and hypersensitivity on feather-picking behavior is unclear, although advances are being made in diagnostic testing for allergies in psittacine patients (Colombini et al. 2000; Macwhirter et al. 1999).

A thorough physical examination is necessary. Feather abnormalities will be confined to areas that the bird can reach. There may be evidence of chewed feathers, damaged soft tissue, missing feathers, or feather regrowth.

Diagnostic testing may include fecal examination, skin scrapings, hematology, biochemical analysis, radiographs, bacterial or fungal culture and sensitivities, feather pulp and skin cytology, feather follicle and skin biopsies, and viral testing (Koski 2002; Rosenthal 1993). Air quality, humidity level, and exposure to toxins, chemicals, or smoke should also be addressed.

Taking a detailed behavioral history for the avian patient is a time-consuming, but extremely important, component of the diagnostic process. Information obtained from the history will aid not only in the diagnoses but also in designing a comprehensive treatment plan. To increase efficiency, clients can complete a questionnaire prior to the appointment, and additional questions can be based on this information. A thorough behavioral history should include information regarding the onset of feather picking, environmental changes associated with the onset of the behavior, duration of the condition, the time of day when the behavior is most intense, progression of signs, housing considerations, social interactions with other birds and human caregivers, a description of the abnormal behaviors, any seasonal patterns that may be apparent, and responses to previous treatments. Additional information should be obtained about the eliciting stimuli, how the behavior is terminated, whether or not the behavior can be in-

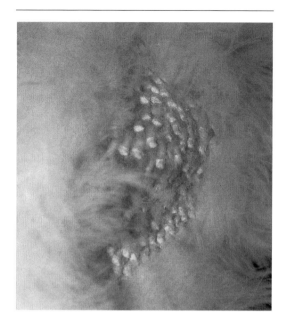

Figure 23.3. Feather chewing in a Sulfur-crested Cockatoo with feather-picking disorder.

terrupted, and how the caregiver reacts to the behavior. Early history information should determine whether the bird was parent- or hand-raised, the source of the bird, the age at weaning, early adverse experiences, previous homes, and contact with other birds and humans during possible sensitive periods of development. Caregivers should be carefully questioned about nutrition, which foods are offered, which are eaten, and the quantities consumed.

CONSEQUENCES OF FEATHER PICKING

Feathers are essential for flight and provide insulation, mechanical and thermal protection, proprioception, and waterproofing (Lucas & Stettenheim 1972; Nett & Tully 2003). The consequences of feather picking may be strictly aesthetic, but more serious sequelae may also result. Molting increases the metabolic demands for the bird, and chronic feather replacement can increase disease susceptibility and alter thermoregulatory ability (Nett & Tully 2003; Rosskopf & Woerpel 1996). Blood loss from traumatized blood feathers and damaged soft tissue can become significant (Galvin 1983). Featherless areas may bruise easily, and secondary infections are also possible. Permanent damage to

the feather follicle may prevent normal regrowth of feathers.

POSTULATED CAUSES OF FEATHER-PICKING DISORDER

The causes of feather-picking disorder have not been determined. Many potential risk factors have been suggested, but the exact etiology remains unknown. The common perception that inappropriate husbandry or boredom is responsible for the development of feather-picking problems raises concerns for caregivers about the quality of life of affected birds.

Boredom is the most commonly cited cause of feather-picking disorder (Galvin 1983; Lawton 1996; Rosenthal 1993). This is an overly simplistic explanation for a complicated disorder that likely develops as a result of multiple factors, including developmental influences, socialization deficits, neurochemical abnormalities, environmental issues, temperament traits, hormonal influences, genetics, undiagnosed medical conditions, and learning factors.

Foraging is an activity that consumes a significant amount of time for free-ranging psittacine birds. Ad libitum provision of food for captive psittacine birds, as well as restrictions in free movement, may predispose some birds to develop behavior problems (Lawton 1996; Rosskopf & Woerpel 1996). Environmental enrichment efforts for avian species have addressed the importance of providing opportunities for foraging (Bauck 1998; VanHoek & King 1997).

Optimal environments for captive psittacine birds should also provide opportunities for the bird to engage in species-typical behaviors, including locomotor activities. Chronic confinement does not provide the necessary opportunities for the bird to engage in normal behaviors.

Inappropriate or inadequate social interactions are also common issues for captive birds and may be problematic for some birds with feather-picking disorder. Pet birds are often isolated from conspecifics and must rely on human caregivers for social interactions. The majority of psittacine species kept in captivity are highly social, living in stable flocks under natural conditions, and may not acclimate well to a solitary lifestyle. Separation anxiety should be considered in birds that engage in feather-picking behavior while alone and in birds that show distress upon being left alone. Undesired exposure or contact with family pets, other birds, natural predators, or family members has also been implicated in some cases of feather picking.

Stress may also cause feather-picking behaviors to develop. Preening is commonly performed as a displacement behavior in situations in which conflicting behavioral systems are activated or in states of motivational ambivalence (Spruijt et al. 1992). Preening has been associated with comfort or dearousal and may therefore be performed in times of stress (Delius 1988). An unpredictable environment may be associated with increased stress (Rosenthal 1993). Crowding can also contribute to stress, as well as poor husbandry. Any abrupt change to the environment should also be considered as a potential stressor and contributing factor. Environmental changes of potential importance may include additions or deletions to the family, changes in the physical environment, schedule changes, housing changes, moving the bird, or climate changes. Rehoming of birds can contribute to stress when important social bonds are broken and new social bonds must be formed.

Exaggerated or prolonged reproductive behavior has been suggested as a possible cause of feather picking (Rosenthal 1993). Reproductive behavior changes can occur on a seasonal basis or throughout the year, particularly in birds that are exposed to unnatural photoperiods. Some avian species naturally remove feathers from their abdomen during the breeding season to enhance contact with their eggs, creating a brood patch (Oppenheimer 1991). Feather removal during the breeding season that involves ventral areas may be associated with reproductive behavior. Feather picking that persists past the breeding season is consistent with a feather-picking problem. Birds that are exposed to prolonged light photoperiods, consume high fat diets, or display sexual behaviors should be considered at risk for feather picking, and these issues should be addressed. According to Rosskopf and Woerpel (1996), cockatoos, macaws, conures, and Grey-cheeked Parakeets are likely to present with reproductively induced feather picking.

Additional considerations for birds suspected of reproductive-related feather picking include inappropriate mate pairings, frustrated mating instincts, lack or loss of a mate, or the presence of other nesting birds in the environment.

Sleep deprivation can have detrimental effects on the welfare of captive birds. Pet birds are often housed in common areas of the home and covered when the caregivers retire for the evening, or at dusk. The high level of vigilance that is characteristic of prey species may prevent adequate rest in these environments. In addition to the stress associated with inadequate rest, exposure to lengthy photoperiods can increase the incidence of undesirable reproductive behaviors.

Psittacine infants are altricial, requiring a relatively long period of maternal care. Newly hatched birds in captive breeding programs are often removed from their parents and weaned by human surrogates in an effort to promote adequate socialization to humans. However, detrimental effects of early maternal deprivation have been documented in other species (Ruppenthal et al. 1976; Suomi et al. 1976) and should be considered in planning captive breeding programs for psittacine birds (Jenkins 2001). If birds reared by human surrogates do not possess adequate coping skills as adults, then alternative rearing methods should be considered. Aengus and Millam (1999) have documented successful socialization of parent-raised Orange-winged Amazon Parrots with neonatal handling. One group was handled daily for 10–30 minutes, while the control group was handled only to obtain their weights. The handled group was significantly tamer than the control group, indicating that brief handling can promote tameness in parent-raised birds.

Iatrogenic causes of feather picking have also been suggested, including feather trauma from sloppy wing trims, small cages, or improperly placed perches (Davis 1991). Birds may also pick at injury sites (Rosenthal 1993).

With chronic feather picking, the initial precipitating causes may no longer be present or relevant, but the abnormal behaviors persist (Cooper & Harrison 1994). Neurochemical abnormalities may exist that support the persistence of these behavioral patterns, even in the absence of stressors and environmental deficits. Based on findings in other species, neurotransmitters of interest would include dopamine, serotonin, and opioids.

COMPARISON TO HUMAN PSYCHIATRIC DISORDERS

Feather-picking disorder has been compared to human disorders involving obsessive-compulsive behavior and loss of impulse control. Obsessive-compulsive disorder (OCD) is classified by *The Diagnostic and Statistical Manual of Mental Disorders,* 4th ed. (DSM-IV) as an anxiety disorder. Obsessive-compulsive disorders are characterized by obsessions, intrusive thoughts or images, and compulsions, repetitive behaviors performed in an attempt to prevent or reduce anxiety. Excessive hand washing is an example of a commonly reported compulsive behavior in humans. Stein (1996) and Stein et al. (1992) have suggested that hand washing in human OCD patients shares behavioral similarities with repetitive grooming behaviors in animals, including feather picking in birds.

Bordnick et al. (1994) discuss the similarities between feather-picking disorder in birds and trichotillomania, or hair pulling, in humans. Trichotillomania is an impulse control disorder characterized by hair removal that results in alopecia. It can involve any region of the body where hair grows. Tension increases as the individual attempts to resist the urge to pull hair. Manipulation of the hair is common, including hair twirling, chewing or mouthing the hair, and manual manipulation of removed hairs. Trichophagia may also occur. Similarly, birds with feather-picking disorder have been reported to chew, manipulate, and sometimes consume removed feathers.

Garner et al. (2003) compared the stereotypic behaviors of captive Orange-winged Amazon Parrots with those of human patients suffering from autism or schizophrenia. Performance of stereotypic behaviors by the parrots correlated with poor performance on a learning task in which the subjects tended to repeat rather than switch incorrect responses for subsequent trials. These responses were consistent with the performance of human patients with basal ganglia dysfunction.

TREATMENT OF FEATHER-PICKING DISORDER

Treatment recommendations should be specific for each individual based on a thorough history and accurate assessment of the contributing factors. Feather-picking disorder can be difficult to treat, and outcomes are often discouraging (Galvin 1983; Harrison 1994). Treatment should address underlying medical issues, nutritional deficiencies, environmental factors, behavior modification, and, in some cases, restraint options.

Housing should address the needs of the bird and provide adequate stimulation as well as a sense of safety. Cages that are kept in busy areas of the home may not provide adequate privacy, while cages kept in lower traffic areas may not provide sufficient stimulation. Cages should be large enough to allow movement, but all birds should have supervised time outside of the cage. Perches should provide stable surfaces in a variety of diameters and materials. Perches should be carefully placed such that feathers are not damaged when the bird turns or moves in the cage.

Air quality can be addressed by providing regular access to fresh air, use of air purifiers and humidifiers, and restricting the bird's exposure to chemicals, scented oils, Teflon, and cigarette smoke. The importance of regular bathing opportunities for healthy skin and feathers has also been discussed (Lawton 1996; Rosskopf & Woerpel 1996).

Most birds will manipulate objects (toys), and personal preferences should dictate the types of toys that are offered. Some toys should provide the bird with an opportunity to chew, such as rawhide, pieces of non-toxic wood, alfalfa cubes, or cardboard. Toys should not overcrowd the enclosure and can be rotated on a regular basis to maintain the bird's interest.

Foraging devices that require captive birds to work for food have been used for environmental enrichment purposes (Coulton et al. 1997). Foraging enrichments that require subjects to manipulate objects, sort through inedible materials, chew through barriers, and open containers were found to reduce feather-picking behavior in amazon parrots (Meehan, Millam, & Mench 2003). In addition to preventing the development of feather-chewing behaviors in the enriched group, the same enrichments were used to reverse the development of feather picking in control birds. Environmental enrichments have been found to compensate for some of the effects of early maternal deprivation in rodent species (Bredy et al. 2003; Francis et al. 2002).

Treatment for feather-picking disorder may involve provision of appropriate social contacts. Meehan, Garner, and Mench (2003) found that isosexual pairing of captive Orange-winged Amazon Parrots (*Amazona amazonica*) effected the development of abnormal behaviors. Pair-housed birds used enrichment devices more than singly housed cohorts and spent less time screaming, less time preening, and were more active. Pair-housing was protective against the development of stereotypic behaviors and neophobia. Local avian groups have attempted to provide opportunities for socialization with other birds through weekly or monthly gatherings of bird owners and their birds.

When reproductive causes are suspected, the environment can be modified to decrease reproductive behaviors. Shorter photoperiods, removal of toys or mirrors that promote masturbation or regurgitation, and separation from other nesting birds have been suggested (Harrison & Davis 1986). Interactions with the caregiver should be limited to activities that do not promote reproductive behaviors. Providing an appropriate mate has also been suggested.

Sleep requirements need to be addressed for affected birds (Galvin 1983; Wilson 1999). A two-cage system, including a day cage and sleeping cage in a quiet room, will provide the bird with a quiet secluded sleeping area. A regular schedule should be maintained, with seasonal variations when appropriate.

Behavior modification exercises have been recommended for the treatment of feather-picking disorder. Positive reinforcement of appropriate behaviors, with food treats, praise, or an object reward, can be used when the bird is playing independently or manipulating appropriate objects. Training sessions to teach commands will provide mental stimulation, increase bird-caregiver interactions, and allow the owner to redirect inappropriate behaviors more effectively (Jenkins 2001). Desensitization and response substitution techniques can also be employed. Desensitization involves benign gradual exposures to stress-inducing stimuli at a rate that does not provoke a stress response. Desensitization techniques can be combined with response substitution in which the bird is directed to perform an appropriate activity that is incompatible with the undesirable behavior, such as performing commands, taking food treats, or playing with a favorite toy.

Acupuncture has been used to treat feather-picking disorder. Worell and Farber (1993) treated 28 birds (12 species) in an open trial. The subjects underwent weekly or biweekly acupuncture treatments, ranging from one to 42 treatments. Some of the subjects responded well to acupuncture treatments, but more studies are needed to assess required duration of treatment, frequency of treatment, and species differences in responses to acupuncture therapy.

The use of restraint devices has been advocated by some and dismissed by others. Most practitioners agree that restraint devices should be fitted in the hospital to ensure that they can be worn safely, and that they should be used only when necessary to prevent serious self-injury (Lawton 1996; Rosskopf & Woerpel 1996). Some birds react violently to restraint devices.

A variety of collars are available, including Elizabethan-style collars, made from radiographic film or plastic, and tube collars made from pipe insulator or acrylic (Figures 23.4, 23.5, 23.6, and 23.7). The author has used a sweater-type restraint device made from a thick cotton tube sock successfully in a variety of species. Cockatoos seem to be particularly accepting of this form of restraint and rarely need to be hospitalized for fittings (Figure 23.8).

PHARMACOLOGICAL AGENTS

Few drugs have been systematically evaluated for adjunctive treatment of feather-picking disorder. They should be used with caution until more information is available about toxicity, dosage requirements, and efficacy. Pharmacological therapies have historically been considered only as a last resort (Johnson-Delaney 1992). Dopamine antagonists, serotonergic agents, opioid antagonists, tricyclic antidepressants, benzodiazepines,

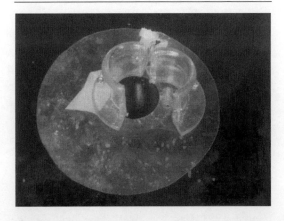

Figure 23.4. Combination collar constructed of acrylic and plastic, weighing approximately 80 grams.

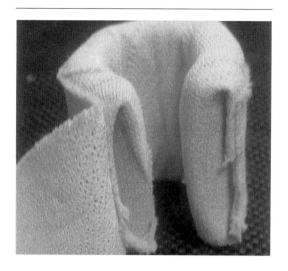

Figure 23.5. Tube collar constructed from pipe insulation weighing less than 10 grams.

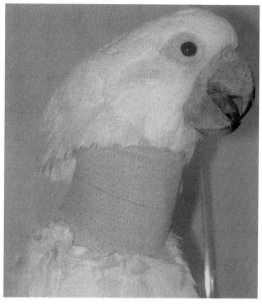

Figure 23.7. Umbrella Cockatoo wearing the collar in Figure 23.5.

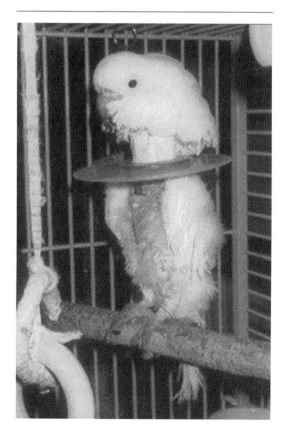

Figure 23.6. Umbrella Cockatoo wearing the collar in Figure 23.4.

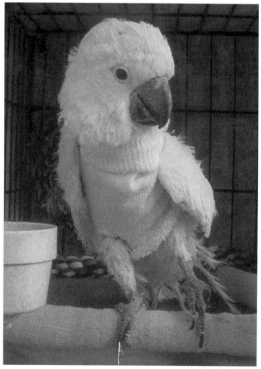

Figure 23.8. Moluccan Cockatoo wearing a sock sweater. See also color section.

Table 23-1   Dosages for drugs used in the treatment of feather-picking disorder

Drug	Dosage
Amitriptyline	1.0–5.0 mg/kg PO q 12–24 h (Lawton)
Butorphanol	0.2–1.0 mg/kg IM[a]
Chorionic gonadotropin (hCG)	500–1,000 IU/kg IM on days 1, 7, 14, 21, then q 28 d[a]
Clomipramine	1 mg/kg PO q 12 h[b]
Diazepam	0.6 mg/kg IM; 1 mg/6 oz water[b] 1.25–2.5 mg/120 ml water[a] 2.5–4.0 mg/kg PO q 6–8 h[a]
Diphenhydramine	2.0–4.0 mg/kg PO q 12 h 0.5 mg/240 ml water[a]
Doxepin	0.5–1.0 mg/kg PO q 12 h[a]
Fluoxetine	0.4 mg/kg PO q 24 h (Lawton) 2.0 mg/kg PO q 12 h[a]
Haloperidol	0.15–0.4 mg/kg PO q 12 h (Iglauer, Rasim) 1.0–2.0 mg/kg IM q 21 d[a]
Hydroxyzine	2.0–2.2 mg/kg PO q 8 h[a] 4 mg/120 ml water[a]
Leuprolide acetate	700–800 mcg/kg IM q 14 d for 3 doses, then q 4 mo
Naltrexone	1.5 mg/kg PO q 12 h (Turner)

[a]Carpenter, Mashima, Rupiper, Exotic Animal Formulary, 2001.
[b]AAHA Exotic Animal Formulary.

and hormonal therapies have been used for the treatment of feather picking, but few controlled studies are available (Table 23-1). Welle (1998) has reviewed the psychotropic drugs used in avian species. Use of psychotropic drugs in psittacine species constitutes extra-label use and informed consent of caregivers is recommended.

Serotonergic agents are the most commonly prescribed pharmacological treatment for trichotillomania in humans and compulsive disorder in non-human species (Christianson & Crow 1996; Diefenbach et al. 2000). Fluoxetine (Prozac) is a selective serotonin reuptake inhibitor that enhances serotonergic function via selective inhibition of neurotransmitter reuptake at the serotonin transporter. Fluoxetine has been used to treat feather picking in birds at doses ranging from 1 to 4 mg/kg q 24 h, but anecdotal reports would suggest that it is not very effective (Jenkins 2001). Fluoxetine, along with behavior and environmental modifications, was used to treat repetitive toe chewing in a Cockatiel at a dose of 1 mg/kg q 24 h (Seibert 2004).

Tricyclic antidepressants enhance serotonergic and noradrenergic transmission by blocking their reuptake into the presynaptic neuron. In addition, they produce anticholinergic and antihistaminic effects. Doxepin (Sinequan) and amitriptyline (Elavil) have been used to treat feather-picking disorder.

Clomipramine is a tricyclic antidepressant with high selectivity for serotonin reuptake inhibition. It was the first medication to be approved by the Food and Drug Administration (FDA) for the treatment of obsessive-compulsive disorder in humans.

Ramsey and Grindlinger (1992) used clomipramine to treat feather-picking disorder in an open trial with 11 psittacine birds. Doses were gradually increased to a maintenance dose of 0.5 mg/kg q 12 h. Only two of the 11 birds responded. A Congo African Grey Parrot (*Psittacus erythacus*) was treated for feather picking and self-mutilation with an initial clomipramine dose of 4 mg/kg q 12 h by Juarbe-Diaz (2000). The dose was eventually increased to 9.5 mg/kg q 12 h. Feather regrowth occurred, and the caregiver felt that the feather picking was adequately controlled three months after the final dosage adjustment.

Ritchie and Harrison (1994) recommended using a low dose of clomipramine initially with a gradual increase over a four- to five-day period. However, they stated that clinical impressions suggest that this drug is rarely effective in controlling mutilation behavior in birds.

A placebo-controlled clomipramine trial in cockatoos with feather-picking disorder revealed significant improvement in treated birds at a dose of 3 mg/kg q 12 h (Seibert et al., in press). No side effects were reported in cockatoos during the trial. However, a Green-winged Macaw being treated by the author with clomipramine at a dose of 3 mg/kg q 12 h died on day 2 of treatment.

Haloperidol (Haldol) is a butyrophenone antipsychotic agent that exerts its behavioral effects by blocking dopaminergic activity. Doses ranging from 0.1–0.4 mg/kg q 12 h have been used effectively (Iglauer & Rasim 1993; Lennox & VanDerHeyden 1993). It is recommended that lower doses be used in cockatoos, African Grey Parrots, and Quaker Parrots (0.05 mg/kg q 24 h). Side effects include sedation, agitation, inappetence, incoordination, severe depression, anorexia, and hyperexcitability. An injectable form is available, haloperidol decanoate, and has been used at a dose of 1 to 2 mg/kg IM q 14–21 d.

Opioid antagonists may improve feather-picking behavior through their ability to block the release of endogenous opioids. Naltrexone (Trexan) was used to successfully treat feather picking at a starting dose of 1.5 mg/kg q 12 h in a variety of species (Turner 1993).

Benzodiazepines have been used for the short-term alleviation of symptoms and to aid in acceptance of restraint devices. Benzodiazepines exert their effects by binding to a site on the GABA receptor and enhancing GABA-ergic activity.

Feather-picking disorder is a complicated syndrome commonly seen in several pet bird species. Multiple etiologies should be considered before developing a treatment plan. Medical conditions, nutritional deficiencies, behavioral abnormalities, and environmental situations must be assessed for each patient. Effective treatment depends on thorough consideration of relevant factors, treatment of underlying or complicating medical issues, correction of environmental deficits, and implementation of behavior modification exercises. The use of restraint devices should be reserved for severe cases involving mutilation of soft tissue. Use of psychoactive medications should include informed caregiver consent and careful consideration of potential risks. Several areas warrant further investigation, such as the impact of early maternal deprivation on adult behavior, the safety of psychoactive drug use in psittacine species, and the risk factors for feather-picking disorder to guide preventive counseling.

REFERENCES

Aengus, W.L., and J.R. Millam. 1999. Taming parent-reared orange-winged amazon parrots by neonatal handling. *Zoo Biology* 18:177–187.

American Psychiatric Association. 1994. *Diagnostic and statistical manual of mental disorders*, 4th ed. Washington, DC: American Psychiatric Association.

Bauck, L. 1998. Psittacine diets and behavioral enrichment. *Sem Avian Exotic Pet Med* 7 (3):135–140.

Bordnick, P.S., B.A. Thyer, and B.W. Ritchie, BW. 1994. Feather picking disorder and trichotillomania: An avian model of human psychopathology. *J Behav Ther and Exp Psychiat* 25 (3):189–196.

Bredy, T.W. R.A. Humpartzoomian, D.P. Cain,and M.J. Meaney. 2003. Partial reversal of the effect of maternal care on cognitive function through environmental enrichment. *Neuroscience* 118 (2):571–576.

Briscoe, J.A., L. Wilson, and G. Smith. 2001. "Nonmedical risk factors for feather picking in pet parrots." Proc Assoc Avian Vet, p. 131.

Christianson, G.A., and S.J. Crow. 1996. The characterization and treatment of trichotillomania. *J Clin Psychiatry* 57 (S8):42–49.

Colombini, S., C.S. Foil, G. Hosgood, and T.N. Tully. 2000. Intradermal skin testing in Hispaniolan parrots (*Amazona ventralis*). *Veterinary Dermatology* 11 (4):271–276.

Cooper, J.E., and G.J. Harrison. 1994. "Dermatology." In *Avian medicine: Principles and application,* ed. B.W. Ritchie, G.J. Harrison, and L.R. Harrison, pp. 607–639. Lake Worth, FL: Wingers Publishing Inc.

Coulton, L.E., N.K. Waran, and R.J. Young. 1997. Effects of foraging enrichment on the behavior of parrots. *Animal Welfare* 6:357–363.

Davis, C.S. 1991. Parrot psychology and behavior problems. *Vet Clin North Am Small Anim Pract* 21 (6):1281–1288.

Delius, J.D. 1988. Preening and associated comfort behavior in birds. *Ann NY Acad Sci* 525:40–55.

Diefenbach, G.J., D. Reitman, and D.A. Williamson. 2000. Trichotillomania: A challenge to research and practice. *Clin Psychol Rev* 20 (3):289–309.

Francis, D.D., J. Diorio, P.M. Plotsky, and M.J. Meaney. 2002. Environmental enrichment reverses the effects of maternal separation on stress reactivity. *Journal of Neuroscience* 22 (18):7840–7843.

Fudge, A.M., and L. McEntee. 1986. "Avian giardiasis: Syndromes, diagnosis and therapy." Proc Assoc Avian Vet, pp. 155–164.

Galvin, C. 1983. "The feather picking bird." In *Current veterinary therapy VIII small animal practice,* ed. by R.W. Kirk, pp. 646–652. Philadelphia: W.B. Saunders Co.

Garner, J.P., C.L. Meehan, and J.A. Mench. 2003. Stereotypies in caged parrots, schizophrenia and autism: Evidence for a common mechanism. *Behav Brain Res* 145 (1–2):125–134.

Harrison, G.J. 1986. Feather disorders. *Vet Clin of North Am Caged Bird Med* 14 (2):179–199.

Harrison, G.J. 1994. "Perspective on parrot behavior." In *Avian medicine: Principles and application,* ed. B.W. Ritchie, G.J. Harrison, and L.R. Harrison, pp. 96–108. Lake Worth, FL: Wingers Publishing Inc.

Harrison, G.J., and C. Davis. 1986. "Captive behavior and its modification." In *Clinical avian medicine and surgery,* ed. G.J. Harrison, pp. 20–28. Philadelphia: W.B. Saunders Co.

Iglauer, F., and R. Rasim. 1993. Treatment of psychogenic feather picking in psittacine birds with a dopamine antagonist. *J Sm Anim Pract* 34:564.

Jenkins, J. 2001. Feather picking and self-mutilation in psittacine birds. *Vet Clin N Amer Exotic Anim Prac* 4 (3):651–667.

Johnson-Delaney, C. 1992. "Feather picking: Diagnosis and treatment." Proc Assoc Avian Vet, p. 82.

Juarbe-Diaz, S.J. 2000. Animal behavior case of the month. *J Am Vet Med Assoc* 216 (10):1562–1564.

Koski, M.A. 2002. Dermatologic diseases in psittacine birds: An investigational approach. *Sem Avian Exotic Pet Med* 11 (3):105–124.

Lawton, M.P.C. 1996. "Behavioural problems." In *BSAVA Manual of Psittacine Birds,* ed. P.H. Beynon, N.A. Forbes, and M.P.C. Lawton, pp. 106–114. Ames: Iowa State University Press.

Lennox, A.M., and N. VanDerHeyden. 1993. "Haloperidol for use in treatment of psittacine self-mutilation and feather plucking." Proc Assoc Avian Vet, pp. 119–120.

Lucas, A.M., and P.R. Stettenheim. 1972. *Avian anatomy: Integument*. Washington, DC: U.S. Government Printing Office.

Macwhirter, P., R. Mueller, and J. Gill. 1999. "Ongoing research report: Allergen testing as a part of diagnostic protocol in self-mutilating psittaciformes." Proc Assoc Avian Vet, pp. 125–128.

Meehan, C.L., J.P. Garner, and J.A. Mench. 2003. Isosexual pair housing improves the welfare of young amazon parrots. *Appl An Behav Sci* 81:73–88.

Meehan, C.L., J.R. Millam, and J.A. Mench. 2003. Foraging opportunity and increased physical complexity both prevent and reduce psychogenic feather picking by young amazon parrots. *Applied Animal Behavior Science* 80 (1):71–85.

Nett, C.S., and T.N. Tully. 2003. Anatomy, clinical presentation, and diagnostic approach to feather picking pet birds. *Compendium* 25 (3):206–218.

Oppenheimer, J. 1991. "Feather picking: Systemic approach." Proc Assoc Avian Vet, pp. 314–315.

Perry, R.A. 1994. "Perspective on parrot behavior." In *Avian medicine: Principles and application,* ed. B.W. Ritchie, G.J. Harrison, and L.R. Harrison, pp. 96–108. Lake Worth, FL: Wingers Publishing Inc.

Ramsey, E.C,, and H. Grindlinger. 1992. "Treatment of feather picking with clomipramine." Proc Assoc Avian Vet, pp. 379–382.

Ritchie, B.W., and G.J. Harrison. 1994. "Formulary." In *Avian medicine: Principles and application,* ed. B.W. Ritchie, G.J. Harrison, and L.R. Harrison, p. 461. Lake Worth, FL: Wingers Publishing Inc.

Rosenthal, K. 1993. "Differential diagnosis of feather picking in pet birds." Proc Assoc Avian Vet, Nashville, TN, pp. 108–112.

Rosskopf, W.J., and R.W. Woerpel. 1991. Pet avian conditions and syndromes of the most frequently presented species seen in practice. *Vet Clinics N Am Sm Anim Pract* 21 (6):1189–1211.

Rosskopf, W.J., and R.W. Woerpel. 1996. "Feather picking and therapy of skin and feather disorders." In *Diseases of cage and aviary birds*, 3rd ed., ed. W.J. Rosskopf and R.W. Woerpel, pp. 397–405. Baltimore: Williams and Wilkins.

Ruppenthal, G.C., G.L. Arling, H.F. Harlow, G.P. Sackett, and S.J. Suomi. 1976. A 10-year perspective of motherless-mother monkey behavior. *Journal of Abnormal Psychology* 85 (4):341–349.

Seibert, L.M. 2004. Animal behavior case of the month. *J Am Vet Med Assoc* 224 (9):1433–1435.

Seibert, L.M., Crowell-Davis, S.L., G.H. Wilson, and B.W. Ritchie. In press. Placebo-controlled clomipramine trial for the treatment of feather picking disorder in cockatoo (*Cacatua*) species. *J Am Anim Hosp Assoc.*

Spruijt, B.M., J.A. Van Hooff, and W.H. Gispen. 1992. Ethology and neurobiology of grooming behavior. *Physiol Rev* 72 (3):825–852.

Stein, D.J. 1996. The neurobiology of obsessive-compulsive disorder. *Neuroscientist* 2 (5):300–305.

Stein, D.J., N. Shoulberg, K. Helton, and E. Hollander. 1992. The neuroethological approach to obsessive-compulsive disorder. *Comp Psychiatry* 33 (4): 274–281.

Suomi, S.J., M.L. Collins, H.F. Harlow, and G.C. Ruppenthal. 1976. Effects of maternal and peer separations on young monkeys. *Journal of Child Psychol Psychiatry* 17 (2):101–112.

Turner, R. 1993. "Trexan (naltrexone hydrochloride) use in feather picking in avian species." Proc Assoc Avian Vet, pp. 116–118.

VanHoek, C.S., and C.E. King. 1997. Causation and influence of environmental enrichment on feather picking of the crimson-bellied conure (*Pyrrhura perlata perlata*). *Zoo Biol* 16 (2):161–172.

Welle, K.R. 1998. "A review of psychotropic drug therapy." Proc Assoc Avian Vet, pp. 121–124.

Welle, K.R. 1999. "Clinical approach to feather picking." Proc Assoc Avian Vet, pp. 119–124.

Wilson, L. 1999. Sleep: How much is enough for a parrot? *Pet Bird Report* 43:60–62

Worell, A.B., and W.L. Farber. 1993. "Use of acupuncture in the treatment of feather picking in psittacines." Proc Assoc Avian Vet, Nashville, TN, pp. 121–126.

24
Psittacine Behavioral Pharmacotherapy

Kenneth M. Martin

INTRODUCTION

Behavioral problems are one of the leading causes of pet relinquishment and/or euthanasia. The use of behavioral drugs has been advised in the past to be considered only as a "last resort."[1] It was believed that once on medication, birds would have to remain on that drug permanently. In reality, appropriate usage of behavioral drugs may mean the difference between a healthy human/bird bond and relinquishment or euthanasia. Psittacines with behavioral disorders often benefit from timely and appropriate use of behavioral drugs. When triggers are identified, and drugs are used as an adjunct to behavioral and environmental modification, birds may be successfully weaned off medication.

MECHANISM OF ACTION

Most behavioral drugs exert their effects through actions on neurotransmitters in the central nervous system. Neurotransmitters are responsible for transmission of impulses between neuronal and non-neuronal cells. Alterations in neurotransmitter levels and receptors can lead to neurological and behavioral disorders. Behavioral drugs can be used to modify these neurotransmitters and result in physiological and behavioral changes. Understanding basic neurotransmitter pathophysiology and how alterations in the levels of neurotransmitters affect behavior is beneficial in selection of behavioral drugs.

Neurotransmitters are released from the presynaptic neuron into the synaptic cleft and act on the postsynaptic cell. Stimulation of neurotransmitter receptors on the postsynaptic cell can have excitatory or inhibitory effects. Continuous stimulation by neurotransmitters or drugs (agonists) can hyposensitize or down-regulate receptors, while receptors that are not stimulated by neurotransmitters or blocked by drugs (antagonists) can become hypersensitive or up-regulated. Some neurotransmitters can also act on distant targets and thus act as neurohormones. Depending on the neurotransmitter, enzymes in the synaptic cleft or in the presynaptic neuron may inactivate these neurotransmitters. Reuptake inhibitors block reuptake and may prolong the effect of the neurotransmitter. This is the basis for the proposed mechanism of action of psychoactive drugs. Specific mechanisms of action are largely unknown.

NEUROTRANSMITTERS

Neurotransmitters of importance are serotonin (5HT or 5-hydroxytryptamine), norepinephrine (NE), epinephrine (E), dopamine (DA), gamma-aminobutyric acid (GABA), and acetylcholine (Ach). Serotonin, norepinephrine, and dopamine are classified as monoamines.

Monoamines may be divided into two classes, catecholamines and indoleamines. They are concentrated in the midbrain, hypothalamus, and limbic system. The catecholamines include norepinephrine, epinephrine, and dopamine. They are derived from the amino acid tyrosine. The indoleamines include serotonin and melatonin and are derived from dietary tryptophan.

Serotonin

Serotonin is found mainly in cells of the midline raphe and plays a role in the sleep-wake cycle, mood and emotion, and the suppression of impulsive behavior. Serotonin is inactivated by reuptake or breakdown by monoamine oxidase (MAO). Serotonin depletion has been associated with depression, increased anxiety, irritability and aggression, and impulsiveness. Increasing or normalizing brain serotonin levels is beneficial in compulsive and stereotypic disorders and some forms of anxiety and aggression. Serotonin excess has been associated with confidence, calmness, flexibility, and resilience. Selective serotonin reuptake inhibitors and tricyclic antidepressants increase serotonin availability by decreasing reuptake.

Norepinephrine

Norepinephrine is formed from the hydroxylation of dopamine. Norepinephrine is broken down by monoamine oxidase A (MAO A) and by catechol-O-methyltransferase (COMT). Norepinephrine depletion has been associated with depression, while excess has been associated with mania. Drugs that inhibit MAO and norepinephrine reuptake are beneficial in treating depression in humans.

Epinephrine

Epinephrine is secreted from the adrenal gland in response to norepinephrine to cause sympathetic effects. There are alpha and beta adrenergic receptors. Alpha adrenergic activation leads to vasoconstriction, increased cardiac contraction, iris dilation, intestinal relaxation, pilomotor contraction, contraction of the bladder and intestinal sphincters, and inhibition of the parasympathetic nervous system.[2] Beta one adrenergic stimulation increases cardiac output, while beta two adrenergic stimulation causes vasodilation, bronchodilation, intestinal relaxation, uterine relaxation, and dilation of coronary blood vessels.[2] Beta blocking drugs are beneficial in reducing the physiological signs of fear.

Dopamine

Dopamine is produced from L-dopa and stored in the presynaptic vesicles. Dopamine is a precursor for norepinephrine. Dopamine is inactivated by monoamine oxidase (primarily MAO B) and by catechol-O-methyltransferase (COMT). Dopamine depletion produces behavioral quieting, depression, and extrapyramidal signs (muscle tremors, tics, and motor restlessness), while dopa-

mine excess has been associated with compulsive and stereotypic behavior.

Gamma-Aminobutyric Acid

Gamma-aminobutyric acid (GABA) is an inhibitory neurotransmitter that is widely distributed in the central nervous system. It is synthesized from the amino acid glutamate. GABA depletion and dysregulation has been associated with seizure activity, Parkinson's disease, and fears and phobias. Benzodiazepines and barbiturates are GABA agonists and are useful in treating these disorders.

Acetylcholine

Acetylcholine is the most widely distributed neurotransmitter in the body and is excitatory in function. Acetylcholine is synthesized from acetate and choline and inactivated by acetylcholinesterase. Acetylcholine activates two different types of receptors referred to as muscarinic and nicotinic receptors. Muscarinic receptors are found in cells stimulated by the postganglionic neurons of the parasympathetic nervous system and postganglionic cholinergic neurons of the sympathetic nervous system.[2] Muscarinic stimulation leads to arteriole vasodilation, decreased heart rate and cardiac output, and stimulation of the digestive system. Nicotinic receptors are found in the synapses between pre- and postganglionic neurons of the sympathetic and parasympathetic nervous system.[2] Depletion of acetylcholine is associated with cognitive decline and Alzheimer's disease. Blockade of muscarinic cholinergic receptors is responsible for anticholinergic side effects (dry mouth, dry eye, pupil dilation, tachycardia, constipation, and urinary retention) of tricyclic antidepressants.

DRUG SELECTION AND CONSIDERATION

There are currently no behavioral drugs licensed for use in psittacine birds. Owners should be informed of use that is considered "extra-label" with respect to the manufacturer's recommendations and sign an appropriate consent form before the drug is dispensed. In addition, many drugs must be compounded before they can be administered to avian patients. The effects of compounding on storage and stability must be considered. Administration of behavioral drugs can also be problematic, depending on the owner's ability to handle the avian patient and/or the bird's failure of oral acceptance of the drug. Taste aversion and the inability of masking bitter-tasting drugs with fruit flavorings may be encountered. Often, drugs may be injected into fruits, such as a grape, or mixed with yogurt or fruit-based baby food to facilitate oral administration.

Dosages and regimens of behavioral drugs are often extrapolated from veterinary and human literature and anecdotal reports in avian species. For many drugs, accurate dosages and controlled studies have not been performed. Dosage variation can be found in the veterinary literature. Whenever possible, drug dosages and regimens given in this chapter will be based on veterinary references (see Table 24-1). Ultimately, the prescribing veterinarian is responsible for appropriate selection, dosage, and administration of behavioral drugs in the specific clinical situation and patient.

Drug selection requires an accurate diagnosis of the behavioral problem and knowledge of drug efficacy and safety in the human and veterinary literature. Veterinarians should become familiar with indications, contraindications, proposed mechanism of action, common side effects, and the potential for adverse effects before using behavioral drugs. The bird species, age, sex, health, the cost of the medication, and ease of administering the medication are important aspects of drug selection. The safest drug that will be effective in treating the behavioral problem should be used first. If drug treatment fails or unacceptable side effects occur, one should consider dosage adjustment, if the drug was used for an adequate duration for effect, and re-evaluate the original diagnosis. The benefit/risk ratio of other drug options may be considered.

Ideally, a complete blood count and general biochemistry should be preformed to rule out underlying medical problems and establish a baseline for future testing. Regular monitoring of blood work should be performed based of the bird's health and the potential for adverse effects from the drug. Medical conditions should be treated concurrently with any behavioral problems. Long after the medical condition has resolved, behavioral disorders may continue. This is especially true for compulsive disorders. In addition, medical conditions lower the tolerable threshold for anxiety-related behavioral disorders.

Behavioral drugs should be used only as an adjunct to behavioral and environmental modification. Lack of concurrent behavioral and environmental modification may lead to drug treatment failure. The drug may become less effective in modifying behavior with time. The first time using a drug with behavioral modification is the best chance for cure. In addition, without concurrent behavioral and environmental modification, the problem is likely to reoccur when the drug is discontinued.

Drug desensitization is often used when the stimulus cannot be controlled or avoided, or when there is overwhelming fear/anxiety or aggression. In this manner, behavioral drugs are used to facilitate learning. The drug is used to decrease arousal and/or anxiety to a level that allows learning to cope with the stimuli or situation. After a sufficient learning period has occurred, the drug should be weaned gradually. Abrupt discontinuance is likely to result in withdrawal syndrome characterized by rebound anxiety and/or aggression and reoccurrence of the behavioral problem. Generally, it is recommended that these drugs be weaned by reducing the total daily dosage by 25% every three weeks while maintaining the same dosing frequency. If during the weaning process behavioral problems reoccur, the dosage should be increased to the previous effective dose and treatment duration should be extended.

DRUG CLASSES

Benzodiazepines

Benzodiazepines (BDZ) potentiate the effects of GABA, an inhibitory neurotransmitter, and are beneficial in treating conditions of fear, phobia, and anxiety, including fear aggression. Benzodiazepines have been used to facilitate social interaction and increase friendliness. Caution should be taken when used in aggression cases. Fear usually is conducive to defensive aggression, and benzodiazepines have the potential to disinhibit aggression, making the aggression more offensive. Benzodiazepines also have anticonvulsant effects for the treatment of acute seizure disorders. They have a rapid onset of action. Side effects include sedation, ataxia, muscle relaxation, increased appetite, paradoxical excitation, and memory deficits. Benzodiazepines may interfere with learning and affect behavioral modification and

Table 24-1 Psittacine behavioral pharmacotherapy

Drug	Class	Dosage	Route	Indications
Diazepam (Valium®, Roche, Nutley, NJ, USA)	BDZ	2.5–4.0 mg/kg q6–8h[34]	PO	Sedation
		1.25–2.50 mg/120 ml water[14]	PO	Acute fears
				Acute anxiety FPD
		0.6 mg/kg q8–12h[5]	IM, IV	Anticonvulsant
Amitriptyline (Elavil®, AstraZeneca, Wilmington, DE, USA)	TCA	1–5 mg/kg q12h[7]	PO	Pruritic FPD
				Chronic anxiety disorders
Doxepin (Sinequan®, Pfizer, New York, NY, USA)	TCA	1–2 mg/kg q12h[7]	PO	Pruritic FPD (preferred drug)
		1–2 mg/lb q 12h[40]		Chronic anxiety disorders
Clomipramine (Anafranil® or Clomicalm®, Novartis, East Hanover, NJ, USA)	TCA, Selective	3–5 mg/kg q12–24h[7]	PO	Compulsive disorder Compulsive FPD Chronic anxiety disorders
Nortriptyline (Pamelor®, Sandoz, East Hanover, NJ, USA)	TCA	2 mg/120 ml drinking water[14]	PO	Chronic anxiety disorders
				Anxiety-induced FPD (seldom used)
Fluoxetine (Prozac®, Eli Lilly, Indianapolis, IN, USA)	SSRI	1–4 mg/kg q24h[7] Dosages have been used up to 20 mg/kg/day[7]	PO	Compulsive disorder Compulsive FPD Global fear, phobia Aggression
Paroxetine (Paxil™, GlaxoSmithKline, Triangle Research Park, NC, USA)	SSRI	1–2 mg/kg q12–24h[16]	PO	Compulsive disorder Compulsive FPD Global fear, phobia Aggression (preferred drug)
Chlorpromazine (Thorazine®, SmithKline Beecham, Philadelphia, PA, USA)	Antipsychotic Low potency	0.1–0.2 mg/kg once[14]	IM	Tranquilization
		1 ml solution X/4 oz drinking water[14]	PO	Compulsive FPD used with Carbamazepine
		0.2–1.0 ml/kg solution X q12–24h[14]	PO	Solution X = 125 mg chlorpromazine/31 ml simple syrup[14]
Haloperidol (Haldol®, OrthoMcNeil, Raritan, NJ, USA)	Antipsychotic DA antag- onist High potency	0.2–0.9 mg/kg q24h[7]	PO	Compulsive FPD
		1–2 mg/kg q4wk[24]	IM	Self-mutilation
		6.4 mg/L drinking water[19]	PO	(preferred drug)
		0.08 mg/kg sid[5] Lower dosage in Quaker Parakeets and cockatoos[41]	PO	
Diphenhydramine (Benadryl®, Parke-Davis, Morris Plains, NJ, USA)	Antihistamine	2–4 mg/kg q12h[24,41]	PO	Pruritic FPD
		0.5 mg/240 ml drinking water[14]		

Table 24-1 Psittacine behavioral pharmacotherapy (*continued*)

Drug	Class	Dosage	Route	Indications
Hydroxyzine (Atarax®, Pfizer, New York, NY, USA)	Antihistamine	2 mg/kg q12h[14]	PO	Pruritic FPD
Phenobarbital (Solfoton®, ECR Pharm, Richmond, VA, USA)	Anticonvulsant	1–7 mg/kg q8–12h[24] 6–10 mg/120 ml drinking water[14]	PO PO	Seizure disorder
Carbamazepine (Tegretol®, Novartis, East Hanover, NJ, USA)	Anticonvulsant	3–10 mg/kg q24h[14] 20 mg/120 ml drinking water[14]	PO PO	Seizure disorder Compulsive/impulsive disorder
Naltrexone (Revia®, DuPont, Wilmington, DE, USA)	Narcotic antagonist	1.5 mg/kg q12h[32]	PO	Acute compulsive FPD
Butorphanol (Torbugesic®, Fort Dodge, IA, USA)	Narcotic agonist	2–4 mg/kg q8h[33]	PO, IM, IV	Moderate/severe pain (preferred drug)
Buprenorphine Buprenex®, Reckitt & Colman, Richmond, VA, USA)	Narcotic agonist	0.1 mg/kg q12h[34]	IM, IV	Moderate/severe pain
Carprofen (Rimadyl®, Pfizer, New York, NY, USA)	NSAID	2–10 mg/kg q24h[34]	SQ, IM, IV	Mild/moderate pain
Ketoprofen (Orudis®, Wyeth-Ayerst, Philadelphia, PA, USA, or Ketofen®, Fort Dodge, Fort Dodge, IA, USA)	NSAID	2 mg/kg q24h[34]	IM	Mild/moderate pain
Chorionic gonadotropin (APL®, Wyeth-Ayerst, Philadelphia, PA, USA)	Hormone	500–1,000 U/kg q4–6wk[35]	IM	Hormonal FPD Chronic egg production Sexual behavior
Leuprolide acetate (Lupron®, Tap Pharmaceuticals, Lake Forest, IL, USA)	Hormone	100–1,000 ug/kg q2wks[36] (for 3 treatments) ≤300g bird—750ug/kg >300g bird—500ug/kg	IM	Hormonal FPD Chronic egg production Sexual behavior (antiandrogenic)
Medroxyprogesterone acetate (Depo-Provera®, Pharmacia & Upjohn, Kalamazoo, MI, USA)	Hormone	5–50 mg/kg q4–6wk[34] 150g bird—0.05mg/g 300–700g bird—0.03mg/g >700g bird—0.025mg/g	SQ, IM	Chronic egg production Sexual behavior (suggest use once)

training. At low dosages, they act as sedatives, at moderate dosages they have anxiolytic effects, and at high dosages benzodiazepines act as hypnotics and facilitate sleep. Tolerance to sedation, ataxia, and muscle relaxation may develop with time. There is the potential for injury to birds from falling when perched. Generally, benzodiazepines appear to be very safe drugs, but idiosyncratic hepatic failure has been reported in cats.[3]

Benzodiazepines are best used for short-term treatment of acute and intermittent behavioral disorders. When not used as a monotherapy, benzodiazepines may be combined with tricyclic antidepressants or selective serotonin reuptake inhibitors. Dosages should be adjusted accordingly. When prescribing benzodiazepines, one must consider that they are controlled substances and have the potential for human abuse.

Diazepam (Valium®)

Diazepam is available as an injectable solution (5 mg/ml) for IM or IV administration or as a solution (1 or 5 mg/ml) for PO administration. It is also available in 2 mg, 5 mg and 10 mg tablets for compounding. Three mg of diazepam is soluble in 1 ml of water. Diazepam is tasteless initially, but a bitter aftertaste soon develops. Diazepam may be used to control seizure disorders. It can be used to treat fears, phobias, anxiety, and possibly fear aggression. Diazepam is helpful in treating acute seizure disorders (0.05–2.0 mg/kg IM or IV).[4] Diazepam may be beneficial in acute anxiety-induced feather picking that is not compulsive in nature (0.6 mg/kg IV, IM).[5] Diazepam may also be useful to facilitate tolerance to Elizabethan collars in acute cases of self-mutilation. When used in combination therapy with tricyclic antidepressants or selective serotonin reuptake inhibitors the starting dosage should be reduced. Caution is warranted in patients with hepatic disease.

Antidepressants

Antidepressant drug classes include tricyclics, selective serotonin reuptake inhibitors, and monoamine oxidase inhibitors. To the author's knowledge, MAO inhibitors have not been used in avian patients. Indications and side effects vary based on sensitivity to and specificity for neurotransmitters. Generally, these drugs are best used to treat chronic anxiety disorders and cannot be used on an "as needed" basis.

Tricyclic Antidepressants

Tricyclic antidepressants (TCAs) block the reuptake of norepinephrine and serotonin and are competitive antagonists at the muscarinic acetylcholine, histamine H_1, and alpha$_1$ and alpha$_2$ adrenergic receptors. Increasing the availability of 5HT, NE, and DA, TCAs are indicated for treating fear, phobia, anxiety, and aggression. Chronic neuropathic pain may also be ameliorated by TCAs. The onset of action is usually delayed, with clinical effects usually seen by three to four weeks. Clomipramine is most selective for serotonin reuptake inhibition, making it the only tricyclic effective in treating canine compulsive disorders.[6] Tricyclic antidepressants produce various degrees of sedation based on anticholinergic and antihistaminic effects. Amitriptyline and doxepin produce the strongest antihistaminic effects, making them useful when sedation and antipruritic effects are desired. Sedation, taste aversion, gastrointestinal upset, and anticholinergic side effects may occur, precluding use. They are contraindicated with alterations of blood glucose, glaucoma, seizures, cardiac disease, and concurrent use of thyroid medication. Exercise caution with concurrent use of serotonergic drugs.

Amitriptyline (Elavil®)

Amitriptyline is available as a 10 mg, 25 mg, 50 mg, 75 mg, 100 mg, and 150 mg tablet for oral administration, as well as an injectable (10 mg/ml) for IM administration. Amitriptyline has been suggested for feather picking, yet is rarely effective.[5] The drug is ineffective in treating disorders of compulsive etiology. It is effective in treating global fear, separation anxiety, and generalized anxiety disorders. Amitriptyline is a potent H_1 blocker secondary to doxepin and may be beneficial in cases of pruritis. Amitriptyline is freely soluble in water or alcohol and has a bitter and burning taste. Amitriptyline inhibits 5HT and NE reuptake. Nortriptyline is the active metabolite. Suggested dosage is 1–5 mg/kg PO bid.[7]

Doxepin (Sinequan®)

Doxepin is available in 10 mg, 25 mg, 50 mg, 75 mg, 100 mg, and 150 mg capsules for oral administration, as well as a 10 mg/ml oral suspension. It is freely soluble in alcohol. Doxepin is a moderate inhibitor of NE and a weak inhibitor of 5HT. Doxepin is the most antihistaminic TCA and may be effective in treating pruritic feather picking. H_1 antagonism of doxepin is 800 times more potent than the antihistaminic effect of diphenhydramine.[1] Doxepin is the most sedating TCA and should be the antipruritic drug of choice. Anecdotal reports in African Grey Parrots and cockatoos suggest the drug is beneficial in reducing agitation, aggression, and fear, while increasing appetite, friendliness, play, and vocalizations at a dosage of 0.5–1.0 mg/kg PO bid.[8] Suggested dosage ranges from 1–4 mg/kg PO bid. Use the lowest effective dosage to control the behavior.

Clomipramine (Anafranil® or Clomicalm®)

Clomipramine is available in 25 mg, 50 mg, and 75 mg oral capsules. Clomicalm® is available in 20 mg, 40 mg, and 80 mg tablets. It is freely soluble in water and bitter tasting. Clomicalm, which is approved for treating separation anxiety in dogs, is contraindicated for treating aggression per drug label and has been known to increase aggression. Clomipramine has been used in human and veterinary patients to effectively control compulsive disorders.[9, 10] In humans, clomipramine was the first drug to be FDA approved for treating obsessive-compulsive disorders. Clomipramine is the most serotonin selective of the TCAs. It may be effective in treating compulsive feather picking and less effective when there is a component of self-mutilation. Sedation and regurgitation may be a common side effect. Regurgitation may be prevented if given with food. Bitter taste may prevent oral administration in some birds. One study found clomipramine (1.0 mg/kg PO sid, or divided bid) effective in only three of 11 feather-picking psittacines treated for four weeks; however, all birds had a positive attitude change.[11] Another placebo-controlled study found clomipramine (3 mg/kg PO bid) effective in eight of 11 treated feather-picking cockatoos (six pickers, five mutilators) at six weeks.[12] Seven of the eight birds began to improve at three weeks, with significantly greater improvement noted at six weeks. One clomipramine treated bird (mutilator) was worse at six weeks, and the remaining two treated birds were unchanged. No adverse events were reported during the study period. A raspberry syrup and 2% carboxymethyl cellulose suspension of clomipramine (4 mg/ml) was used. This study suggests the drug may be beneficial at higher dosages and for a longer duration of treatment. Suggested dosage is 3–5 mg/kg PO sid to bid.[7]

Nortriptyline (Pamelor®)

Nortriptyline is available as a 10 mg, 25 mg, 50 mg, and 75 mg capsule or as a 10 mg/5 ml suspension for oral administration. Nortriptyline has been used in humans to treat depression. It may be beneficial in some cases of feather picking that are anxiety induced. Hyperactivity is a common side effect and dosage should be adjusted accordingly. Suggested dosage is 1 ml (10 mg/5 ml suspension) per 4 ounces drinking water or 2 mg/120 ml drinking water.[13, 14]

Selective Serotonin Reuptake Inhibitors

Selective serotonin reuptake inhibitors (SSRIs) increase the availability of serotonin by blocking reuptake. They are indicated for compulsive disorders, fear, phobia, anxiety, and aggression. Because of their mood-stabilizing effect, SSRIs should be the drugs of choice for affective or anxiety-induced aggression. SSRIs are believed to be the least likely drugs to disinhibit aggression. Onset of action is believed to be delayed, reaching peak in three to four weeks. Disorders of compulsive etiology may take longer to respond. SSRIs have a safer side effect profile than the TCAs, with minimal anticholinergic effects. Side effects may include sedation and gastrointestinal signs such as anorexia and nausea. Contraindications include seizures and alterations in blood glucose. Caution needs to be exercised when used concurrently with serotonergic drugs.

Fluoxetine (Prozac®)

Fluoxetine is available in 10 mg, 20 mg, and 40 mg capsules, 10 mg and 20 mg tablets, and in a 4 mg/ml mint-flavored liquid for oral administration. Approximately 50 mg is soluble in 1 ml of water. Fluoxetine is odorless and tasteless. Fluoxetine is highly selective for serotonin and has little effect on other neurotransmitters, such as norepinephrine and dopamine. Fluoxetine is the least sedating SSRI, yet in some cases may lead to increased anxiety and agitation. Norfluoxetine is the active metabolite. Fluoxetine (2–3 mg/kg sid to 3 mg/kg bid) was evaluated in 24 feather-picking psittacines of various species.[15] In all 12 psittacines that completed the trial, significant improvements were noted after two weeks. All birds relapsed after four weeks, yet responded positively to a dosage increase at that time. Benefits only lasted a limited time, requiring increased dosage. Temporary ataxia and lethargy were reported. Suggested dosage is 1–4 mg/kg PO sid adjusted to effect. Dosages up to 20 mg/kg/day have been used.[7]

PAROXETINE (PAXIL™)
Paroxetine is available in a 10 mg, 20 mg, 30 mg, and 40 mg tablet, as well as a 2 mg/ml orange-flavored suspension for oral administration. Paroxetine is a highly selective 5HT reuptake inhibitor. Minimal anticholinergic effects have been noted with usage, making it more sedating than fluoxetine. Paroxetine is beneficial in treating compulsive disorder, social phobia, and panic and anxiety disorders in people and animals. The author has found paroxetine extremely beneficial in treating phobic psittacines. It is the author's preferred drug for treating compulsive feather picking. Suggested dosage is 1–2 mg/kg PO sid to bid.[16]

Antipsychotics

Antipsychotics have also been referred to as neuroleptics or dopamine receptor antagonists. Antipsychotics have been used in humans to treat schizophrenia and other psychotic disorders, such as mania, severe agitation, and violent behavior.[17] Antipsychotics are classified based on chemical structure and potency. Low-potency antipsychotics are commonly used in veterinary medicine as tranquilizers. High-potency antipsychotics (e.g., haloperidol) are probably more effective in treating behavioral disorders. The antipsychotic haloperidol has been used experimentally to reduce compulsive behavior in many animal species.[10] High-potency dopamine antagonists have been used successfully to treat compulsive feather-picking disorders in psittacids.[18–20] Potential side effects include hypotension, decreased seizure threshold, bradycardia, ataxia, extrapyramidal signs such as muscle tremors or tics, and motor restlessness. Low-potency antipsychotics (e.g., chlorpromazine) have more non-neurological (cardiotoxic, epileptogenic) side effects and are more sedating. High-potency antipsychotics (e.g., haloperidol) cause more neurological side effects and are least sedating.

Chlorpromazine (Thorazine®)

Chlorpromazine, a phenothiazine, is available in a 2 mg/ml (syrup) oral suspension, 25 mg/ml injection, and 10 mg, 50 mg, 100 mg, and 200 mg tablets. One gram is soluble in 1 ml of water and 1.5 ml of alcohol. Idiosyncratic aggression has occurred in dogs with the use of the phenothiazine acepromazine. Dosages necessary to treat aggression suppress all other forms of behavior, including social and exploratory behavior. Phenothiazines are a poor choice for aggression in animals. In addition, phenothiazines lack specificity as dopamine antagonists and interact with serotonin and norepinephrine. Chlorpromazine's major effect is sedation. Anticholinergic side effects and extrapyramidal reactions (Parkinson's-like side effects) may occur. Ataxia, regurgitation, and drowsiness have been reported in birds. Chlorpromazine has been suggested for feather-picking birds.[14] It is suggested to discontinue usage within 30 days. Efficacy reportedly diminishes in 14–30 days when given orally. In cockatoos, it has been suggested for use once IM in combination with the anticonvulsant carbamazepine.[14]

Haloperidol (Haldol®)

Haloperidol, a butyrophenone, is available as a 2 mg/ml solution for oral administration and a 50 or 100 mg/ml injectable decanoate for IM administration. Haloperidol is colorless, odorless, tasteless, and water soluble. Haloperidol has been effective in treating compulsive and aggressive states in people and animals. Haloperidol has been used effectively to treat compulsive feather picking.[18–20] It appears to work best in cockatoos and in cases of self-mutilation, suggesting different etiologies in various species.[21] The effect of the injectable decanoate may last three to four weeks. Quaker Parakeets and Umbrella and Moluccan Cockatoos appear to be sensitive, therefore lower dosages should be used (0.08 mg/kg sid).[5] Anorexia, ataxia, or vomiting may occur but usually resolve in 24–48 hours.[18] Dosage should be increased or decreased 0.01 ml every two days to effect. Successful long-term usage (seven to nine years) to control feather picking has been reported in a Moluccan Cockatoo and Yellow-naped Amazon Parrot with few side effects.[18] Similarly, two African Grey Parrots with feather-picking disorder were successfully treated with haloperidol for approximately seven months.[19] Anecdotal reports of death in a Hyacinth Macaw and Red-bellied Macaw suggest caution in these species.[20]

OTHER AGENTS

Antihistamines

Antihistamines block the physiologic effects of histamine. H_1 receptors are responsible for pruritus, increased vascular permeability, release of histamine mediators, and recruitment of inflammatory cells.[22] Antihistamines are beneficial in the treatment of pruritus, self-trauma, and anxiety. H_1 receptor antagonists have sedative, antinausea, anticholinergic, antiserotinergic, and local anesthetic effects.[22] Caution with concurrent anticholinergic agents, CNS depressants, and patients with hepatic disease is indicated. Paradoxical excitation and anxiety are rare side effects.

Diphenhydramine (Benadryl®)

Diphenhydramine is available in 25 mg and 50 mg capsules for oral administration as well as a 10 or 50 mg/ml injectable for IM or IV administration. One gram is soluble in 1 ml of water or 2 ml of alcohol. Diphenhydramine has antihistaminic, sedative, and antidepressant activity. Atropine-like anticholinergic side effects may occur. In humans it has been used to treat neuroleptic-induced parkinsonism.[17] Diphenhydramine may be beneficial in pruritic feather-picking birds. Suggested dosage is 2–4 mg/kg PO bid, or 0.5 mg/240 ml drinking water.[14]

Hydroxyzine (Atarax®)

Hydroxyzine is available in a 10 mg, 25 mg, 50 mg, and 100 mg tablet, as well as a 2 mg/ml solution for oral administration. It is available as an injection (25 mg/ml) for IM administration. It is very soluble in water and freely soluble in alcohol. Hydroxyzine may also inhibit mast cell degranulation. Hydroxyzine has been used as an anxiolytic agent and may be beneficial in pruritic feather-picking birds. One case report suggested hydroxyzine combined with eicosapentaenoic acid (DermCaps) was benefical in treating a feather-picking Red-lored Amazon Parrot.[23]

Suggested dosage is 2.2 mg/kg PO tid, or 4 mg/100–120 ml drinking water.[14]

Anticonvulsants

Anticonvulsants have few behavioral applications unless there is an epileptic component. Occasionally, it is difficult to differentiate compulsive disorders from focal seizures. Response to therapy may be diagnostic. Benzodiazepines have also been used as anticonvulsants for status epilepticus. They are not preferred for long-term management of seizure disorders. Side effects of barbiturates are similar to those of benzodiazepines but with a lower therapeutic index. Caution is indicated with concurrent CNS drugs (antipsychotic and antidepressant) because of increased CNS and respiratory depression, and in patients with hepatic disease.

Phenobarbital (Solfoton®)

Phenobarbital is available as a 15 mg, 16 mg, 30 mg, 60 mg, and 100 mg tablet, a 3 mg/ml elixir, and 4 mg/ml solution for oral administration. One gram is soluble in approximately 1,000 ml of water and 10 ml of alcohol. It is beneficial in treating seizure disorders. It has sedative, antispasmodic, and anticholinergic effects. Side effects may include depression, vomiting, and ataxia. Phenobarbital is a controlled substance with human abuse potential. Suggested dosages vary from 1–7 mg/kg PO bid to tid.[24, 25] One should use the lowest dosage that controls the disorder. Alternately, 6–10 mg/120 ml drinking water or 2–3.2 mg/kg PO bid has been suggested for amazon parrots and idiopathic epilepsy.[14]

Carbamazepine (Tegretol®)

Carbamazepine is available in a 100 mg and 200 mg tablet or as a 20 mg/ml suspension for oral administration. Structure is similar to the tricyclic antidepressant imipramine. Carbamazepine has been used to treat seizures, depression, mania, and explosive aggressive states in people.[17] In birds it may be useful in the treatment of compulsive disorders and aggression due to anxiety or frustration. Carbamazepine is slightly sedating, mildly anticholinergic, and does not cause muscle relaxation. Contraindications include renal, hepatic, cardiovascular, or hematological disorders. Carbamazepine has been suggested by some to be the preferred drug for psittacine feather picking.[14] Usually, the drug is combined with chlorpromazine or haloperidol for the initial two weeks of treatment. Suggested dosage is 3–10 mg/kg PO sid or 20 mg/120 ml drinking water.[14]

NARCOTIC ANTAGONISTS

Narcotic antagonists have been used to treat stereotypies in zoo and companion animals.[26–29] In humans, it has been used to treat self-injurious behavior and addictions. Opiate peptides are released during stress and activate the dopamine system, which may lead to compulsive and stereotypic behaviors.[31] Endogenous opioids may induce analgesia and block pain, allowing self-mutilation to occur. Therefore, narcotic antagonists may be effective in reducing compulsive and stereotypic behaviors of recent origin. Clinical suppression of compulsive disorder may be short-lasting and only beneficial in acute presentations.[27–30]

Naltrexone (Revia®)

Naltrexone is a synthetic opiate antagonist that is available in 50 mg oral tablets. 100 mg of naltrexone is freely soluble in 1 ml of water. Caution is indicated in patients with hepatic disease. In one study, naltrexone was effective in reducing feather picking in 26 of 42 cases. The use of restraint collars in the study makes it difficult to critically assess the effectiveness of the drug.[21] A 50 mg tablet can be mixed with 10 cc sterile water and is apparently stable if refrigerated for up to three months. Suggested dosage is 1.5 mg/kg or three to four drops oral bid for a Sulfur or Umbrella Cockatoo-sized bird.[32]

NARCOTIC AGONISTS

Narcotic agonists, or opiates, are useful in treating moderate to severe pain in birds. Birds may respond to pain by trying to escape, becoming restless and anxious, vocalizing and struggling, or becoming aggressive. Acute pain may also manifest as ruffled feathers and immobility. Behavioral signs of chronic pain may include inappetence, weight loss, lack of grooming or overgrooming a painful site, or feather picking over a specific body area or region.[33] In cases of self-injurious behavior and mutilation, a trial with an effective pain reliever may be warranted. Recent studies suggest that kappa opioids, such as butorphanol, may be more effective analgesics in birds than mu agonists, such as buprenorphine.[33] Respiratory, cardiac, and CNS depression may be increased with concurrent use of other CNS depressants. Opiates are controlled substances with the potential for human abuse.

Butorphanol (Torbugesic®)

Butorphanol, a kappa opioid, is available as a 1 mg/ml, 2 mg/ml, and 10 mg/ml injectable for IM administration. Butorphanol (1–3 mg/kg) has been found to be an effective analgesic in African Grey Parrots, cockatoos, and Hispaniolan Parrots.[33] One study found the drug an ineffective analgesic at 1 mg/kg for amazon parrots. Dosages of 6 mg/kg may have hyperalgesic effects in some birds. Suggested dose is 2–4 mg/kg IV, IM, or PO tid.

Buprenorphine (Buprenex®)

Buprenorphine, a mu agonist, is available as a 0.3 mg/ml injection. One study in African Grey Parrots found no significant analgesic effect with large doses. Suggested dosage is 0.1 mg/kg IV or IM bid.[34]

Nonsteroidal Anti-inflammatory Drugs

Nonsteroidal anti-inflammatory drugs (NSAIDs) are analgesic, anti-inflammatory, and antipyretic. Carprofen and ketoprofen are the most commonly used NSAIDs in avian medicine for mild to moderate pain.[32] NSAIDs are synergistic and more effective when combined with other analgesic agents. In mammals, gastrointestinal ulceration and bleeding may result from drug-induced inhibition of prostaglandin synthesis. Use caution in dehydrated patients because of increased renal complications. Information on dosages in birds has been established empirically.

Carprofen (Rimadyl®)

Carprofen is available as a 50 mg/ml injectable for IM, IV, or SC administration, or as a 25 mg, 50 mg, 75 mg, and 100 mg tablet for oral administration. Carprofen is insoluble in water and freely soluble in ethanol. Carprofen at 1 mg/kg SQ has been shown an effective analgesic in broiler chickens, reaching peak plasma levels in one to two hours and raising pain thresholds for at least 90 minutes.[33] Carprofen is a specific COX-2 inhibitor, making its primary effect anti-inflammatory, and thus sparing prostaglandins.

Suggested dosage is 2–10 mg/kg IV, IM, or SQ sid.[34]

Ketoprofen (Orudis® or Ketofen®)

Ketoprofen is available for IM, IV, or SC injection (100 mg/ml), as well as a 12.5 mg, 25 mg, 50 mg, and 75 mg capsule for oral administration. Ketoprofen is practically insoluble in water and freely soluble in alcohol. Suggested dosage is 2 mg/kg IM sid.[34]

Hormones

Hormones have historically been used to treat some forms of anxiety and aggression in animals. In birds, they have a non-specific calming effect and have been advocated for treating dominance and/or sexual aggression among birds and plucking.[35] Progestins are antiandrogenic, cause CNS depression, and increase appetite. Severe side effects include diabetes mellitus, bone marrow suppression, adrenocortical suppression, and carcinomas.

Chorionic Gonadotropin (APL®)

Human chorionic gonadotropin (hCG) is available for IM injection (500 units/ml, 1,000 units/ml, and 2,000 units/ml). The drug has been used to inhibit egg laying. It has been reported moderately successful for aggressive and feather-plucking female birds. It has been reported less successful in male birds with the exception of Eclectus males.[35] Dosage protocols suggest 500–1,000 units/kg IM.[35] If no response is seen within three days, the dosage may be repeated. If no response after a second injection, the drug is unlikely to be effective. Injections may be repeated every four to six weeks. Often the drug is less effective with time, requiring a shorter dosing frequency or making usage impractical.

Leuprolide Acetate (Lupron®)

Leuprolide is available as an injection (5 mg/ml). It is a luteinizing hormone (LH)-releasing hormone that has an effect on lowering follicle-stimulating hormone (FSH), LH, testosterone, and estrogen through negative feedback. The drug has been used to treat chronic egg laying, cystic ovarian and oviduct disease, egg yolk peritonitis, granulomas of the ovary and oviduct, cloacal prolapse, continued ovulation after salpingohysterectomy, feather picking, aggression, and persistent sexually induced regurgitation. Anecdotal reports suggest 73% overall improvement, with resolution in 89% of chronic egg-laying psittacids.[36] Dosage recommendations vary from 100–1,000 g/kg IM every two weeks for three treatments.[36]

Medroxyprogesterone Acetate (Depo-Provera®)

Medroxyprogesterone is available as a 100 mg/ml and 400 mg/ml injectable. It has been used for excessive egg production in Cockatiels and to deter sexual behavior, including feather plucking. Side effects, such as lethargy, inappetence, weight gain, polyuria and polydipsia, hepatopathy, and death, preclude routine usage.[35] Suggested dosage is 5–50 mg/kg IM or SQ every four to six weeks—150g bird—0.05mg/g, 300–700g bird—0.03mg/g, and >700g bird—0.025mg/g.[34]

COMBINATION THERAPY

Behavioral drugs are occasionally used in combination to enhance their effectiveness. The most sensible choice is the combination of benzodiazepines with antidepressants. Benzodiazepines may be added to antidepressants when the effectiveness of the antidepressant is waning. In addition, benzodiazepines are useful because of their rapid onset of action when waiting for the delayed effect of antidepressants. Caution should be taken because concurrent administration may lead to increased CNS depression. The dosage of the benzodiazepine should be lowered to avoid this complication. In humans, one study found that combined administration of fluoxetine and alprazolam, a benzodiazepine, resulted in a 30% increase in the plasma benzodiazepine concentrations.[37]

Fluoxetine and amitriptyline have been used concurrently in human and canine patients. Fluoxetine potentiates the effects of amitriptyline and the intermediate metabolite nortriptyline.[38] Caution should be taken with concurrent usage of tricyclic antidepressants and specific serotonin reuptake inhibitors (SSRIs and TCAs) because of the risk of serotonin syndrome. Serotonin syndrome is a serious and potentially fatal condition. In order of appearance as the condition worsens, signs include diarrhea; restlessness; extreme agitation, hyperreflexia, and autonomic instability with possible rapid fluctuations in vital signs; myoclonus, seizures, hyperthermia, uncontrollable shivering, and rigidity; and delirium, coma, status epilepticus, cardiovascular collapse, and death.[17] Treatment is often supportive.

Phenothiazines may be combined with benzodiazepines or SSRIs with additive sedative effects. Phenothiazines and TCAs should not be used in conjunction because both have sedative and anticholinergic effects. The anticonvulsant carbamazepine has been used in combination with antipsychotics (chlorpromazine and haloperidol) during the initial treatment (first two weeks) of compulsive feather-picking disorders and self-mutilation.[14] Combined administration of paroxetine and phenobarbital may result in a decreased plasma concentration of paroxetine.[39]

CONCLUSIONS

Behavioral pharmacotherapy is a beneficial adjunct to behavioral and environmental modification in many situations. Most avian patients will benefit from timely and appropriate use of behavioral drugs. Behavioral results are often expedited, and outcomes are often improved with concomitant use of drugs. Unfortunately, scientific literature for use in treating behavioral problems of birds is limited at this time and consists primarily of anecdotal reports and uncontrolled studies. At present, studies are often of small sample size and varied species, making it difficult to draw statically significant conclusions. Further clinical trials are necessary.

REFERENCES

1. Johnson-Delaney, C. 1992. Feather picking: Diagnosis and treatment. *Journal of the Association of Avian Veterinarians* 6 (2):82.
2. Guyton, A.C. 1991. *Basic neuroscience: Anatomy & physiology,* 2nd ed. Philadelphia: W.B. Saunders, p. 277.
3. Center, S.A., T.H. Elston, P.H. Rowland, D. Rosen, B.L. Reitz, I.E. Brunt, I. Rodan, J. House, S. Banks, L. Lynch, L. Dring, J. Levy. 1996. Fulminant hepatic failure associated with oral administration of diazepam in 11 cats. *Journal of Veterinary Emergency and Critical Care* 6:618–625.
4. Quesenberry, K. 1994. "Avian neurological disorders." In *Saunders manual of small animal practice,* ed. S.J. Birchard and R.G. Sherding, pp. 1312–1316. Philadelphia: W.B. Saunders.
5. Ritchie, B.W., and G.J. Harrison. 1994. "Formulary." In *Avian medicine: Principles and applica-*

tion, B.W. Ritchie, G.J. Harrison, and L.R. Harrison, pp. 457–478. Lake Worth, FL: Wingers Publishing, Lake Worth, Florida.
6. Hewson, C.J., J.M. Parent, P.D. Conlon, A.U. Luescher, R.O. Ball. 1998. Efficacy of Clomipramine in the treatment of canine compulsive disorder. *Journal of the American Veterinary Medical Association* 213:1760–1766.
7. Seibert, L.M. 2003. "Psittacine feather picking." Proceedings, Western Veterinary Conference.
8. Johnson, C.A. 1987. "Chronic feather picking: A different approach to treatment." Proceedings, First International Conference on Zoological and Avian Medicine, pp. 125–142.
9. Luescher, A.U. 2002. "Compulsive behaviour." In *BSAVA manual of canine and feline behavioural medicine,* ed. D. Horwitz, D. Mills, and S. Heath, pp. 229–236. Quedgeley, Gloucester, England: BSAVA.
10. Luescher, A.U. 1998. "Compulsive behavior: Recognition and treatment." Proceedings, Am Assoc Zoo Vet/Am Assoc Wildlife Vet, pp. 398–402.
11. Ramsey, E.D., and H. Grindlinger. 1994. Use of clomipramine in the treatment of obsessive behavior in psittacine birds. *J Assoc Avian Vet* 8:9–15.
12. Seibert, L.M., S.L. Crowell-Davis, G.H. Wilson GH, and B.W. Ritchie. 2004. Placebo-controlled clomipramine trial for the treatment of feather picking disorder in cockatoos. *Journal of the American Animal Hospital Association* 40:261–269.
13. McDonald, S.E. 1989. Summary of medications for use in psittacine birds. *Journal of the Association of Avian Veterinarians* 3 (3):120–127.
14. Carpenter, J.W., T.Y. Mashima, and D.J. Rupiper. 2001. *Exotic animal formulary,* 2nd ed. Philadelphia: W.B. Saunders, pp. 171–174.
15. Mertens, P.A. 1997. "Pharmacological treatment of feather picking in pet birds." Proceedings, First International Conference on Veterinary Behavioral Medicine, Birmingham, England, pp. 209–211.
16. Martin, K.M. 2004. "Behavioral approach to psittacine feather picking." Proceedings, Association of Avian Veterinarians.
17. Sadock, B.J., and V.A. Sadock. 2001. *Kaplan & Sadock's pocket handbook of psychiatric drug treatment,* 3rd ed. Philadelphia: Lippincott Williams & Wilkins, p. 198.
18. Lennox, A.M., and N. VanDerHeyden. 1999. "Long-term use of haloperidol in two parrots." Proceedings, Association of Avian Veterinarians, pp. 133–137.
19. Iglauer, F., and R. Rasim. 1993. Treatment of psychogenic feather picking in psittacine birds with a dopamine antagonist. *Journal of Small Animal Practice* 34:564–566.

20. Lennox, A.M., and N. VanDerHeyden. 1993. "Haloperidol for use in treatment of psittacine self-mutilation and feather plucking." Proceedings, Association of Avian Veterinarians, pp. 119–120.

21. Welle, K.R. 1998. "A review of psychotropic drug therapy." Proceedings, Annual Conference of the Association of Avian Veterinarians, pp. 121–123.

22. Scott, D.W., W.H. Miller, and C.E. Griffin. 1995. "Dermatologic therapy." In *Muller & Kirk's small animal dermatology,* 5th ed., pp. 211–218. Philadelphia: W.B. Saunders.

23. Krinsley, M. 1993. Use of Dermcaps liquid and hydroxyzine hcl for the treatment of feather picking. *Journal of the Association of Avian Veterinarians* 7 (4):221.

24. Gould, W.J. 1995. Caring for pet birds' skin and feathers. *Veterinary Medicine* 90 (1):53–63.

25. Bennett, R.A. 1996. "Common avian emergencies." Proceedings, Fifth International Veterinary Emergency and Critical Care Symposium, pp. 698–703.

26. Kenny, D.E. 1994. Use of naltrexone for the treatment of psychogenically induced dermatoses in five zoo animals. *Journal of the American Veterinary Medical Association* 205:1021–1023.

27. Dodman, N.H., and L. Shuster. 1998. *Psychopharmacology of animal behavior disorders.* Oxford, England: Blackwell Science, pp. 209–211.

28. Brown, S.A., S. Crowell-Davis, T. Malcom, P. Edwards. Naloxone-responsive tail-chasing in a dog. *Journal of the American Veterinary Medical Association* 1987:190;884–886.

29. Dodman, N.H., L. Shuster, S.D. White, M.H. Court, D. Parker, and R. Dixon. 1988. Use of narcotic antagonists to modify stereotypic self-licking, self-chewing, and scratching behavior in dogs. *Journal of the American Veterinary Medical Association* 193:815–819.

30. White, S.D. 1990. Naltrexone for the treatment of acral lick dermatitis in dogs. *Journal of the American Veterinary Medical Association* 196:1073–1076.

31. Landsberg, G., W. Hunthausen, and L. Ackerman. *Handbook of behavior problems of the dog and cat,* 2nd ed. Philadelphia: W.B. Saunders, p. 138.

32. Turner, R. 1993. "Trexan (naltrexone hydrochloride) use in feather picking avian species." Proceedings, Association of Avian Veterinarians, pp. 116–118.

33. Paul-Murphy, J. 2003. "Managing pain in birds." Proceedings, Managing Pain Symposium.

34. Doolen, M. 1996. "Appendix—Formulary." In *BSAVA manual of psittacine birds,* ed. P.H. Beynon, N.A. Forbes, and M.P.C. Lawton, pp. 228–234. Ames: Iowa State University Press.

35. Lightfoot, T.L. 2001. "Feather 'Plucking.'" Proceedings, Atlantic Coast Veterinary Conference.

36. Zantop, D.W. 2000. "Using leuprolide acetate to manage common avian reproductive problems." Proceedings, International Conference on Exotics (2,3), p. 70.

37. Lasher, T.A., J.C. Fleishaker, R.C. Steenwyk, and E.J. Antal. 1991. Pharmacokinetic pharmacodynamic evaluation of the combined administration of alprazolam and fluoxetine. *Psychopharmacology* 104:323–327.

38. Mills, D.S., and B.S. Simpson BS. 2002. "Psychotropic agents." In *BSAVA manual of canine and feline behavioural medicine,* ed. D. Horwitz, D. Mills, and S. Heath, pp. 237–244. Quedgeley, Gloucester, England: BSAVA.

39. Aranow, R.B., J.I. Hudson, H.G. Pope, T.A. Grady, T.A. Laage, I.R. Bell, and J.O. Cole. 1989. Elevated anti-depressant plasma levels after addition of fluoxetine. *Am J Psychiatry* 146:922–913.

40. Jenkins, J.R. 2001. "Feather picking and self-mutilation in psittacine birds." In *Veterinary clinics of North America: Exotic animal practice,* ed. T.L. Lightfoot, pp. 651–667. Philadelphia: W.B. Saunders.

41. Tully, T.N. "Formulary." In *Avian medicine and surgery,* ed. R.B. Altman, S.L. Clubb, G.M. Dorrestein, and K. Quesenberry, pp. 671–673. Philadelphia: W.B. Saunders.
Drug solubility was obtained from Plumb, D.C. 1999. *Veterinary drug handbook,* 3rd ed. Ames: Iowa State University Press.

25

Behavior of Captive Psittacids in the Breeding Aviary

G. Heather Wilson

INTRODUCTION

Psittacine birds have been kept in captivity since at least the fifth century B.C. In the 1800s, British records showed that several different species were bred successfully in captivity. However, it wasn't until modern methods of travel, such as the commercial airplane, arose that larger psittacine birds began to be propagated in captivity in earnest. In the 1970s, importation of psittacine birds for the purpose of captive breeding was a lucrative industry. These birds were usually wild-caught animals that were arbitrarily thrown together in pairs or in colonies and expected to reproduce. When they did not, it was generally assumed that something was medically wrong or that the birds were past fertile age, and since replacement breeder imports were readily available, little attention was given to solving the mysteries of poor production. In the early 1980s, the Association of Avian Veterinarians was established, providing a forum for ideas on the improvement of avian health and aviculture. In the early 1990s, with the passage of the Wild Bird Conservation Act, the flow of imported parrots slowed to a trickle. This necessitated more advanced avicultural practices to increase domestic production and greater attention was given to the husbandry and behavioral issues behind infertility. The realization dawned among aviculturists and veterinarians alike that birds must not only be healthy but also "happy" in order to reproduce consistently. Unfortunately, there have been relatively few studies of free-ranging or captive psittacine birds that might better define their normal behavior and promote reproductive efficiency (Millam 1994; Styles 2001). Most of what is thought to be known today is anecdotal infor-

mation and observations made by aviculturists, avian veterinarians, and a few behaviorists.

SOCIALIZATION

It has long been discussed among aviculturists that for many psittacine species, wild-caught pairs make better breeding stock than domestically bred birds. Although there have been no studies to confirm this, the observation may have some validity. Proper socialization is critical to breeding success among birds. Birds learn variable socialization skills at different stages of their lives. These stages are known as sensitive or critical periods (Smith 1999). Obviously, a wild-caught adult parrot will have experienced the most normal social development through these stages. However, it is possible to reproduce proper socialization forums for young parrots in captivity and these birds may be more adapted to the stress of living in close proximity to humans and appear to reach puberty earlier, making them potentially better breeding stock. Indeed, recent anecdotal reports from aviculturists with F2, 3, and 4 generation birds support this premise. Ideally, young birds that are intended for breeding should be parent-raised and then placed in flights with other juveniles of the same species so that flock socialization may occur. If hatchlings and fledglings are not properly socialized with their own species, then poor mating success or other problems may result later in life (Meehan et al. 2003; Immelmann 1972; Rajecki et al. 1977). Critical periods vary based on species and the type of learning that occurs. For example, filial imprinting and sexual imprinting occur during different critical periods (Smith 1999; Vidal

1980). Young cockatoos may not recognize parental vocalization until approximately five weeks after hatching (Rowley 1980). There are some species that may breed successfully after being hand-raised and kept as a companion animal without proper flock socialization, such as amazons and many of the smaller species. However, there are others that will very rarely breed under these conditions, such as African Greys.

Most psittacine birds are social species and spend the non-breeding season in flocks, although some birds, like the Kakapo, may be solitary. During the breeding season, most free-ranging psittacine birds break off from the flock in pairs, although some nest in colonies, such as Patagonian Conures and Quaker Parakeets. Although most larger parrots do form long-term pair bonds and are monogamous, there are some exceptions, such as the Kea, which is polygamous. Free-ranging male amazon parrots have been documented to break up a nesting pair and then mate with the hen (Wiley 1980). In Asiatic Parakeets, such as the Indian Ringneck, and Eclectus Parrots, the pair bonds only last for one reproductive season. There have been two reports of breeding and nesting behavior in captive Cockatiel flocks that demonstrate pairs, triads, and extra-pair mating do occur (Seibert & Crowell-Davis 2001; Harrison 1995). This same behavior has been recorded in free-ranging Echo Parakeets (Thorsen et al. 1998).

COURTSHIP BEHAVIOR

Courtship is an important prelude to breeding in all avian species. Allopreening and allofeeding may be seen in bonded pairs throughout the year but often escalate prior to breeding (Figures 25.1a and b). Previous observations suggest that in amazon parrots, lovebirds, and the genus *Melopsittacus,* the preening is confined to the head and neck region, while in *Aratinga, Brotogeris, Ara,* and *Cacatua* the area preened includes the head, wings, and tail (Harrison 1995). A receptive hen will signal her readiness to mate by leaning forward and fanning her tail. Amazons and some other species mount from the side, placing one foot on the hen's back, but in Cockatiels, lovebirds, lories, and many other species the male mounts by placing both feet on the hen's back.

If a new pair is to be introduced, it is generally advisable to put both birds simultaneously in a new cage. If this is not possible, altercations may

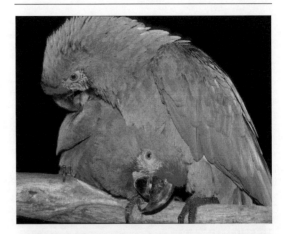

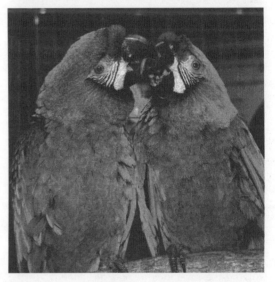

Figure 25.1a and 25.1b.   A bonded pair of Military Macaws engaged in allopreening and allofeeding. See also color section.

be decreased by timing the introduction to coincide with the non-breeding season, allowing the hen to occupy the breeding cage and the cock a smaller cage hung low on the outside of the larger cage, and performing wing, beak, and nail trims on the male prior to introduction into the hen's cage.

Psittacine birds have complex methods of communication, including color, posturing, and vocalization. Vocalization may play an integral part in the courtship of some species. It has been theorized that contact call imitation in adult Budgerigars contributes to pair bond formation and maintenance (Hile et al. 2000). Vocalizations were found to be distinct among pairs of Puerto Rican Amazon Parrots in the wild (Wiley 1980).

In most species, the cock is generally dominant to the hen. In one study of the agonistic and affiliative behaviors of a flock of 12 captive Cockatiels that were colony housed, males were shown to rank significantly higher than females in the social hierarchy based on dyadic agonistic interactions (Seibert & Crowell-Davis 2001). However, there are exceptions to this scenario, as with psittaculid parakeets and Eclectus Parrots. In these species the hen is thought to be dominant and it is preferable to keep an older cock with a younger hen for optimal breeding success and to prevent damage to the male. In all psittacine birds commonly kept in captivity, it is the hen that chooses a male deemed suitable for mating. When birds are forced paired, aggression or lack of breeding success may occur. Recent observations suggest improved breeding success when members of a species or genera are flocked together in the non-breeding season and allowed to choose

their own mates and are then paired off for the breeding season into separate cages (Figure 25.2).

CAGING AND NEST SELECTION

When considering cage design and nest box construction, the natural behavior as well as the health of the species should be considered. For example, is the species predominately arboreal, such as most amazons, or does it spend a significant portion of its time in terrestrial activity, like many of the Australian cockatoos? This may provide guidance in selecting either a suspended welded-wire enclosure or one that allows access to the ground, despite increased health risks associated with this type of caging (Figure 25.3). Additionally, most parrots have evolved as a prey species, therefore the ability to "escape" at least a short distance is critical for the psychological comfort of most of these birds. Cages that provide perches that are high above human heads, and that allow for some flight distance, will result in birds that are less stressed and more likely to perceive the enclosure as "safe" nesting territory (Figure 25.4).

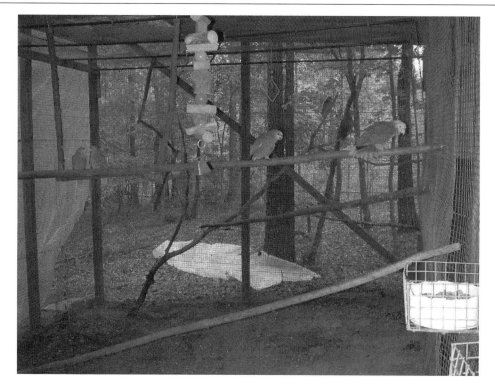

Figure 25.2. Flocking birds of the same species or genera in the non-breeding season may increase production by allowing voluntary mate selection. See also color section.

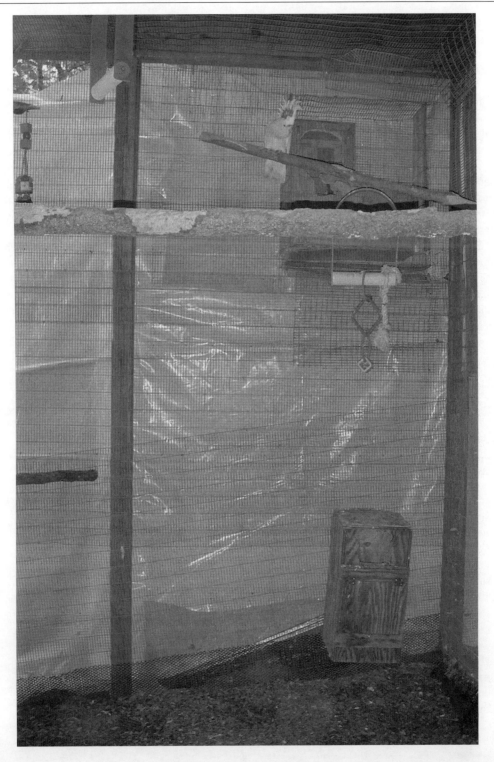

Figure 25.3. An example of a captive environment that allows some natural behaviors, such as ground foraging, which can improve breeding success in some species such as this Major Mitchell Cockatoo.

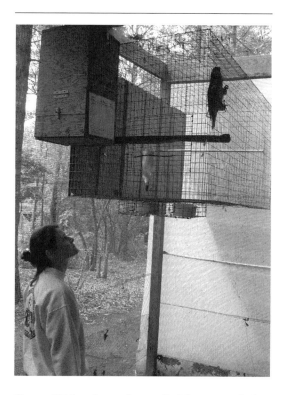

Figure 25.4. An enclosure that is suspended high above the ground, like this nesting Blue-fronted Amazon pair's cage, can decrease stress and increase chick production.

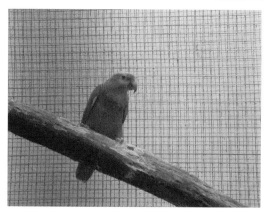

Figure 25.5. Inappropriate perching, as demonstrated by the slick, overly wide branch this Red-lored Amazon is trying to balance on, can interfere with breeding success.

Appropriate perching is also vital to reproductive success. Secure wooden branches that allow the bird to wrap its foot approximately halfway around the diameter are usually ideal. Wooden perches naturally provide good footing, are easily replaceable and provide good nesting material and safe chewing substrate (Figure 25.5).

It has been proposed that nest box presentation is the most effective stimulus for eliciting egg laying in psittacine birds (Millam 1994). A wide variety of nest boxes have been promoted in aviculture. Sometimes providing a choice of a couple of different styles to birds may help increase nest satisfaction and thus production. Most parrots are not nest builders (although there are some exceptions, such as lovebirds and Hanging Parrots) but rather nest in cavities, usually in trees, in the wild. Therefore, wooden boxes with dark inner cavities are usually preferred. Many species, such as some macaws, prefer either broad perches or horizontal boxes that allow them to mate in the nest. Others,

such as African Greys or the *Poicephalus* species, may prefer the "boot" type box that allows decreased light penetration into the egg-laying area. Still others, like many cockatoo species, may prefer the "grandfather clock" or vertical type box that would more closely approximate the length of a tree trunk (Figure 25.6). Many species excavate down a tree trunk nest several feet before feeling safe enough to lay and captive nests must approxi-

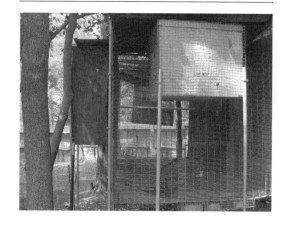

Figure 25.6. A choice of nest box styles and materials may help encourage a pair to go to nest. This pair of Hyacinth Macaws routinely "work" the grandfather-style box early in the season and then lay eggs in the horizontal box later in the season.

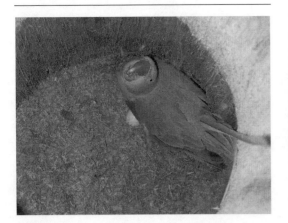

Figure 25.7. Deep, dark natural nesting cavities, such as this hollowed out palm log, are often preferred nesting sites, as demonstrated by this Alexandrine Parakeet hen on five fertile eggs. See also color section.

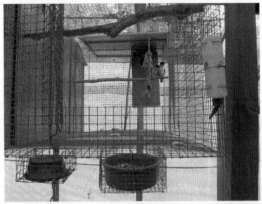

Figure 25.8. Keeping the nesting box away from high traffic areas, such as the path traveled when doing daily feeding, may increase breeding success. See also color section.

mate this (Figure 25.7). Additionally, some aviculturists prefer a "T" type box, especially with aggressive cockatoos, with two holes that allow the hen to escape aggressive advances from the cock. Nest boxes should be placed on the cage in such as way as to minimize disruptions (i.e., away from food bowls and general foot traffic) but allow easy inspection from outside the cage (Figure 25.8).

Nest substrate may also play a vital role in increased production. While some species may be content to nest on recycled paper products, others may need more natural bark chips or wood that can be chewed down to the proper consistency. There have been many observations that suggest not only may this be stimulatory for the pair but that it may also help to decrease mate aggression in some species, as the cock is initially busy preparing the nesting cavity and therefore gives the hen more time to reach breeding condition. Having a narrow entrance to the box that must be chewed open to allow the pair access may also serve this same purpose.

The location of the cage in relation to other cages has also been shown to affect breeding behavior. From a health aspect, it is important not to house species from different continents in the same air space. This premise may also have some important psychological impact. For example, African Greys are a relatively quiet species and breeding success has been shown to increase when these birds are housed away from noisier birds, such as amazons or cockatoos. There may even be problems when housing birds within the same genus together. For example, most cockatoos, which are a highly territorial species, need larger breeding space. For these birds, as well as other species like African Greys, visual barriers between cages kept in close proximity may increase reproductive success in captivity (Figure 25.9). Alternatively, some conures (*Aratinga* or *Pyrrhua*) or Budgerigars are communal and don't appear to be disrupted by visual contact with neighboring pairs. In fact, having other mating pairs of the same species in the vicinity is thought to stimulate breeding for many species. These birds may even be propagated in colony breeding situations, although it is advisable to have an equal number of males and females (Figure 25.10).

Ideally, cages should be located outdoors to allow access to a natural photoperiod and full-spectrum light. Circadian rhythms affect body temperature, hormone output, metabolism, and reproductivity (Ryan 1999). In birds, there are at least three distinct input pathways for light to act on circadian rhythms (Campbell & Murphy 1998). Although some species may reproduce despite lack of natural photoperiod, it probably does play a supportive role in the breeding success of most pairs (Millam 1994). It has been shown that spermatogenesis in the Budgerigar can be arrested by reducing the birds' photoperiod to eight hours of daylight or less (Humphreys 1975). In most cases, even breeding pairs that are imported

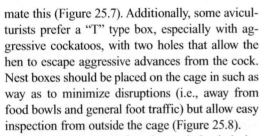

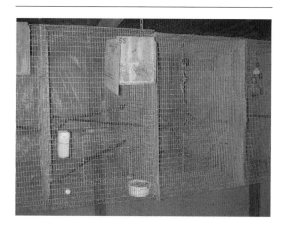

Figure 25.9. Complete visual barriers between the cages of territorial species, such as these lovebirds, can improve production.

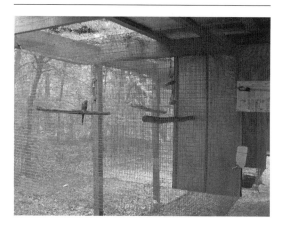

Figure 25.10. Conure species may only require visual barriers around the next box itself.

into the United States and housed in outdoor aviaries will adjust their breeding season to the spring and summer months of the Northern Hemisphere. There are some exceptions to this, such as Eclectus Parrots, which may breed year-round, and Alexandrine Parakeets and some *Poicephalus* parrots, which may breed in the winter (Figure 25.11). Interestingly, it has been noted that in the wild, Eclectus Parrots do not exhibit breeding seasonality but rather breed whenever a nesting site becomes available (Sparks & Soper 1990). Stimulation of egg laying and increase in plasma luteinizing hormone (LH) secretion was found to be highest in Cockatiel hens provided

with full mate contact, nest box access, and appropriate photostimulation (Shields et al. 1989). It has also been shown that the plumage of most parrots reflects near ultraviolet (UVA) wavelengths (300–400 nm) and exhibits UVA-induced fluorescence. This appears to play a role in mate selection, possibly making access to full-spectrum light important in facilitation of pair bonding (Pearn et al. 2001).

Environmental stimuli that may serve as cues to the onset of the avian breeding season are not limited to light alone. Circannual rhythms, which control when certain species of birds know to migrate or mate, are probably controlled by other factors, such as temperature, humidity, nutrition, and social interaction. All these variations are more difficult to control in captive indoor settings and can affect breeding success (Millam 1994).

PARENTING

In most species, it is the hen that is responsible for incubation of the eggs. There are some exceptions to this, such as Cockatiels, macaws, and conures, in which the cock incubates during the day and the hen at night. In all psittacine species studied thus far the cock assists in the rearing of the young (Figure 25.12). Some species or individuals appear to have better parenting skills than others and cross-fostering is commonly employed in aviculture. It is advisable to remain within the species if this is a common practice, both from a disease perspective and behavioral development. This is just one reason why aviaries that concentrate on one genus or species are often more successful than those that collect multiple species and attempt to propagate all of them. A flock average of five fledged chicks/pair/year is considered an optimum production rate that neither "wears out" breeding pairs nor underutilizes them.

BEHAVIORAL ABNORMALITIES

Most psittacine birds, whether imported or domestically bred, kept as companion animals or used as breeding stock, are not considered domesticated but rather captive wild animals. Additionally, unlike some other companion species, such as dogs or cats, psittacine birds are a prey species. The forced proximity of captive parrots to humans and the effectively curtailed ability in most cases of these animals to flee when threatened have produced a wide variety of behavioral problems. Most of these will be addressed else-

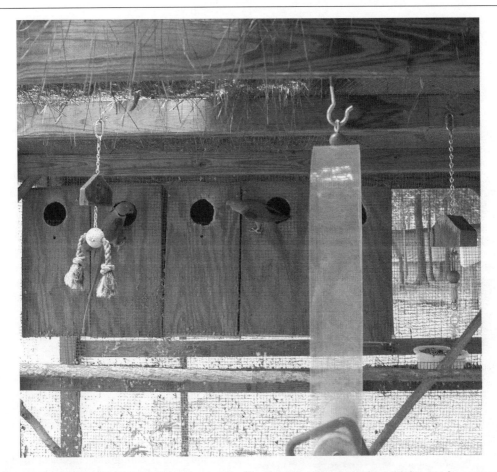

Figure 25.11.   Large flights, like this Alexandrine Parakeet enclosure, with multiple nest boxes may improve fertility in colonial species.

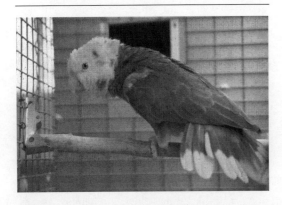

Figure 25.12.   A Double Yellow-headed Amazon Parrot displaying normal territorial aggression in defense of the nest box where the hen is on eggs. See also color section.

where in this text. However, there are some behavioral abnormalities that impair effective reproduction that must be mentioned here. These include destruction of eggs, nest abandonment, excessive aggression toward mates or chicks, and stereotypical behaviors that consume the individual to the exclusion of breeding.

Enclosure size, placement, and height as mentioned previously may all play a role in preventing or alleviating these deviant behaviors. Additionally, proper nutrition (also described in another chapter) plays a critical role and should be tailored to each species or individual. Environmental enrichment is also vital and should be given the same attention in either breeding or companion birds. Disruptions by human or other predators may precipitate these maladaptive behaviors and should be kept to a minimum (Figure 25.13).

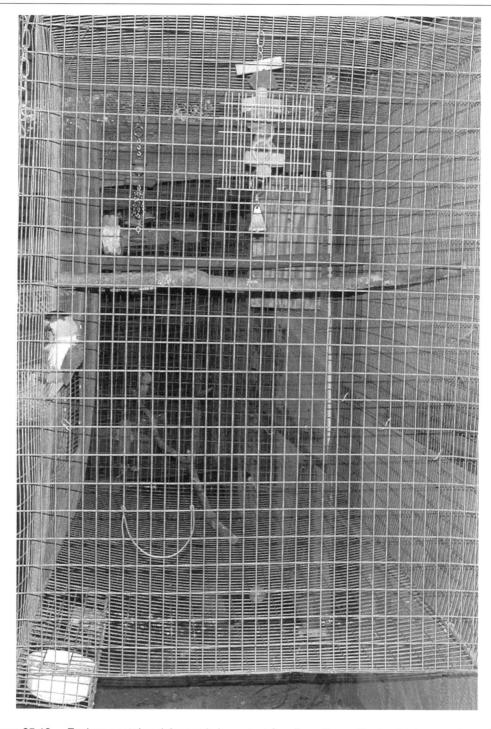

Figure 25.13. Environmental enrichment is important for all captive psittacine birds, even those in breeding aviaries.

CONCLUSION

As the reproductive lifespan of birds imported in the 1970s and 1980s draws to a close, the successful reproduction of their progeny becomes more critical to the perpetuation of aviculture. Given the importance of normal reproductive behavior in facilitating fertility and hatchability in psittacine birds, it is hoped that aviculturists and avian veterinarians will continue to demonstrate support in the study of these fascinating and complex creatures.

REFERENCES

Campbell, S.S., and P.J. Murphy. 1998. Extraocular circadian phototransduction in humans. *Science* 279:396–398.

Harrison, G.J. 1995. "Perspective on parrot behavior." In *Avian medicine: Principles and application,* ed. B.W. Ritchie, G.J. Harrison, and L. Harrison, pp. 96–105. Lake Worth, FL: Wingers Publishing.

Hile, A.G., T.K. Plummer, and G.F. Striedter. 2000. Male vocal imitation produces call convergence during pair bonding in budgerigars, *Melopsittacus undulatus. Anim Behav* 59 (6):1209–1218.

Humphreys, P.N. 1975. Ultrastructure of the budgerigar testis during a photoperiodically induced cycle. *Cell Tissue Research* 159 (4):541–550.

Immelmann, K. 1972. "Sexual and other long term aspects of imprinting in birds and other species." In *Advances in the study of behavior,* ed. D.S. Lehrman, R.A. Hinde, and E. Shaw, pp. 147–174. New York: Academic Press.

Meehan, C.L., J.P. Garner, and J.A. Mench. 2003. Isosexual pair housing improves the welfare of young amazon parrots. *Applied Animal Behavior Science* 81:73–88.

Millam, J.R. 1994. "U.C. Davis amazon breeding project." Proc Assoc Avian Vet, pp. 403–408.

Pearn, S.M., A.T. Bennett, and I.C. Cuthill. 2001. Ultraviolet vision, fluorescence and mate choice in a parrot, the budgerigar *Melopsittacus undulatus. Proc R Soc Lond B Biol Sci* 268 (1482):2273–2279.

Rajecki, D.W., S.J. Suomi, E.A. Scott, and B. Campbell. 1977. Effects of social isolation and social separation in domestic chicks. *Developmental Psychology* 13 (2):143–155.

Rowley, I. 1980. Parent-offspring recognition in a cockatoo, the galah, *Cacatua roseicapilla. Austr J Zool* 28 (3):445–456.

Ryan, T. 1999. "Use of light in aviculture and avian medicine." Proc Assoc Avian Vet, pp. 179–186.

Seibert, L.M., and S.L. Crowell-Davis. 2001. Gender effects on aggression, dominance rank, and affiliative behaviors in a flock of captive adult cockatiels (*Nymphicus hollandicus*). *Applied Animal Behavior Science* 71:155–170.

Shields, K.M., J.T. Yamamoto, and J.R. Millam. 1989. Reproductive behavior and LH levels of cockatiels (*Nymphicus hollandicus*) associated with photostimulation, nest-box presentation, and degree of mate access. *Hormones and Behavior* 23 (1):68–82.

Smith, I.L. 1999. "Basic behavioral principles for the avian veterinarian." Proc Assoc Avian Vet, pp. 47–55.

Sparks, J., and T. Soper. 1990. *Parrots: A natural history.* New York: Facts on File.

Styles, D.K. 2001. "Captive psittacine behavioral reproductive husbandry and management: Socialization, aggression control, and pairing techniques." Proc Assoc Avian Vet (Avian Specialty Advanced Program), pp. 3–14.

Thorsen, M., R. Shorten, G. Buchanan G, et al. 1998. "Echo parakeet management report from the Mauritian Wildlife Foundation." Proc Internatl Avicult Soc, pp. 1–31.

Vidal, J.M. 1980. The relations between filial and sexual imprinting in the domestic fowl: Effects of age and social experience. *Anim Behav* 28 (3):880–891.

Wiley, J.W. 1980. "The Puerto Rican parrot (*Amazona vitatta*): Its decline and the program for its conservation." Proc ICBP Parrot Working Group Meeting, pp. 133–159.

26
Housing and Management Considerations for Problem Prevention

Andrew U. Luescher and Liz Wilson

PARROTS AS PETS

Parrots are wild animals. Most species, although now domestically bred, are no more than one or two generations away from their wild ancestors. This not only means that parrots still have the behavioral repertoire of the wild birds but most of all that they become socially mature. Our domestic companion animals, and especially dogs, make good pets because they are neotenized. That means they retain juvenile characteristics into adulthood and never become socially mature when compared to their wild relatives. They stay babies and readily accept our caregiving all their lives.

Parrots, on the other hand, become socially mature. That is the time when many people start having problems with them. We believe that reaching social maturity is much more important for the development of behavior problems than attaining sexual maturity. The two are not the same, and sexual maturity may be achieved earlier than social maturity. This is obvious in human teenagers, in puppies, and likely applies to parrots as well. If the owner has not put a great deal of effort into earning the parrot's trust and affection, and has not communicated clear contingencies relative to the bird's behavior (i.e., set consistent rules), behavior problems often ensue.

This is often accepted as a fact of life. One of the authors (Luescher) remembers discussing different species with a breeder and being told that one species was better as a pet because it stayed nice longer, implying that sooner or later

all parrots lost their pet qualities. This does not need to be the case, as many happy long-term relationships between owners and parrots last. We hope that this and other chapters in this book will help set the groundwork for a happy, long-lasting, and enjoyable relationship between parrots and owners.

Parrots are highly intelligent and remember for a long time (see chapter 13). Parrots are a prey species and their first reaction to novel stimuli will be fear and avoidance. This is important to remember when new toys or other cage furniture, house decorations, or other pets are introduced. As a prey species they are very intolerant of physical or emotional abuse. In nature, physical restraint would likely mean death for a parrot and is therefore very frightening for pet birds unless they have been desensitized to it. If they are physically or emotionally abused even just once, it can take a very long time for them to overcome their fear and distrust.

Parrots are high-input companions and need a stable and consistent environment. Most species are also very long-lived. Before deliberating what species to obtain, potential owners should ask themselves if they are really ready and willing to have a bird. They should think about being able to provide the necessary environment and care for a long time to come. If they are young and plan on having children, they may not be able to make that commitment. Certain rules have to be followed to accommodate a parrot in a young family.[1]

Because parrots are high-input companions, an owner should generally only get one bird at a time (the exception may be when an owner wants to pair-house two birds of a small species, is willing and able to work with each separately, and can accept that there may be some territorial or mate-related aggression later on). There is a tendency in the United States for the number of birds per bird-owning households to increase. We suppose with all the different, beautiful species available, a collector instinct is easily awakened in many owners. Recently one of the authors (Luescher) talked to people who bought 14 parrots in five months. As long as they are all babies, all seems well. However, it is not humanly possible (unless maybe for a professional trainer who can devote all day to the birds) to train all these birds to the point that there won't be any problems once they become adults. A parrot needs daily one-on-one attention and training if he or she is to make a good pet.

Parrots are often obtained for the wrong reasons. Many birds are impulse bought because of their beauty, their potential ability to talk, their cuteness as babies, and their apparent ability to make the owner feel "cool." Many people have no idea what they are getting into when they bring home a parrot. Most people do not understand what kind of work is involved when they purchase their first parrot, and well over half of owners would not replace their parrot if it died.

The reality is that most humans are not prepared—physically or psychologically—to share their life with a wild animal. People generally want a pet animal that considers them (the human) to be the center of the universe, an animal that offers unconditional love. Indeed, dogs are the only animals on this planet that fulfill these requirements. Parrots do not fulfill these obligations. Parrots are not dogs with feathers, nor are they feathered children. They are simply themselves, and they are unable to make the compromises that the average human expects from a companion animal.

CHOICE OF SPECIES

Generally, most people are attracted to the large and expensive species because of the status they convey. At avicultural meetings the influence and credibility of people seem to be directly correlated to the price of their birds. However, few peo-

ple are capable of offering a Hyacinth Macaw or Moluccan Cockatoo the accommodation and care it needs. Most people would be better off with a small species such as a Budgie, Cockatiel, or Quaker Parakeet. Most of all, these small birds are better off as pets because they can be provided with more room, more appropriate play gyms, and so forth. They also are not as intimidating, make less of a mess, and do less damage when they bite or chew. Their pet quality is equal to or better than that of many large and expensive birds. Small birds are therefore less likely to be relegated to a solitary, deprived life in the garage or basement.

When choosing a species, size, manageability, personality, and ability to cope with life as a solitary bird should be the key factors. The amount and kind of noise a bird makes will in part depend on the species, as will the amount of dust. Talking ability and beauty are certainly factors to consider as well, but they should be considered secondary to the others. A plain-colored bird that does not talk may be more likely to provide lasting joy than a beautiful talking bird that becomes emotionally unstable because the owner can't manage it.

CAGING

Parrots will naturally use different habitats for different activities. They often forage in areas that are quite different from the place where they roost. Therefore, pet parrots should have at least two cages, one for the night and one for the day. Using the two-cage system or "multiple habitat housing" has several advantages. It forces the owners to take the bird out of its cage and handle it at least twice a day. It likely reduces cage territoriality. It makes it much easier to place the bird in the cage before leaving for work and makes life much more interesting and more natural for the bird.

The night cage doesn't need to be big and can be sparsely furnished, but it has to provide security, that is, near a wall, not too low, maybe partly sheltered. The night cage should be placed in a quiet room away from the main living/activity area, where it will be dark after 9 or 10 P.M., so that the bird can get a regular and sufficient dark period.

The day cage needs to be as large as possible. In particular, the day cage should be horizontal rather than vertical. In a vertically oriented cage, the bird will sit at the top most of the time and move around little. In horizontal cages, it can move around without having to give up height and may therefore be much more active. A horizontal cage also allows for arrangement of toys and other furniture in places where they are not likely to be soiled. For small species, it may even allow some flight inside the cage. If fitted with a proper-size door, it will also allow enough elbow room for the owner to train the up and down commands in the cage. Cages should be rectangular rather than round. Round cages allow no corner to sit in for a nervous bird. They are also usually rather high but small in diameter. The round, tall "tower" design is the most misguided cage design. Unfortunately, most cages offered in most pet stores are not suited for housing birds.

Cage placement is an important issue, as this can dramatically influence a parrot's stress levels and, therefore, the stress levels of the humans around it. The ideal location is dependent on the personality of the particular bird. An extroverted parrot that is caged away from human activities is likely to scream excessively as it calls to other "flock members." Anxious, high-strung parrots may show stress behaviors like feather destruction if caged in the middle of a high traffic area, especially if the cage shares a wall with a door. If so, the bird is continually jolted by people appearing abruptly. Many birds enjoy a window view, but cage placement directly in front of a window can cause stress if the animal cannot hide or avoid direct sunlight.

In general, the day cage should therefore be located where there is an appropriate amount of activity for the bird's personality. However, it should be placed against a wall so that the bird has at least one direction toward which it does not need to be vigilant. Threatening stimuli should be avoided. For some birds, these may include apparently innocuous things such as clocks or pictures. The cage should be placed so that the bird does not get surprised and startled by a person suddenly entering its visual field. By placing the cage partially against a window and partially against a solid wall, the bird is allowed the choice to be exposed to the outside or not and to avoid direct sunlight. This appears critical to decreasing stress in the companion parrot.

Cages can be made easily and cheaply from galvanized wire. In a species that is not generally a strong chewer, and if the cage is big enough and furnished with enough things that are more attractive to chew on, this may be an acceptable solution. Zinc toxicity is a concern, at least in some species, and with poor-quality galvanization.[2] However, it has to be kept in mind that most breeder birds are kept in galvanized cages, usually without problem.

Having a play gym on top of the cage is discouraged because it makes the cage dark and may be conducive to territorial aggression (the play gym being the same area as the cage). It also tempts the owner to let the bird in and out of the cage on its own and discourages regular handling. The bird can also not enjoy any change in scenery if it is only either in or on top of the cage. If it always remains in the same constant environment, it may become overreactive to any change.

Cages should open wide: the door should cover almost the whole front. Otherwise it will be more difficult to remove a bird, and the bird will not be taken out as often. Also, small doors make training the parrot in the cage (training to step up and down in the cage) difficult. Thus, owners tend to just open the door and let the bird leave and enter the cage of its own free will. However, this will likely cause problems with territorial aggression.

Commonly, many cage companies equip their cages with huge perches that are too large for any but the largest psittacine species. Appropriately sized perches will allow a bird to wrap its feet most of the way around, thereby providing a stronger, safer grip. Due to its resistance to psittacine beaks, companies often use manzanita for perches, and this wood creates problems for many parrots. Extremely smooth and slippery, it can increase the potential for accidents. Natural branches with bark provided as roosts provide more foot comfort due to softness and irregular thickness and provide a substrate for chewing. Natural branches can be arranged so that the food and water, as well as the perches themselves, don't get soiled. While contamination with wild bird droppings is a concern, one of the authors (Luescher) knows of many large breeding facilities, including Loro Parque, that provide fresh branches on a regular basis without problems. Some trees are toxic in themselves or sprayed with toxic chemicals, so only branches of known origin and species, without obvious contamination with bird droppings, should be used. Soft wood provides much more recreational qualities than non-destructible hardwood. Trees that one of the authors (Luescher) has experience with are pine, soft maple, tulip, and various poplar species, as well as wild grapevines.

Cages need to be designed so they can be cleaned and sanitized easily. Flooring where the droppings fall through (cage grates) is probably preferable for most species.

For prey species, hiding places are also important, and parrots should be allowed the choice to be invisible to others in the environment. Hiding places can entail anything from branches attached with electrical ties or cotton string to the outside of the cage to produce a pseudo thicket (M.S. Athan, personal communications, 2000), to a sheet thrown over one corner, to wooden shelters attached to the side of the cage. Enclosed shelters can work well for young parrots, but they are often perceived as nests as parrots mature. Mature parrots can be accommodated with incomplete shelters such as a three-sided and roofed construction with a perch but lacking a front and floor (see chapter 18 on aggression).

Cage height is important. If caged too low, an insecure parrot can become seriously frightened. If caged too high, some individuals may be more fearful and more difficult to handle. Many parrots appear most comfortable when allowed to perch at human chest or shoulder level.

PLAY GYMS

Play gyms can be bought for lots of money but are often uninteresting and provide a very limited number of roosting places. Play gyms are much more interesting when large, with varied types of perches, and destructible (or holding lots of destructible toys). Unfortunately, many commercially available play gyms are small due to price considerations, and they are made out of indestructible material such as manzanita, plastic, or even stainless steel.

Play gyms can easily be made (at least for small species) from under-bed plastic storage trays and branches or vines. Plastic storage trays of various sizes are useful. Four fresh branches are each placed with the thick end in one corner, leaned toward each other, and tied together above the center of the tray (Figure 26.1). They provide novelty, interesting shape, and destructibility to the bird at a minimal price. Since they are very

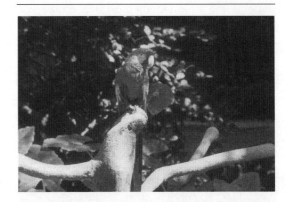

Figure 26.1.   A beautiful Scarlet Macaw (*Ara macao*) at Palmitos Park.

cheap, a number of them can be set up in several rooms of the house, so it will be possible to take the bird along from room to room and have a designated place for him or her. One can be placed on a side table beside the dining room table, and the bird can be trained to stay on it while the family eats, receiving his or her own treats on the play gym.

A particularly nice play gym or indoor tree can be made from a chimney flue and natural branches. On a vinyl floor cover (or the like), the chimney flue is placed upright. The branches are then stuck into it like into a vase (no water is added, of course). Soon, the birds will climb up and down in their tree and remove all the leaves and small twigs. The floor underneath will soon look like a forest floor but can easily be cleaned up. Their enjoyment is well worth the trouble. A similar idea is to use a Christmas tree stand and put a branch in it. Obviously, all these gyms have to be stable, especially for large species and when children or other pets are around. Once these play gyms don't look good any more, the branches can be used to start a fire in the fireplace, and new branches are brought in.

ROUTINE

Birds like routine. This does not mean that things have to happen at the same time each day. In fact, it is a good thing to get the bird used to some variation in routine from an early age, so that it is less stressful for them when the routine is broken. However, they like important events, such as feeding or being taken out of the cage, to happen at the same place in the routine. This way, events become predictable. Just as important is that the birds learn that at certain times in the routine they are not getting any attention, and they will be content being ignored at those times.

As a basic routine, birds should be removed from the night cage in the morning, taken along through the house to some of their play gyms, maybe have breakfast with the owners (but they should also be trained that sometimes they can't participate in meals, for when guests are over), and eventually be placed in the day cage. To facilitate placing the bird into the cage, a treat or foraging device should be placed in the cage. Using a separate day and night cage makes it much easier anyway to remove a bird from its cage and to place it into the other cage. In the evening a similar routine should be practiced, and the bird should be placed in the night cage at a fairly regular time.

Parrots, especially youngsters, need a sufficiently long dark period each night—probably as many as ten hours. Many companion parrot species are equatorial in origin, and therefore evolved in an ecosystem that provided 12 hours of darkness, year-round. As previously mentioned, due to their social nature, parrots are often caged in high traffic areas, and this often puts them in the same room with the family TV. When questioned about sleep, owners generally count the hours from the cage being covered until it is uncovered the following morning. However, logic indicates that a prey species is unlikely to sleep deeply when a predator (human) is moving near its roost. As a consequence, the real measure of the bird's sleep period is the time between the last person leaving the room at night and the time the first person arises in the morning. Behavioral manifestations of sleep deprivation would include hyperactivity, aggression, excessive screaming (especially after sunset), and feather destruction.[3]

The feeding schedule contributes to routine as well. Free choice feeding is the most common method of feeding pet birds. While this is probably the simplest method and assures adequate access to food, it is not really natural. Wild parrots spend a substantial part of their time foraging for food. The activities involved in their foraging behavior are the same behaviors we associate with play behavior in pet birds. Chewing, manipulat-

ing, and investigating are all part of the process of finding food. In captivity, birds have enormous quantities of calorie-dense food placed in easily accessible bowls at all times. Dr. Ted Lafeber often recommended meal-feeding pet birds.[4] He felt that meal-feeding might encourage greater activity by allowing birds to "forage" when food was not directly in front of them. In addition, he felt that when given some time with no food in front of them, birds might be somewhat more adventurous about trying new food items. A compromise may be found by offering pellets free choice and fresh items in the morning and evening, when the birds' foraging activities naturally peak.

Other factors that can be important regarding feeding schedules regard the freshness of the food. Fresh food items can spoil after a few hours and sometimes will attract insects. The health implications of this are obvious, but also some birds will be very upset when they see flies or other insects flying around their food dishes.

TOYS

Toys are a valuable means of encouraging development in pet birds. The activities involved in toy play can promote learning, relieve stress, and occupy idle time.

Natural branches keep birds better occupied and meet their motivation to forage and chew more than commercial toys. Some commercial toys with tassels are conducive to facilitate redirected social grooming and therefore may help meet this special need. Foraging devices are very useful. Some are commercially available but they can also be homemade. Seeds can be pressed into a squash or placed between the leaves of a half of a cabbage. They could also be strewn between large pebbles. However, size is important. One of the authors (Luescher) tried this with too small a pebble size. His house looked like a gravel pit when he came home because the birds flung all the pebbles out of the cages. Sometimes a whole ear of sweet corn in the husks can be provided. Large chunks of vegetables and fruit can be given on skewers (see Figures 26.2 to 26.14).

Safety has to be kept in mind with toys. Some toys with threads can result in a bird strangling itself. Also, toys with rings or large chain links, through which the bird can put its head, should be avoided. To keep toys interesting, they should be

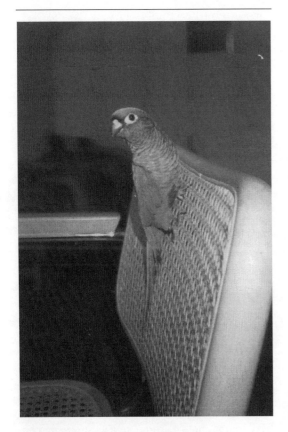

Figure 26.2. A Maroon-bellied Conure (*Pyrrhura frontalis*). See also color section.

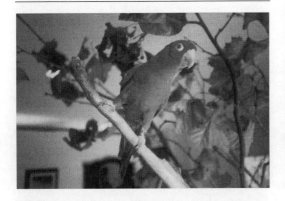

Figure 26.3. A Red-masked Conure (*Aratinga erythrogenys*). See also color section.

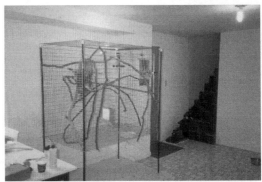

Figure 26.4. A homemade, roomy cage for two larger conures (Sharp-tailed Conures, *Aratinga acuticaudata*).

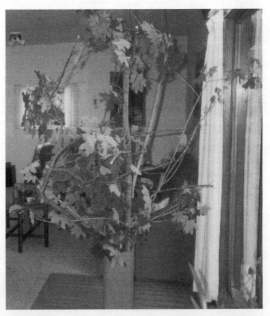

Figure 26.5. An appropriate play gym for small to medium-sized birds, made from a chimney flue and natural branches. See also color section.

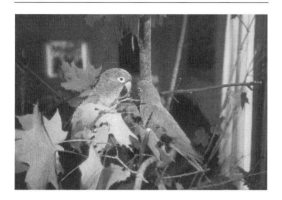

Figure 26.6. Two Sharp-tailed Conures (*A. acuticaudata*) enjoying natural branches. See also color section.

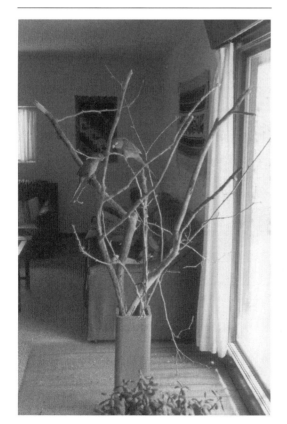

Figure 26.7. A play gym made from a chimney flue and natural branches after the birds spent some time on it. See also color section.

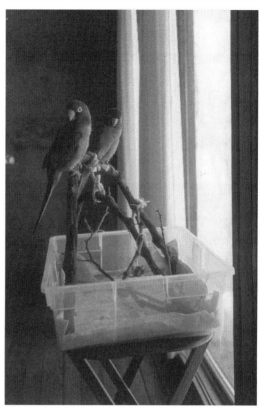

Figure 26.8. A smaller play gym made from a storage container and wild grape vines. See also color section.

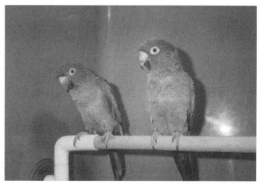

Figure 26.9. Some birds enjoy joining the owner in the shower on a commercially available shower perch. See also color section.

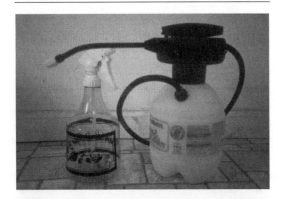

Figure 26.10. Two different devices to spray parrots. The regular spray bottle on the left is adequate for individual birds. The pressure sprayer on the right is most suitable for larger numbers of birds.

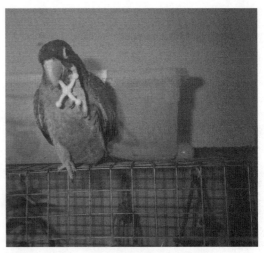

Figure 26.12. A Mitred Conure (*Aratinga mitrata*) with a "foot toy," a toy commercially available for cats. See also color section.

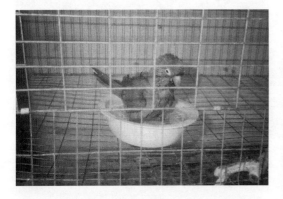

Figure 26.11. Some birds prefer to wet themselves by taking a bath in a water dish. In a large cage, a water dish can be positioned so that fecal contamination is minimized.

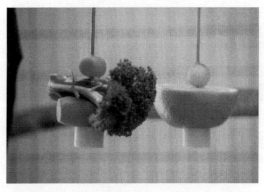

Figure 26.13. Large pieces of fruits and vegetables provided on a skewer encourage foraging.

rotated (i.e., only a few provided at once and exchanged for others every few days). Toys toward which the bird redirects social preening should stay in the cage permanently, however, as long as the bird is not aggressive when near them.

GROOMING

In most situations, the wing feathers of pet birds will have to be clipped for safety reasons. Overly aggressive and cosmetically pleasing grooming styles can, however, be devastating for a bird. Clipping style should be individually adjusted to each bird so that the bird can still fly, although not upward. Clipping should always be symmetrical to allow the bird to control the direction of the flight. Clipping too severely can result in traumatic falls and loss of self-confidence. It can also increase the danger that the parrot may fall into or onto something harmful or become a victim of another pet, such as a dog.

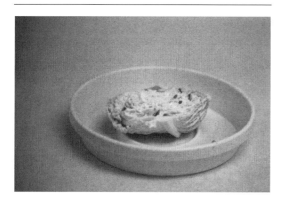

Figure 26.14. Half of a Savoy cabbage with seeds strewn in between its leaves.

TRAINING AND INTERACTION

Petting, cuddling, kissing, and allowing birds onto the shoulders are activities that will tend to encourage an inappropriate pair bond between owner and bird. Conversely, some activities encourage a bird to flock bond. Toy play, training, verbal games, dancing, and exercise are all activities that encourage a healthier bond. Time spent on a perch with the family without being held is an extremely valuable activity for pet birds. This can encourage the bird to be more independent. As flock animals, wild parrots spend very little time alone. The protective presence of the flock gives them a much-needed sense of security in the dangerous world in which they exist. Nonetheless, confident pet parrots tolerate a certain amount of "alone time" well.

Training is discussed extensively in chapter 15. The only thing that shall be emphasized here is that training goes a long way toward problem prevention. Trained birds can be controlled better and are more likely to stay out of trouble. Most importantly, training makes the interaction between owner and bird much more consistent, predictable, and stress-free. A relationship based on teaching and learning is much healthier than one based on petting, cuddling, and, inadvertently, sexual stimulation. The basic commands used in bird training are the "up" and "down" commands. They should be practiced many times every day, and the bird should be rewarded most times for performing the behaviors throughout its life. If a bird is in full flight, it should also be trained to "come" reliably when told. In addition, many tricks can be taught (for the bird, all trained behaviors are tricks). Training should start early in life, ideally with the breeder, and continue for the rest of the parrot's life on a daily basis. No treats should be given to a parrot without a specific purpose. Giving treats outside of a training context (in the widest sense, including, e.g., a desensitization procedure) will result in missed opportunities to train, make the interaction between owner and parrot less consistent and thus more stressful, and result in begging.

REFERENCES

1. Doane, B.M., and T. Qualkinbush. 1994. *My parrot, my friend.* New York: Howell Book House, p. 20.
2. Holz, P., J. Phelan, R. Slocombe, A Cowden, M. Miller, and B. Gartrell. 2000. Suspected zinc toxicosis as a cause of sudden death in orange-bellied parrots (*Neophema chrysogaster*). *J Avian Med Surg* 14:37–41.
3. Wilson, L. 1999. Sleep: How much is enough for a parrot? *Pet Bird Report* 43:60–63.
4. Lafeber, T.J. 1998. *Let's celebrate pet birds.* Odell, IL: Lafeber Co.

27
Captive Parrot Welfare

Cheryl Meehan and Joy Mench

INTRODUCTION

The issue of captive parrot welfare is both timely and ethically significant. Parrots are kept in a variety of captive situations including breeding facilities, wholesale/retail facilities, zoos, shelters, sanctuaries, entertainment venues, and conservation programs. In addition, the pet parrot industry has grown tremendously over the past decade, and parrots are now the third most popular companion animals in the United States (AVMA 2002). Recent estimates from the American Veterinary Medical Association reveal that there are 10.1 million parrots in 4.6 million homes in this country alone (AVMA 2002). As they become more and more popular, it is becoming increasingly evident that ensuring a good state of welfare for captive parrots is not an easy task.

Parrots and other birds whose environmental and behavioral needs are not met in captivity may engage in a variety of distressing abnormal behaviors, including incessant screaming, stereotypic pacing, and feather picking that becomes so extreme that the bird denudes itself and even causes skin or tissue injury (Grindlinger 1991; Davis 1991; van Hoek & ten Cate 1998; Meehan & Mench 2002; Meehan et al. 2002). These birds may also become excessively fearful or aggressive, directing their aggression toward family members or family friends. Improper care and environmental conditions may also result in psychological and physiological problems including acute illness, injury, and even sudden death. Considering the life span of many birds (Budgerigars may live 15 years, Cockatiels 25–30 years, and large parrots up to 70 years), problems like these may prove to be overwhelming for companion bird owners, leading to the bird being abused, neglected, sold, given away, released, or relin-

quished to a shelter or sanctuary. A 2001 census of ten parrot rescue and sanctuary organizations compiled by the Gabriel Foundation revealed that there were over 2,000 parrots and small birds housed at these organizations (J. Murad, personal communication, 2001), and there is anecdotal evidence of an escalation in the numbers of birds being relinquished by private owners. For captive parrots, there are now many of the same overpopulation problems as for dogs and cats—too many unwanted animals and not enough qualified homes. Part of the problem is that there is not enough information available to parrot owners regarding parrot welfare, including what parrots need in order to maintain good welfare and how poor welfare can be assessed and improved.

The main objective of this chapter is to examine some of the welfare problems facing parrots in a companion context in order to gain an understanding of their causes and potential solutions. Many of the principles discussed in this chapter will also be relevant to parrots housed in zoos, aviaries, and other captive settings. First, however, we will discuss some of the concepts associated with the study of animal welfare in general.

WHAT IS ANIMAL WELFARE?

In the last few decades, there has been increasing discussion about human ethical obligations toward animals, which has been reflected in a growing body of legislation, particularly in Europe, designed to protect the welfare of farm, laboratory, and companion animals. Although it is beyond the scope of this chapter to provide details of the various ethical theories about human-animal relationships that have been proposed, all are based on a common assumption: that animals have interests (e.g., an interest in avoiding pain and suffering) that deserve consideration by humans. This assumption is now also widely accepted by most people, at least in developed countries, although there is still considerable disagreement about the nature of animals' interests and how they should be weighed against human interests.

This ethical concern for the quality of life of animals has led to the development of the field of animal welfare science. The goal of this field is to develop methods for assessing and improving the welfare of animals in a variety of settings including laboratories, zoos, farms, shelters, and private homes. Welfare is viewed as something intrinsic to the individual animal, that is, the animal's state of being well or "faring" well. That state of well-being has both a physical and psychological component and can be influenced by many factors including the animal's housing, care, physical health, and interactions with humans.

There are three broad approaches to the scientific study of animal welfare (Duncan & Fraser 1997). "Feelings-based" approaches equate an animal's welfare with its subjective experience. Proponents of this approach place primary emphasis on the reduction of pain and suffering and the provision of comfort and pleasure. Dawkins (1988, p. 209) sums up the spirit of this approach with this quote: "To be concerned about animal welfare is to be concerned with the subjective feelings of animals, particularly the unpleasant subjective feelings of suffering and pain." Observation of behaviors such as avoidance, aggression, and vocalizations can be used to gain information about the internal experiences of animals with respect to fear, pain, and distress. Determination of what animals prefer and what they would rather avoid are also important for evaluating subjective feelings.

A second approach, known as the "functioning-based" approach, uses the biological state of the animal as the main criteria by which to judge welfare. Normal functioning of biological and behavioral systems is essential to good welfare from this perspective. Thus, disease, injury, failure to reproduce, and the performance of abnormal behaviors are considered evidence of compromised welfare.

A third approach operates under the assumption that in order to provide good welfare for a captive animal we should allow it to perform all "natural" behaviors and raise it in an environment that is as close to a natural environment as possible. Research approaches appropriate to this view include using the behavioral repertoire of animals in the wild as a guide for evaluating the welfare of captive counterparts of the same or similar species. Thus, from this perspective, parrots in captivity that are unable to perform behaviors such as locomotion, social interaction, and foraging for food would have compromised welfare.

These different approaches to conceptualizing and assessing animal welfare are not necessarily mutually exclusive. For example, problems that affect the functioning of animals can also affect their feelings: a parrot that injures itself when feather picking will have reduced biological functioning and also experience pain as a result of the injury. However, there are other situations in which the relationships among indicators of welfare are not straightforward. Laying hens kept in cages without nests pace and vocalize frantically before laying their eggs, which is an indicator of distress, but show no obvious impairment of reproduction or health (Appleby et al., in press).

Fraser et al. (1997) suggest that the three approaches can most usefully be integrated by understanding that all animals possess adaptations that have arisen during the course of evolution. In the wild, these adaptations are reflected in an animal's normal behavioral repertoire. Some adaptations, however, may not be necessary in the captive environment because their original function is achieved in some other way. For example, adaptations used to regulate body temperature during cold weather are not necessary if animals are kept in comfortable, temperature-controlled environments. Depriving the animal of the ability to perform the behavior associated with such an adaptation will not affect the animal's quality of life unless the behavior is also motivated by a strong affective (emotional) experience, like hunger or a desire to escape. In this situation, the animal's feelings, and hence its welfare, will be compromised even if its biological functioning is not. For example, captive animals are sometimes feed restricted because otherwise they become obese due to lack of exercise. While this actually promotes good physical health, the animal still feels hungry and may even develop abnormal behaviors, like chewing on cage bars or ingesting non-food items (pica), in an attempt to diminish its hunger.

Welfare problems can also arise if animals lack the adaptations necessary for particular features of the captive environment. Atmospheric ammonia levels can be high in farm and laboratory environments, but most animals do not have evolutionary adaptations to environmental pollutants and may show no avoidance reactions to high ammonia environments, even though exposure eventually results in damage to the eyes and respiratory system, and hence impairment of biological functioning. Lastly, welfare problems can arise when animals possess the appropriate adaptations, but the adaptations are inadequate to the degree of challenge imposed within the captive environment. In this case, there is likely to be a high correspondence between feelings and functioning (e.g., feeling hot and showing signs of heat stress). These examples illustrate how important it is to assess multiple measures and responses to gain the most accurate picture of the animal's welfare.

THREATS TO PARROT WELFARE

The main threats to the welfare of captive parrots fall into three categories: husbandry, environment, and human interactions. Husbandry-related threats include such things as poor nutrition (for a full discussion, see chapter 6), unsanitary conditions, lack of veterinary care, improper light/dark cycles, inappropriate temperature, and lack of opportunity for bathing. Environmental issues include lack of space, threats to safety such as dangerous objects, improper bar spacing or potential for escape, improper perch size, barren cages, social isolation, and lack of opportunity for privacy. Threats due to human interactions include abuse, neglect, improper taming/training techniques, and sexual bonding between parrots and human companions.

In most cases, these threats will manifest themselves in the parrots through physical, psychological, or behavioral indicators associated with poor welfare. Physical indicators include disease, injury, parasites, obesity, and malnutrition. Apathy and anhedonia (loss of interest in things the parrot once enjoyed such as favorite foods and toys) are potential psychological indicators of poor welfare. Behavioral indicators include abnormal behaviors such as stereotypy (repetitive, invariant performance of a behavior, such as pacing), feather picking, incessant screaming, and excessive aggression or fearfulness. Sometimes these indicators are observed shortly after the threat to welfare has been imposed. For example, an injury may result immediately after an unsafe toy is placed in the cage. However, other indicators of poor welfare may not be obvious for days, weeks, or even years. During the intervening time, the parrot may be attempting to cope with the threat and may show no outward signs of poor welfare. For example, sick birds often do not show any signs of illness until they are in an advanced disease state, and birds may live for long periods of time in barren conditions before developing abnormal behaviors. Despite the fact that outwardly these parrots appear and act normally, biological and behavioral changes may be occurring that will eventually result in overt signs of poor welfare. At that point, reversing these changes, and thus returning the parrot to a state of good welfare, may be difficult or impossible. For this reason, it is imperative that owners thoroughly understand the threats to their parrots' welfare and strive to eliminate these threats from their parrots' lives as soon as possible. Prevention of poor welfare is the best solution to poor welfare.

While there are many threats to companion parrot welfare, space does not permit a thorough discussion of them all. As such, the remainder of this chapter will be focused on the behavioral effects of environmental threats to welfare. We will address the connection between the captive environment and several of the most common behavioral problems experienced by parrots. We will also provide information that will assist companion parrot owners with the design of a captive environment that can successfully prevent abnormal behaviors from occurring, and sometimes even decrease or abolish already-established abnormal behaviors.

THE CAPTIVE ENVIRONMENT AND PARROT WELFARE

As previously mentioned, animals have evolved to respond adaptively through behavior to changes in their environment. They have also evolved the ability to change their environment to meet their needs and goals. In the course of evolution, animals have been selected, in considerable part, based upon the strength of these abilities. In the wild, behavioral skills are used regularly in the course of capturing or gathering food, avoiding predators, finding or creating shelter, and choosing or attracting mates. In captivity, most needs of animals are met without their direct participation—food arrives at regular intervals pre-killed, cooked, or peeled; shelter is provided and often is immutable; social groups are selected by humans; and predators are kept away by bars and glass. On one hand, a controlled environment may seem ideal as it provides freedom from food scarcity, predation, and extreme climatic changes. But at the same time, many captive environments are quite limited with respect to space, complexity and behavioral opportunity when compared to the environments of free-living individuals. This is the paradox of life in captivity—in an attempt to reduce exposure to environmental pressures, we prevent parrots from exhibiting many of their natural behaviors, creating a mismatch between the parrot and its environment. If this mismatch is significant, normal behavioral expression is prevented and abnormal behaviors can develop instead.

In order to understand how the captive environment might affect the welfare of parrots, it is necessary that we first understand the behavior of parrots in the wild and how this diverges from the behavior of parrots in captivity. It is also necessary to understand parrots in the context of domestication to appreciate how behaviorally close captive parrots are to their wild counterparts.

PARROTS IN THE WILD

In the wild, parrots are constantly engaged with their environment whether it is via social interactions, foraging activities, territory defense, nest selection, or predator avoidance. When brought into captivity and placed under close environmental control, the opportunity to perform many of these behaviors is reduced.

Two of the most severely constrained classes of behavior in captive parrots are foraging and locomotion. Parrots in the wild regularly travel several miles between feeding sites, and once they arrive engage in a rich suite of local search, food selection, and food manipulation behaviors. For example wild Puerto Rican Amazons (*Amazona vittata*) spend approximately four to six hours per day foraging and are known to ingest the fruit, leaves, bark, vines, and/or other portions of at least 58 species of indigenous plant material (Snyder et al. 1987). A study performed in 1985 by Magrath and Lill characterized the activity

budget of a wild psittacine, the Crimson Rosella, in its native Australian habitat. Although the activity budget differed seasonally, young Rosellas in this study spent a mean time of 67% in feeding/foraging and only 7% of their time resting. It is likely that other parrot species invest similar amounts of time in feeding behavior. In some cases the investment is made in searching for food and in some cases in processing it. For example, the Gang-gang Cockatoo (*Callocephalon fimbriatum*) habitually feeds on the very well-protected nuts of the eucalyptus tree, expending a considerable portion of its time simply exposing the edible portion of the item (Bauck 1999). In contrast, most parrots in captivity do not travel between feeding sites, do not have to select different foods to balance their diet, and have little opportunity to manipulate objects to obtain food. Thus, captive Orange-winged Amazon Parrots (*Amazona amazonica*) spend only 30–72 minutes a day in feeding behaviors when fed a pelleted diet (Oviatt & Millam 1997). Many captive feeding methods allow minimal environmental interaction and greatly reduce the amount of work and energetic cost involved in feeding activities. Because of the importance of these behaviors in the repertoire of wild parrots, it is possible that captive parrots are highly motivated to search for, access, and process food items.

Wild parrots also exploit a complex physical environment and, in addition to flight, show a number of physical and behavioral adaptations to this habitat. For instance, they utilize their grappling beak and grasping feet to negotiate treetops and unstable fruit-bearing branches, are adept climbers of vertical surfaces, and are equally graceful traversing the underside of branches (Sparks & Soper 1990). In captivity, parrots are rarely able to fly and are usually severely constrained in the other locomotor behaviors they can perform due to the design of their cage environment.

For most species of parrot, sociality is a constant feature throughout the lifetime of an individual, although the characteristics of social groupings can change daily and seasonally. For example, during the breeding season, wild amazon parrots tend to form small groups consisting of a pair and their young, but outside of the breeding season they can become highly gregarious and flock size can grow significantly (Gilardi &

Munn 1998). The social environment of a parrot also changes during development. As nestlings, parrots are restricted to social interactions with parents and clutchmates. As the birds fledge and become more independent, social interactions increase in diversity and complexity as the young birds are introduced into larger groups. In captivity, companion and laboratory parrots are often socially isolated from conspecifics, although parrots in zoos may be afforded more opportunity for social interaction.

It is evident from this review that foraging, varied locomotion, and social interactions are integral components of the behavioral repertoire of wild parrots. The next section demonstrates why these same behaviors are important to captive parrots as well.

PARROTS AND DOMESTICATION

Domestication is a process of adaptation to captivity that includes both genetic changes occurring over generations as well as environmentally induced developmental events (such as taming) that occur within the lifetime of an individual (Price 1984). Because of their long lifespan (up to 70 years or more), and the recent growth in popularity of parrots as pets, many parrots currently in captivity were born to wild parents or are among the first few generations of captive born. Unlike cats and dogs, which have been bred to live as human companions for thousands of years, pet parrots are only a few generations out of the wild. Thus, although parrots may live in a variety of captive situations, they can't be considered domesticated. Since parrots are very early along in the domestication process, it is likely that the capacity to perform the behaviors seen in wild counterparts remains (Price 1999). Even long-domesticated species such as Norway rats (Boice 1981), rabbits (Vastrade 1986), and pigs (Wood-Gush et al. 1983) behave in a manner that is nearly identical to that of their wild ancestors when housed in "semi-natural" conditions. Although pet parrots are very similar behaviorally and biologically to their wild counterparts, the typical captive environment is a far cry from the environments parrots inhabit in the wild.

Recognizing that the wild can't be re-created inside a cage, the challenge to those interested in improving parrot welfare by improving their environment is twofold: first, to determine which en-vironmental elements are critical to normal behavioral development and second, to develop practical methods of introducing these elements in the captive context, a process referred to as environmental enrichment.

ENVIRONMENTAL ENRICHMENT

The concept of environmental enrichment evolved from a recognition that restrictive and barren captive environments can impair behavioral and physiological development and concomitantly reduce welfare. Shepherdson (1998, pg. 1) broadly defines environmental enrichment as "an animal husbandry principle that seeks to enhance the quality of captive animal care by identifying and providing the environmental stimuli necessary for optimal psychological and physiological well-being."

Common environmental enrichment strategies involve changing the types of food or the methods by which food is provided, providing social stimulation, changing structural features of animals' enclosures to provide cover or to encourage locomotion, or exposing animals to novelty to facilitate exploration. In mammals, appropriate enrichment has been shown to have many beneficial effects, including facilitating a more normal and diverse behavioral repertoire, decreasing stress, improving immune function, improving learning ability, and decreasing fearfulness and the performance of abnormal behaviors (e.g., Renner & Rosenzweig 1987; Carlstead & Shepherdson 1999; Bayne et al. 2002; Newberry 1995).

Although environmental enrichment is a potentially promising strategy for improving the welfare of captive and companion parrots, little is known about the elements necessary for effective environmental enrichment for avian species in general, and particularly for parrots (e.g., Birchall 1990; Shepherdson 1993; King 1993). In fact, avian species are hugely under-represented when it comes to innovations and research regarding environmental enrichment (King 1993). The mammalian bias present in the field of environmental enrichment may be due to the closer evolutionary relationship between humans and other mammals, the popular appeal of megavertebrates such as carnivores and primates, or the perceived lack of intelligence possessed by avian species (King 1993). Whatever the reason, birds in captivity are potentially suffering due to lack of attention to their environmental enrichment needs or due to misguided attempts at enrichment that are not based on scientific research.

In order to develop an enrichment program that will improve the welfare of captive parrots, it is necessary to first identify those behaviors that are most important to optimal behavioral development. Principles of environmental enrichment developed through research with other species can be used to inform the design of enrichment programs for parrots. What is critical is that the enrichments be biologically relevant to the animal and be demonstrated to have positive effects on welfare. For example, enrichment strategies that take into consideration the motivational state and behavioral skills of the particular species in question are generally more successful than strategies that are not based on species-appropriate hypotheses (Newberry 1995). Thus, providing singly housed rhesus monkeys with a foraging/grooming board consisting of a piece of Plexiglass covered with artificial fleece with particles of food treats rubbed into it improves welfare by increasing foraging and grooming behaviors and reducing the performance of abnormal behaviors (Bayne et al. 1991), while providing sticks and dog toys has no effect on the performance of abnormal behaviors in the same species (Line et al. 1991). Similarly, the species-specific strategies of introducing live fish into the pool for fishing cats and hiding food in a brush pile in the enclosure for leopard cats significantly reduce the performance of abnormal behaviors (Shepherdson 1993).

For some animals, the physical design of the cage, rather than the feeding methods, must be modified to reduce abnormal behaviors. Again, these modifications must be relevant to the animal to be effective. For example, provision of cover prevents stereotypies in young bank voles (Cooper et al. 1996), although increased cage space does not (Odberg 1987). Weidenmayer (1997) was successful in preventing nearly all development of stereotypy in gerbils reared with access to a burrow as long as the burrow was paired with a tunnel-shaped entrance, which created a configuration similar to that of a wild gerbil burrowing system.

For species that have evolved in a social milieu, social stimulation may provide the most effective form of environmental enrichment because social stimulation has dynamic qualities and is seldom

constant or completely predictable (e.g., Novak & Suomi 1988; Mendl & Newberry 1997). Although most species of parrots are social in the wild (Sparks & Soper 1990), companion parrots are not often socially housed. In fact, recommendations in the popular literature on parrot care suggest that pet parrots not be pair-housed because they will become less desirable as pets (e.g., Blanchard 1999), although this has not been demonstrated empirically. However, it has been suggested that isolation from conspecifics may contribute to the development of many abnormal behaviors including excessive screaming, stereotypies, fearfulness, and aggression (e.g., Westerhof & Lumeij 1987; Lantermann 1993), so social enrichment may, in fact, be an effective tool for improving the welfare of companion parrots.

From a naturalistic standpoint, re-creating social groups of parrots that are seasonally and developmentally appropriate in a captive setting would be considered the best approach to social housing. However, naturalistic social environments necessarily involve increased risk of infection as well as potential injury or stress due to aggressive encounters. In addition, the goals and restrictions of most captive situations are not compatible with the space, resource, and husbandry requirements of naturalistic social groupings. Thus, pair-housing has been used in many contexts and with many species as an alternative to naturalistic social environments or individual housing in an attempt to enrich the captive environment and improve welfare (e.g. Barnett et al. 1984; Hughes et al. 1989; Reinhardt 1991; Chu et al., in press). Pair-housing can be a practical alternative to single-housing for parrots because the space requirements per pair are not extensive and normal husbandry practices do not need to be changed significantly.

There has been very little research on behavioral aspects of parrot welfare and of effective environmental enrichment. In the following sections, we therefore discuss some experimental evidence derived from studies conducted at our Orange-winged Amazon Parrot colony at the University of California, Davis, that suggests that enriching three aspects of the captive environment can have significant positive effects on parrot welfare. The three forms of enrichment tested in the studies outlined are providing foraging opportunity, increasing the physical complexity of the cage, and allowing for social contact. The foraging enrichments we utilized required the parrots to perform behaviors such as chewing through barriers, sorting through inedible material, maneuvering objects through holes, or opening containers in order to access the food items. Physical enrichments provided alternate perching sites, climbing or swinging opportunities, or movable objects that could be manipulated with the beak and/or feet. In the cases where social enrichment was utilized, some parrots were housed in same-sex, same-age, non-related pairs, while others were singly housed. We found that these three forms of enrichment successfully prevented and reversed the performance of several common abnormal or undesirable behaviors and, as such, improved the welfare of the parrots involved. The behaviors studied were psychogenic feather picking, fearfulness, aggression toward human handlers, stereotypic behavior, and screaming.

Psychogenic Feather Picking

Many owners of companion parrots have been faced with the frustrating dilemma of how to help a feather-picking bird. In fact, it has been estimated that one in ten captive parrots performs self-directed psychogenic feather-picking behavior (Grindlinger 1991). It takes just one look at a parrot denuded or with self-inflicted skin and feather damage for it to become obvious that there is great cause for concern. Psychogenic feather-picking behavior develops or persists in the absence of medical causes, and observational evidence suggests that it may be associated with a number of management factors such as inadequate diet, social isolation, and lack of environmental stimulation (e.g., Mertens 1997). However, despite the severity and prevalence of this problem, there has been very little research on the environmental correlates of feather picking.

Although there have been few systematic studies of feather-picking behavior in psittacines, there has been a significant amount of research on feather pecking, a similar behavior commonly performed by domestic fowl (Mench & Keeling 2001). In chickens feather pecking is generally directed at other birds, while in parrots picking is generally self-directed, but this difference may simply reflect differences in management. Chickens are generally socially housed, while parrots are often caged alone. When parrots are housed in social groups, feather picking can also be directed at cagemates or nestlings.

Feather pecking by chickens is strongly associated with the performance of foraging behavior (e.g., Nicol et al. 2001; Klein et al. 2000; Huber-Eicher & Wechsler 1997, 1998; Blokhuis 1986). In chickens, normal foraging behavior consists of pecks directed at both edible and inedible substrates, but if chickens are housed such that ground pecking is prevented, then pecks may instead be directed at the feathers of conspecifics (Blokhuis 1986; Huber-Eicher & Wechsler 1997). Chickens may also consume the feathers that they manage to pull out (McKeegan & Savory 1999). Provision of non-nutritive foraging material such as long straw and polystyrene blocks is effective in both preventing and reducing feather-pecking behavior by chicks (Huber-Eicher & Wechsler 1997). In addition, hens provided with foraging material show significantly lower rates of feather pecking than those kept without foraging material (Wechsler & Huber-Eicher 1997). Thus, feather pecking is considered by many to be redirected foraging behavior (e.g., Hoffmeyer 1969; Blokhuis 1989; Huber-Eicher & Wechsler 1997; Wechsler & Huber-Eicher 1997).

Given the putative role of foraging behavior in the development of feather pecking by chickens, it is possible that a similar relationship exists between foraging behavior and feather picking in parrots. This may mean that captive parrots are highly motivated to perform the behaviors associated with food procurement in the wild and that this motivation may persist despite the fact that captive feeding methods meet their nutritional needs. There is some evidence that captive parrots prefer to access food utilizing their foraging skills even when "free" food is available (Coulton et al. 1997). Thus, the act of foraging may be a behavioral need for parrots and the absence of foraging opportunity may result in frustration and redirection of foraging-like activities toward the feathers.

In our study of Orange-winged Amazon Parrots (Meehan et al. 2002), one group of young birds (between four and five months old) was given the opportunity to utilize their foraging skills to access food while the other was not. Both groups of parrots were given pellets, fruits, nuts, seeds, and vegetables daily; the difference was in the manner of presentation. The "control" group received these foods cut up and served in a dish,

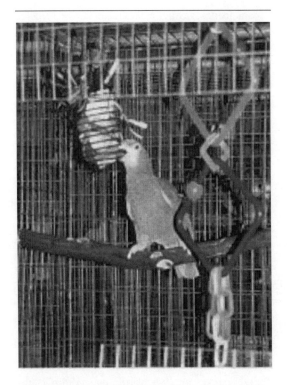

Figure 27.1. Examples of the enrichments utilized in the U.C. Davis experiments. See also color section.

as is common practice with captive parrots, while the "enriched" group received these foods in specially designed feeders (see Figure 27.1). These feeders significantly increased the diversity of feeding behaviors the parrots performed as well as increased the amount of time they spent in feeding activities. Parrots in the enriched group also received enrichments that increased the physical complexity of the cage. Plumage condition served as an indirect measurement of feather-picking behavior.

The effect on feather-picking development was dramatic. Over the course of the one-year study, six of eight parrots in the control group developed feather-picking behavior (as evidenced by significant decreases in feather score), while none of the birds in the enriched group showed any signs of developing the disorder (as evidenced by stability or improvement in feather score). Thus, this study demonstrates that presenting food in a manner that requires parrots to utilize their foraging skills and increasing the physical complexity of

the cage are effective in the prevention of feather-picking behavior. This is excellent news to owners of young parrots as it provides a method of preventing the development of this problematic behavior. However, a second component of the study was required to determine if this method is effective in reversing established feather picking.

In the second phase of the study, the parrots that had once been in the control condition were given access to the feeding devices and physical enrichments used in the original study. After four months, all six parrots that had feather picked showed significant improvements in feather condition, indicating that feather-picking behavior had significantly decreased. These results suggest that making appropriate changes to the environment can effectively treat parrots with established feather-picking behavior. The parrots in this study had been performing the behavior for about one year before it was reversed, however, and it remains to be seen if the same course of action will be effective with parrots that have performed this behavior for several years.

Taken as a whole, these results support the hypothesis that a captive environment that does not support the appropriate expression of foraging behaviors can contribute to the development of psychogenic feather-picking behavior. By providing foraging devices and physical enrichments it is possible to both prevent and reverse this disorder. Since we introduced foraging and physical enrichments together, rather than separately, it is difficult to tell the relative importance of each type of enrichment from our study. It is possible that the combination of physical and foraging enrichments is necessary for the preventative and reversal effects on feather picking we observed. However, since the foraging enrichments were used for significantly greater periods of time than the physical enrichments, our data certainly demonstrate a link between foraging opportunity and the development and performance of feather picking in parrots.

Fearfulness and Aggression

Hyperaggressiveness and excessive fear reactions are often identified as indicators of poor welfare. Excessive aggression can result in injury and can inhibit social interactions within groups of parrots or between captive parrots and their caretakers. In addition, fear is generally considered an undesirable emotional state (Jones 1997) and exaggerated fear reactions such as escape attempts and panic can result in wasted energy or injury (Jones & Waddington 1992). Parrots that are excessively fearful or aggressive are much more difficult to care for and as a result are more likely to be abused, neglected, or relinquished by owners who become frustrated by this behavior.

For parrots, novelty is often a potent stimulus for excessive fearful or aggressive reactions. Unpredictable yet benign environmental changes such as new people, new surroundings, or introduction of new toys or food items can induce screaming, biting, cowering, shaking, and fleeing. It has been shown in other birds and mammals that the degree of fearful and aggressive reactions is associated with the quality of the captive environment, in that animals reared in barren environments with little exposure to novelty and little opportunity for environmental interaction often display exaggerated responses compared to animals reared in more complex environments. For example, rats reared in environments lacking complexity show an increased fear response to novel situations and increased aggression toward novel individuals (Fernandez-Teruel et al. 1997; Escorihuela et al. 1994; Renner 1987), while chickens reared in this type of environment show increased fear responses to novel places and novel objects (Jones 1982; Jones & Waddington 1992).

Environmental enrichment that increases exposure to novelty during development has been successfully employed to modulate fear responses in both birds and mammals as evidenced by increased activity in novel environments (Fernandez-Teruel et al. 1997; Escorihuela et al. 1994; Renner 1987) and decreased fear responses to novel objects (Jones 1982; Jones & Waddington 1992). There is also evidence that enrichment of the physical environment reduces fearfulness of humans (e.g., Jones & Waddington 1992; Nicol 1992; Pearce et al. 1989).

Fear reactions to novel objects may be exaggerated in parrots whose cage environment is barren or unchanging, and environmental enrichment may reduce fear reactions to novelty by exposing parrots to an environment where novelty is experienced on a consistent basis. We compared the responses of parrots from enriched and barren conditions to novel objects (Meehan & Mench 2002). In one study, the enrichments used provided foraging opportunity and increased the physical complexity of the cage. Parrots in the enriched condition received a novel combination of one foraging and one physical enrichment each week for 16 weeks. In a second study, the responses to novel objects of parrots reared in pairs were compared with those of parrots that were singly housed (Meehan et al. 2003). In this study, all parrots received the physical and foraging enrichment protocol previously described, leaving social enrichment as the variable of interest. To test for the effect on fearfulness of novelty in their environment, a novel object was placed in the parrot's home cage in a position that required the bird to approach the object in order to interact with it.

In the first study, parrots from the enriched condition had significantly shorter latencies to interact with novel objects than did parrots from the barren cages. Parrots from the barren cages usually responded initially to the novel object by retreating from it. They would then engage in a series of approach/retreat sequences, eventually contacting the object. The initial reaction of the parrots in the enriched condition was also to retreat from the object. However, shortly after they had retreated and visually inspected the object they would begin to interact with the object without the approach/retreat sequences characteristic of the control group. Thus, the latency to interact with the novel object was significantly shorter in the enriched group than it was in the control group. The data suggest that the accelerated approach toward novel objects in the enriched group reflects decreased fearfulness of the object rather than an increased tendency to engage in exploratory behavior, since the parrots in the enriched condition also had shorter overall duration of interaction and shorter bout lengths of interaction with the objects.

Pair-housing also had an effect on fear responses to novel objects. The single parrots had significantly longer latencies to interact with the novel objects than the paired parrots (when the paired parrots were tested together as a pair). Thus, having a social partner present appears to ameliorate the fear-evoking effect of a novel stimulus. The fear-diminishing effect of a social partner has been observed in chickens (Jones & Merry 1988), monkeys (Coe et al. 1982), and rats (Taylor 1981). In each of these cases, as in our study, a decreased fear response to novelty is observed when the animals are tested with a social partner as compared to when they are tested alone. Thus, in addition to an inanimate enrichment protocol, pair-housing is recommended as an effective method for creating a dynamic cage environment and reducing fearfulness of environmental novelty in captive parrots.

Interactions with Human Handlers

In most situations where companion parrots are kept, positive interactions with humans are valued. Parrots that are excessively fearful of or aggressive toward humans are generally not considered desirable as pets, in aviculture, as research subjects, or as part of zoo exhibits. However, biting and aggression are some of the most commonly reported complaints by parrot owners. Aggressive or fearful responses toward humans may be due to a variety of experiential or developmental factors, including trauma and hormonal changes. In addition, how parrots are housed may contribute to this behavior. While the popular parrot literature suggests that housing parrots together in pairs, rather than singly, may negatively impact their interactions with human handlers (e.g., Blanchard 1999), recent experimental evidence suggests that pair-housing of young parrots in same-sex pairs may actually improve, rather than hinder, interactions with human handlers (Meehan et al. 2003).

Responses to familiar and unfamiliar human handlers were tested in parrots that were housed either individually or in same-sex pairs (Cramton 1998; Aengus & Millam 1999). Testing involved extending a finger toward the parrot, touching the parrot's back, touching the parrot's head, offering food, and observing flight distance when the parrot was placed next to the handler. Two familiar handlers as well as two unfamiliar handlers tested each parrot. The familiar handlers were people who had been working regularly in handling sessions with the parrots, while the unfamiliar handlers were people who were trained in parrot handling but who had never interacted directly with the test parrot.

Pair-housing did not cause parrots to behave more aggressively or fearfully to human handlers. In fact, parrots from both groups showed an improvement in responses to familiar handlers over the course of the year, and overall there was no difference in responses between the two groups.

This suggests paired parrots are equally suitable as pets in this regard as singly housed parrots.

When tested with unfamiliar handlers, there was a difference in responses between the two groups. In this case, the singly housed parrots responded more aggressively and fearfully than did the paired parrots. This difference in response might be explained by the fact that the paired parrots had more opportunities to explore changes in their environment and thus were more likely to respond inquisitively rather than fearfully to the novel human stimulus. In addition, social interaction and play facilitate behavioral flexibility and enhance the ability to transfer learning tasks (e.g., Morgan 1973; Morgan et al. 1975; Einon et al, 1978). Thus, because paired parrots had the opportunity to interact with a pairmate and spent more time in play activities than the single parrots, they may have been better able to transfer the learning experience of the regular handling sessions to the experience with the novel human. This ability is relevant to many captive contexts because parrots are likely to encounter novel humans, such as visitors or veterinarians, regularly.

Stereotypic Behavior

Stereotypies are defined as behavior patterns that are repetitive, invariant, and have no obvious goal or function (Mason 1991). While the precise etiology of these behaviors is not yet understood, it has been suggested that stereotypies develop in animals housed in environments that are suboptimal in one or more dimensions (Mason 1991). For example, in many species, stereotypic behaviors are significantly more evident in environments that do not provide sufficient sensory stimulation (Mason 1991), opportunity to interact with objects or conspecifics (Carlstead 1998), or that leave the animal with little control over its surroundings (Markowitz & Aday 1998).

Stereotypy development may be related to the frustration of specific motivational systems. For example, a number of experiments demonstrate a relationship between stereotypies and restriction of feeding or foraging behaviors, locomotion, or social contact. Feed restriction is closely associated with stereotypy performance in pigs (Terlouw et al. 1991), chickens (Savory et al. 1992), and sheep (Mardsen & Wood-Gush 1986). However, feeding-related stereotypies can occur even when food intake is not restricted. In these cases, it is thought that motivation to perform foraging behaviors underlies stereotypy performance. This idea is supported by evidence that, in both mammals and birds, stereotypy performance is reduced when opportunities to work in order to locate, access and consume food items are provided (e.g., Keiper 1969; Kastelstein & Wiepkema 1989; Line et al. 1989; Carlstead et al. 1991).

Some stereotypies are thought to develop from frustrated locomotor behavior. Hediger (1955) suggested that the stereotyped pacing common to zoo animals might develop from normal patrolling behaviors that are thwarted due to limited space. Increasing the complexity of the cage environment and providing opportunity for additional perching and swinging behaviors reduced stereotypic route tracing in Canaries (Keiper 1969), suggesting that this behavior might be related to frustrated locomotor behaviors.

Finally, motivation for social contact may underlie some forms of stereotypy. For example, frustrated motivation for maternal contact is thought to be associated with some primate stereotypies such as rocking and self-clasping (Marriner & Drickamer 1994), and providing horses with either a mirror or social contact reduces stereotypic weaving behaviors (Nicol 1999).

Thus, there is ample evidence that the frustration of highly motivated behaviors is involved in the development and performance of some forms of stereotypy. However, developmental evidence suggests that stereotypy is not simply a behavioral response to an inappropriate environment but rather the product of an abnormal developmental process resulting in both physiological and behavioral impairment. For example, stereotypies change over time in both form (Meyer-Holzapfel 1968; Cronin et al. 1984; Mason 1993) and frequency (e.g., Mason 1993; Würbel et al. 1998; Powell et al. 2000). In addition, stereotypies may become more difficult to reverse over time (Kiley-Worthington 1977; Cronin et al. 1984; Cooper et al. 1996) and eventually may become established in the behavioral repertoire of animals such that they remain unchanged even when the environment is modified. Thus, the fact that the nature and form of stereotypy change with time, even when the captive environment remains constant, indicates that stereotypy is the result of environmentally induced qualitative changes in the animal (Garner 1999; Würbel 2001).

Similar behaviors are also extremely common in a number of human mental disorders. Stereotypies are performed by approximately 70% of chronic schizophrenic patients (Owens et al. 1982) and are core symptoms of both Tourette's syndrome and autism (American Psychiatric Association 1994). Recent evidence suggests that, like in human patients, stereotypy in caged animals reflects a general disinhibition of behavioral control mechanisms (Garner & Mason 2002; Garner et. al. 2003). Thus, it is possible that stereotypies seen in captive animals are the result of environmentally induced neurological deficits similar to those seen in human psychiatric disorders.

The frequency of stereotypy in the captive parrot population at large has not been estimated. Many parrot owners are not aware of this class of abnormal behavior since stereotypies are often difficult to recognize without prior experience and training. In addition, parrots may only perform stereotypies when they are alone (which is why videotaping is necessary for stereotypy research), and thus owners may never witness their parrots performing stereotypies. While the stereotypies performed by parrots take many forms, they can, for the most part, be classified into three main categories: oral stereotypies, locomotor stereotypies, and object-directed stereotypies. Oral stereotypies include such behaviors as spot pecking, sham chewing, bar biting, or tongue rolling. Locomotor stereotypies include route tracing and pacing. Object-directed stereotypies involve repetitive, invariant manipulation of objects such as toys, feeders, and waterers. The degree to which these behaviors are invariant in their repetitions is illustrated in the following series of pictures captured from a videotape of a parrot performing a route trace (see Figure 27.2).

There have been few studies of stereotypy in parrots, but those that have been completed implicate both lack of foraging opportunity and limited physical complexity in the cage environment in the development of these behaviors. When parrots are housed in cages that lack foraging opportunity and physical complexity, stereotypy reliably develops. For example, 96% of parrots in a colony housed in these conditions performed stereotypy, and individuals spent between 5% and 85% of their active time performing these behaviors (Meehan 2002).

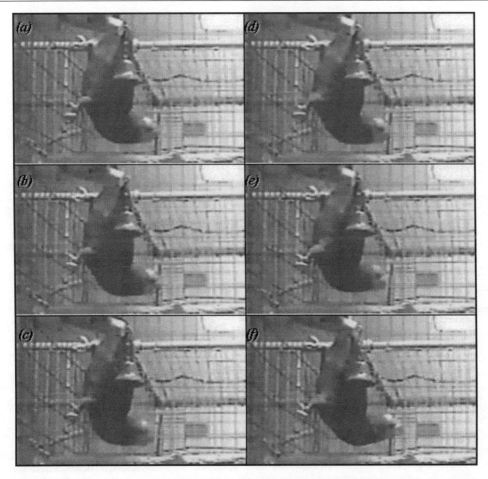

Figure 27.2. The invariance of stereotypy. These frames are taken from a sequence of video in which the corner flipping stereotypy was repeated six times. Note the identical foot positions and body posture. (a) Frame 40, (b) Frame 105, (c) Frame 162, (d) Frame 219, (e) Frame 267, (f) Frame 319. The frame rate is 15 frames per second, giving a mean ± SD interval of 3.72 ± 0.43 seconds between frames. Reproduced with permission from Behavioral Brain Research.

Enriching the environment with foraging devices and increasing the physical complexity of cages significantly decreased the development of stereotypy in young Orange-winged Amazon Parrots (Meehan et al., submitted). Parrots in the control condition spent significantly more of their active time performing stereotypies than did parrots in the enriched condition. However, the degree of environmental modification used in this study was not sufficient to completely prevent the development of stereotypic behavior. At the end of 48 weeks the parrots in the enriched condition performed stereotypies an average of 4% of their active time. This is a common outcome of studies examining the role of specific environmental factors in stereotypy development (e.g., Odberg 1987; Würbel et al. 1998; Powell et al. 2000). For example, increasing the physical complexity of cages with twigs prevents most, but not all, stereotypy development in young voles (Odberg 1987). Similarly, the combination of feeding sunflower seeds and increasing physical complexity has a significant effect on the amount of time deer mice spend performing stereotypy but does not eliminate the development of these behaviors altogether (Powell et al. 2000). These results indicate that additional research is necessary to determine the specific environmental qualities needed to completely eliminate stereotypy from the behavioral repertoire of parrots.

Parrots in the control condition developed both locomotor and oral stereotypies, while those in the enriched condition developed almost exclusively locomotor stereotypies. This suggests that specific forms of stereotypy may be associated with the absence of specific environmental elements (Mason & Mendl 1997). In this case, if oral stereotypies were associated with frustration of foraging behaviors, then the foraging enrichments may have successfully eliminated this frustration. If the development of locomotor stereotypies was associated with limited space, prevention of flight, or lack of social contact, then this would explain why these behaviors were not prevented by the physical enrichments we provided. There is evidence in Canaries that the development of oral stereotypies is related to lack of opportunity to perform foraging behaviors, while the development of locomotor stereotypies is related to a lack of space and physical complexity (Keiper 1969). Thus, additional experiments assessing the effectiveness of increased flight space and social housing are needed to determine appropriate environmental remedies for locomotor stereotypy.

Screaming

The vocal behavior of captive animals is increasingly utilized as an index of welfare (e.g., Weary et al. 1998; Grandin 1998, 2001). For example, Boinski and colleagues (1999) found that the rate of alarm vocalizations was positively correlated with the amount of time male capuchins performed stereotypic and redirected behaviors and negatively correlated with the amount of normal behavior performed. In addition, a positive relationship between fecal cortisol levels and vocalization rate was found, indicating that monkeys that vocalized more may have been more stressed. Finally, modification of the cage environment in the form of toys and foraging materials resulted in a significant decrease in monkeys' vocalization rate.

Incessant screaming is the second (after messiness) most common complaint of parrot owners (Kidd & Kidd 1998) and is one of the precipitating factors for parrot neglect and relinquishment (Reynolds 1998). Much communication between parrots is vocal, and some authors have suggested that loud, high-pitched squawks are used as alarm calls when individuals are in danger or distress (Alderton 1992) or as a contact call between group members (Sparks & Soper 1990). However, when these vocalizations become prolonged and repetitive, they are considered abnormal and may be indicative of boredom (Davis 1991) or, similar to capuchin monkeys, stress (Boinski et al. 1999).

We found that housing young amazons in same-sex pairs effectively reduces the amount of time spent in prolonged vocalizations (loud vocalization bouts lasting more than two seconds) when compared with singly housed parrots of the same age. Over the course of one year, paired parrots spent an average of 4.1% of their active time screaming, while singly housed parrots spent an average of 9.5% of their active time screaming (Meehan et al. 2003). It is important to note that all parrots in this study had visual and vocal contact with other parrots, but only the paired parrots could interact physically. More research in this area is necessary to provide a basis for interpreting the significance of differences in vocal patterns with respect to welfare. However, the fact that social housing impacts the degree to which young parrots perform prolonged vocalizations indicates that lack of physical interaction with social partners may be a factor in the development of this behavior. This finding is of great practical importance because it suggests that pair-housing is an effective way to ameliorate the performance of this common and frustrating behavioral problem.

PRACTICAL CONSIDERATIONS FOR IMPROVING PARROT WELFARE THROUGH ENVIRONMENTAL ENRICHMENT

This chapter has highlighted some of the impacts that environmental enrichment can have on the behavioral development of companion parrots. Effective environmental enrichment can improve the welfare of parrots by increasing the performance of behaviors such as foraging, locomotion, and social interaction, while concomitantly reducing or eliminating the performance of abnormal behaviors such as feather picking, screaming, and stereotypy. While enrichment strategies must take into consideration the behavior and ecology of the species in question as well as the age and history of the individual parrot, there are several important principles of environmental enrichment that will apply across all contexts.

Enrichment must provide a dynamic captive environment. This means that the parrots must be given the opportunity to act, react, and interact within their home environs. Providing novel enrichments on a consistent basis can help to accomplish this goal. Even the most wonderfully enriched cage loses its effectiveness when parrots are exposed to it for long periods of time. The exact timing of enrichment rotation will depend on the context and the particular parrot. Some parrots will require a day or so of habituation to novel enrichments and, in this case, weekly rotation would be advised. On the other hand, some parrots are extremely inquisitive and would be excellent candidates for daily introduction of novel items. Social companions also can provide a dynamic quality to the environment. Ideally, all parrots should have the opportunity to interact physically with other parrots in compatible social groups. However, more research is needed to determine the best approach to providing social enrichment to parrots throughout their lifespan.

The life-history stage of parrots should be taken into consideration when planning to introduce social enrichment. If parrots are introduced to social groups prior to reaching sexual maturity, it is possible that the compatibility of these groups may change as the parrots mature. If the onset of sexual maturity results in reduced compatibility or aggression, then social groupings may need to change as the parrots age. Older parrots may be more suited to mixed-sex groups. In fact, there is some evidence that forming larger, mixed-sex groups of parrots who are sexually mature can be accomplished successfully. An informal study was conducted at U.C. Davis with five pairs of parrots ranging in age from five to eight years old. These parrots had been pair-housed for three years in male/female pairs but had not successfully reproduced during any of the three breeding seasons in which they were paired. A large flight cage was constructed and attached to the home cages of the pairs, which allowed researchers to control access to the flight cage. The flight was furnished with the same foraging and physical enrichments described earlier and access was provided to all ten parrots simultaneously. The parrots were monitored regularly to assess levels of aggression and decrease the risk of injury. After several weeks of interaction, all par-

rots, with the exception of one male (who was removed from the group) co-existed peacefully in the large cage. The parrots utilized the enrichments extensively, despite the fact that they had no prior experience with these types of devices. At this point, nest boxes were introduced and the parrots were allowed to "self-select" pairmates. There was some aggression involved in this process, but the parrots were closely monitored and the aggression was not severe enough to cause injury or warrant separation. Interestingly, two of the original pairs were maintained, one new pair was formed, and one threesome (one male and two females) was formed. Of these, three pairs laid eggs and two successfully reared chicks. Of the pairs that raised chicks, one was an original pair and one was a newly formed pair. It should be noted that social enrichment is an important component of parrot husbandry whether or not the parrots in question are to be used for breeding purposes. Young parrots are very motivated to interact with conspecifics and will cross barriers to access social partners, while they will not cross these same barriers to access food or toys (C. Meehan, unpublished data).

A successful environmental enrichment program can significantly improve environmental quality and positively affect the welfare of captive parrots. In order to be successful, an enrichment protocol must be well-conceived and must provide parrots the opportunity to utilize their considerable behavioral skills. A combination of foraging, physical, and social enrichment is recommended for all parrots held in captivity. Environmental enrichment of this sort results in decreased screaming, feather picking, and stereotypy; increased physical activity and play behavior; reduced fear responses to novelty; and improved reproductive success without imparting significant risk of illness and injury or jeopardizing the ability of parrots to relate positively with humans. Thus, by providing an environment rich with opportunities to perform a wide variety of behaviors, owners can make marked improvements in the welfare of their parrots. Creating a dynamic, enriched environment in captivity requires significantly more time and creativity than housing parrots in barren cages. However, raising a parrot that is physically healthy, behaviorally active, and free from distressing abnormal behaviors is well worth the effort.

REFERENCES

Aengus, W.L., and J.R. Millam. 1999. Taming parent-reared orange-winged amazon parrots by neonatal handling. *Zoo Biology* 18:177–187.

Alderton, D. 1992. *Parrots.* London: Whittet Books.

American Psychiatric Association 1994. *Diagnostic and statistical manual of mental disorders,* 4th ed. Washington, DC: American Psychiatric Association.

American Veterinary Medical Association. 2002. *U.S. pet ownership and demographics sourcebook.* Schaumburg, IL: Center for Information Management, pp. 1–2.

Appleby, M.C., B.O.Hughes, and J.A. Mench. In press. *Poultry behaviour and welfare.* Wallingford, Oxon, U.K.: CAB International.

Barnett, J.L., G.M. Cronin, C.G. Winfield, and A.M. Dewar 1984. The welfare of adult pigs: The effects of five housing treatments on behaviour, plasma corticosteroids and injuries. *Applied Animal Behavior Science* 12:209–232.

Bauck, L. 1999. Nutritional problems in pet birds. *Semin Avian Ex Pet Med* 4:3–8.

Bayne, K.B., B.V. Beaver, J.A. Mench, and D.B. Morton. 2002. "Laboratory animal behavior." In *Laboratory animal medicine,* 2nd ed., pp. 1240–1264. New York: Academic Press.

Bayne, K., H. Mainzer, S. Dexter, G. Campbell, F. Yamada, and S. Suomi. 1991. The reduction of abnormal behaviors in individually housed rhesus monkeys (*Macaca mulatta*) with a foraging/grooming board. *American Journal of Primatology* 23:23–36.

Birchall, A. 1990. Who's a clever parrot, then? *New Scientist,* 24 February, pp. 38–43.

Blanchard, S. 1999. "The pet bird report." www.petbirdreport.com/myths.html.

Blokhuis, H.J. 1986. Feather pecking in poultry: Its relation with ground pecking. *Applied Animal Behaviour Science* 16:63–67.

Blokhuis, H.J. 1989. The development and causation of feather pecking in the domestic fowl. Ph.D. thesis, Agricultural University, Wageningen, the Netherlands.

Boice, R. 1981. Captivity and feralisation. *Psychological Bulletin* 89:407–421.

Boinski, S., S.P. Swing, T.S. Gross, and J.K. Davis. 1999. Environmental enrichment of brown capuchin (*Cebus apella*): Behavioral and plasma and fecal cortisol measures of effectiveness. *American Journal of Primatology* 48:49–68.

Carlstead, K. 1998. "Determining the causes of stereotypic behaviors in zoo carnivores." In *Second nature: Environmental enrichment for captive animals,* ed. D.J. Shepherdson, J.D. Mellen, and M. Hutchins, pp. 172–183. Washington, DC: Smithsonian Institution.

Carlstead, K., J. Seidensticker, and R. Baldwin. 1991. Environmental enrichment for zoo bears. *Zoo Biology* 10:3–16.

Carlstead, K., and D. Shepherdson. 2000. "Alleviating stress in zoo animals with environmental enrichment." In *The biology of animal stress: Basic principles and implications for welfare,* ed. G.P. Moberg and J.A. Mench, pp. 337–354. Wallingford, Oxon, U.K.: CABI Publishing.

Chu, L-r., J.P. Garner, and J.A. Mench. In press. A behavioral comparison of New Zealand white rabbit (*Oryctolagus cuniculus*) housed individually or in pairs in standard cages. *Applied Animal Behaviour Science.*

Coe, C.L., D. Franklin, E.R. Smith, and S. Levine. 1982. Hormonal responses accompanying fear and agitation in the squirrel monkey. *Physiology and Behavior* 29:291–294.

Cooper, J.J., F. Odberg, and C. Nicol. 1996. Limitations on the effectiveness of environmental improvement in reducing stereotypic behaviour in bank voles (*Clethrionomys glareolus*). *Applied Animal Behaviour Science* 48:237–248.

Coulton, L.E., N.K. Warran, and R.J. Young. 1997. Effects of foraging enrichment on the behaviour of parrots. *Animal Welfare* 6:357–363.

Cramton, B. 1998. Master's thesis. Department of Avian Science. University of California, Davis.

Cronin, G.M., P.R. Wiepkema, and G.J. Hofstede. 1984. "The development of stereotypies in tethered sows." In *Proceedings of the International Congress on Applied Ethology in Farm Animals,* ed. J. Unshelm, G. van Putten, & K. Keeb, pp. 97–100. Darmstadt, Germany: KTBL.

Davis, C.S. 1991. Parrot psychology and behavior problems. *Veterinary Clinics of North America: Small Animal Practice* 21:1281–1288.

Dawkins, M.S. 1988. Behavioral deprivation: A central problem in animal welfare. *Applied Animal Behaviour Science* 20:209–225.

Duncan, I.J.H., and D. Fraser. 1977. "Understanding animal welfare." In *Animal welfare,* ed. M.C. Appleby and B.O. Hughes, pp. 19–32. Wallingford, Oxon, U.K.: CAB International.

Einon, D.F., M.J. Morgan, and C. Kibbler. 1978. Brief periods of socialization and later behavior in the rat. *Developmental Psychobiology* 11:213–225.

Escorihuela, R.M., A. Tobena, and A. Fernandez-Teruel. 1994. Environmental enrichment reverses the detrimental action of early inconsistent stimulation and increases the beneficial effects of postnatal handling on shuttlebox learning in adult rats. *Behavioural Brain Research* 61:169–173.

Fernandez-Teruel, A., R.M. Escorihuela, B. Castellano, B. Gonzalez, and A. Tobena. 1997. Neonatal handling and environmental enrichment effects on emotionality, novelty/reward seeking and age-related cognitive and hippocampal impairments: Focus on the Roman rat lines. *Behavior Genetics* 27:513–526.

Fraser, D., D.M. Weary, E.A. Pajor, and B.N. Milligan. 1997. A scientific conception of animal welfare that reflects ethical concerns. *Animal Welfare* 6:187–205.

Garner, J.P. 1999. The aetiology of stereotypy in caged animals. Ph.D. thesis, University of Oxford, U.K.

Garner, J.P., and G.J. Mason. 2002. "Cage stereotypy, psychiatric task performance, behavioural flexibility, and apparent cognitive ability in songbirds: The impact of environmental enrichment." In *The 2nd International Symposium on Comparative Cognitive Science,* ed. T. Matsuzawa, p. 72. Kyoto University, Kyoto and Inuyama, Japan.

Garner, J.P., C.L. Meehan, and J.A. Mench. 2003. Stereotypies in caged parrots, schizophrenia and autism: Evidence for a common mechanism. *Behavioural Brain Research* 145 (1–2):125–134.

Gilardi, J.D., and C.A. Munn. 1998. Patterns of activity, flocking and habitat use in parrots of the Peruvian Amazon. *Condor* 100 (4):641.

Grandin, T. 1998. The feasibility of using vocalization scoring as an indicator of poor welfare during cattle slaughter. *Applied Animal Behaviour Science* 56:121–128.

Grandin, T. 2001. Cattle vocalizations are associated with handling and equipment problems at beef slaughter plants. *Applied Animal Behaviour Science* 71:191–201.

Grindlinger, H. 1991. Compulsive feather picking in birds. *Archives of General Psychiatry* 48:857.

Hediger, H. 1955. *The psychology and behaviour of animals in zoos and circuses.* London: Butterworths.

Hoffmeyer, I. 1969. Feather pecking in pheasants—an ethological approach to the problem. *Danish Review Game Biology* 6:1–36.

Huber-Eicher, B., and B. Wechsler. 1997. Feather pecking in domestic chicks: Its relation to dustbathing and foraging. *Animal Behaviour* 54:757–768.

Huber-Eicher, B., and B. Wechsler. 1998. The effect of quality and availability of foraging materials on feather pecking in laying hen chicks. *Animal Behaviour* 55:861–873.

Hughes, H.C., S. Campbell, and C. Kenney. 1989. The effects of cage size and pair housing on exercise of beagle dogs. *Laboratory Animal Science* 39 (4):302–305.

Jones, R.B. 1982. Effects of early environmental enrichment upon open-field behavior and timidity in the domestic chick. *Developmental Psychobiology* 15:105–111.

Jones, R.B. 1997. "Fear and distress." In *Animal welfare,* ed. M.C. Appleby and B.O. Hughes, pp. 75–87. New York: CAB International.

Jones, R.B., and B.J. Merry. 1988. Individual or paired exposure of domestic chicks to an open field: Some behavioral and adrenocortical consequences. *Behavioral Processes* 16:75–86.

Jones, R.B., and D. Waddington. 1992. Modifications of fear in domestic chicks*, Gallus gallus domesticus*, via regular handling and early environmental enrichment. *Animal Behaviour* 43:1021–1034.

Kastelstein, R.A., and P.R. Wiepkema. 1989. A digging trough as occupational therapy for Pacific walruses (*Odobens rosmarus divergens*) in human care. *Aquatic Mammals* 15:9–17.

Keiper, R.R. 1969. Causal factors of stereotypies in caged birds. *Animal Behaviour* 17:114–119.

Kidd, A.H, and R.M. Kidd. 1998. Problems and benefits of bird ownership. *Psychological Reports* 83:131–138.

Kiley-Worthington, M. 1977. *Behavioural problems of farm animals.* London: Oriel Press.

King, C.E. 1993. Environmental enrichment: Is it for the birds? *Zoo Biology* 12:509–512.

Klein, T., E. Zeltner, and B. Huber-Eicher. 2000. Are genetic differences in foraging behaviour of laying hen chicks paralleled by hybrid-specific differences in feather pecking? *Applied Animal Behaviour Science* 70:143–155.

Lantermann, W. 1993. Social deprivation in amazon parrots. *Kleintierpraxis* 38:511–520.

Line, S.W., H. Markowitz, K.N. Morgan, and S. Strong. 1989. Evaluation of attempts to enrich the environment of singly caged non-human primates. In *Animal care and use in behavioral research: Regulations, issues and applications,* ed. J. Driscoll, pp. 103–117. Beltsville, MD: Animal Welfare Information Center, National Agricultural Library.

Line, S.W, K.N. Morgan, and H. Markowitz. 1991. Simple toys do not alter the behavior of aged rhesus monkeys. *Zoo Biology* 10:473–484.

Magrath, R.D., and A. Lill. 1985. Age related differences in behavior and ecology of crimson rosellas during the non-breeding season. *Austr Wildl Res* 12:299–306.

Mardsen, D., and D.G.M. Wood-Gush. 1986. A note on the behaviour of individually penned sheep regarding their use for research purposes. *Animal Production* 42:157–159.

Markowitz, H., and C. Aday. 1998. Power for captive animals: Contingencies and nature. In *Second nature: Environmental enrichment for captive animals,* ed. D.J. Shepherdson, J.D. Mellen, and M. Hutchins, pp. 47–58. Washington, DC: Smithsonian Institution.

Marriner, L.M., and L.C. Drickamer. 1994. Factors influencing stereotyped behavior of primates in a zoo. *Zoo Biology* 13:267–275.

Mason, G.J. 1991 Stereotypies: A critical review. *Animal Behaviour* 41:1015–1037.

Mason, G.J. 1993. Age and context affect the stereotypies of caged mink. *Behaviour* 127 (3–4):191–229.

Mason, G.J., and M. Mendl. 1997. Do the stereotypies of pigs, chickens and mink reflect adaptive species differences in the control of foraging? *Appl Anim Behav Sci* 53:45–58.

McKeegan, D.E.F., and C.J. Savory. 1999. Feather eating in layer pullets and its possible role in the aetiology of feather pecking damage. *Applied Animal Behaviour Science* 65:73–85.

Meehan, C.L. 2002. Environmental enrichment and behavioral development of orange-winged amazon parrots (*Amazona amazonica*): Applications to animal welfare. PhD diss., University of California, Davis.

Meehan, C.L., J.P. Garner, and J.A. Mench. 2003. Isosexual pair housing improves the welfare of young amazon parrots. *Applied Animal Behaviour Science* 81 (1):73–88.

Meehan, C.L., J.P. Garner, and J.A. Mench. Submitted. Environmental enrichment and cage stereotypy in orange-winged amazon parrots (*Amazona amazonica*): Insights into developmental processes. *Developmental Psychobiology.*

Meehan, C.L., and J.A. Mench. 2002. Environmental enrichment effects fear and exploratory responses in young amazon parrots. *Applied Animal Behaviour Science* 79 (1):77–90.

Meehan, C.L., J.R. Millam, and J.A. Mench. 2003. Foraging opportunity and increased physical complexity both prevent and reduce psychogenic feather picking by young amazon parrots. *Applied Animal Behaviour Science* 80 (1):71–85.

Mench, J.A., and L.J. Keeling. 2001. The social behaviour of domestic birds. In *Social behaviour in farm animals,* ed. L.J. Keeling and H.W. Gonyou, pp. 177–211. Wallingford, Oxon, U.K.: CAB International.

Mendl, M., and R.C. Newberry. 1997. "Social conditions." In *Animal welfare,* ed. M.C. Appleby and B.O.Hughes, pp. 191–203. New York: CAB International.

Mertens, P.A. 1997. "Pharmacological treatment of feather picking in pet birds." In *Proceedings of the First International Conference on Veterinary Behavioral Medicine,* ed. D.S. Mills and S.E. Heath, pp. 209–213. Potters Bar, U.K.: UFAW.

Meyer–Holzapfel, M. 1968. "Abnormal behaviors in zoo animals." In *Abnormal behavior in animals,* ed. M.W. Fox, pp. 476–503. London: Saunders.

Morgan, M.J. 1973. Effects of pre-weaning environment on learning in the rat. *Animal Behaviour* 21:429–442.

Morgan, M.J., D.F. Einon, and D. Nicholas. 1975. Effects of isolation rearing on behavioral inhibition in the rat. *Quarterly Journal of Experimental Psychology* 27:615–634.

Newberry, R.C. 1995. Environmental enrichment: Increasing the biological relevance of captive environments. *Applied Animal Behaviour Science* 44:229–243.

Nicol, C.J. 1992. Effects of environmental enrichment and gentle handling on behaviour and fear responses of transported broilers. *Applied Animal Behaviour Science* 33:367–380.

Nicol, C.J. 1999. Understanding equine stereotypies. *Equine Veterinary Journal,* Supplement 28:20–25.

Nicol, C.J., A.C. Lindberg, A.J. Phillips, S.J. Pope, L.J. Wilkins, and L.E. Green. 2001. Influence of prior exposure to wood shavings on feather pecking, dustbathing and foraging in adult laying hens. *Applied Animal Behaviour Science* 73:141–155.

Novak, M.A., and S.J. Suomi. 1988. Psychological well-being of primates in captivity. *American Psychologist* 10:765–773.

Odberg, F.O. 1987. The influence of cage size and environmental enrichment on the development of stereotypies in bank voles (*Clethrionomys glareolus*). *Behavioural Processes* 14:155–173.

Oviatt, L.A., and J.R. Millam. 1997. Breeding behavior of captive orange-winged amazon parrots. *Exotic Bird Report* 9:6–7.

Owens, D.G.C., E.C. Johnstone, and C.D. Frith. 1982. Spontaneous involuntary disorders of movement—their prevalence, severity, and distribution in chronic-schizophrenics with and without treatment with neuroleptics. *Archives Of General Psychiatry* 39:452–461.

Pearce, G.P., A.M. Patterson, and A.N Pearce. 1989. The influence of pleasant and unpleasant handling and the provision of toys on the growth and behaviour of male pigs. *Applied Animal Behaviour Science* 23:27–37.

Powell, S.B., H.A. Newman, T.A. McDonald, P. Bugenhagen, and M.H. Lewis. 2000. Development of spontaneous stereotyped behavior in deer mice: Effects of early and late exposure to a more complex environment. *Developmental Psychobiology* 37: 100–108.

Price, E.O. 1984. Behavioral aspects of animal domestication. *Quarterly Review of Biology* 59, 1–32.

Price, E.O. 1999. Behavioral development in animals undergoing domestication. *Applied Animal Behaviour Science* 65:245–271.

Reinhardt, V. 1991. Group formation of previously single-caged adult rhesus macaques for the purpose of environmental enrichment. *Journal of Experimental Animal Science* 34:110–115.

Renner, M.J. 1987. Experience-dependent changes in exploratory behavior in the adult rat (*Rattus norvegicus*): Overall activity level and interactions with objects. *Journal of Comparative Psychology* 101: 94–100.

Renner, M.J., and M.R. Rosenzweig. 1987. *Enriched and impoverished environments: Effects on brain and behavior.* New York: Springer-Verlag.

Reynolds, M. 1998. The welfare of pet parrots. *Psittascene* 10:1–3.

Savory, C.J., E. Seawright, and A. Watson. 1992. Stereotyped behaviour in broiler breeders in relation to husbandry and opioid receptor blockade. *Applied Animal Behaviour Science* 32:349–360.

Shepherdson, D.J. 1993. "Environmental enrichment: An overview." Proceedings, Annual Conference of the American Association of Zoological Parks and Aquariums, pp. 100–103.

Shepherdson, D.J. 1998. "Tracing the path of environmental enrichment in zoos." In *Second nature: Environmental enrichment for captive animals,* ed. D.J. Shepherdson, J.D. Mellen, and M. Hutchins, pp. 1–12. Smithsonian Institution.

Snyder, N.F.R., J.W. Wiley, and C.B. Kepler. 1987. *The parrots of Luquillo: Natural history and conservation of the Puerto Rican parrot.* Los Angeles: Western Foundation of Vertebrate Zoology.

Sparks, J., and T. Soper. 1990 *Parrots: A natural history.* New York: Facts on File.

Taylor, G.T. 1981. Fear and affiliation in domesticated male rats. *Journal of Comparative Physiological Psychology* 95:685–693.

Terlouw, E.M.C., A.B. Lawrence, and A.W. Illius. 1991. Influences of feeding level and physical restriction on development of stereotypies in sows. *Animal Behaviour* 42:981–991.

van Hoek, C.S., and C. ten Cate. 1998. Abnormal behavior in caged birds kept as pets. *Journal of Applied Animal Welfare Science* 1:51–64.

Vastrade, F.F. 1986. The social behavior of free-ranging domestic rabbits (*Oryctolagus Cuniculus L.*). *Applied Animal Behaviour Science* 16:165–177.

Weary, D.M., L.A. Braithwaite, and D. Fraser. 1998. Vocal responses to pain in piglets. *Applied Animal Behaviour Science* 56:161–172.

Wechsler, B., and B. Huber-Eicher. 1997. The effect of foraging material and perch height on feather pecking and feather damage in laying hens. *Applied Animal Behaviour Science* 58:131–141.

Weidenmayer, C. 1997. Causation of the ontogenetic development of stereotypic digging in gerbils. *Animal Behaviour* 53:461–470.

Westerhof, I., and J.T. Lumeij. 1987. "Feather picking in the African grey parrot." Proceedings of the European Symposium on Bird Diseases, Beerse, Belgium. Netherlands Association of Avian Veterinarians, pp. 98–103.

Wood-Gush, D.G.M., A. Stolba, and C. Miller 1983. "Exploration in farm animals and animal husbandry." In *Exploration in animals and humans,* ed. J. Archer & L.I.A. Birke, pp. 198–209. London: Van Nostrand Reinhold.

Würbel, H. 2001. Ideal homes? Housing effects on rodent brain and behaviour. *Trends in Neurosciences,* 24(4):207–211.

Würbel, H., R. Chapman, and C. Rutland 1998. Effect of feed and environmental enrichment on development of stereotypic wire-gnawing in laboratory mice. *Applied Animal Behaviour Science,* 60:69–81.

Index